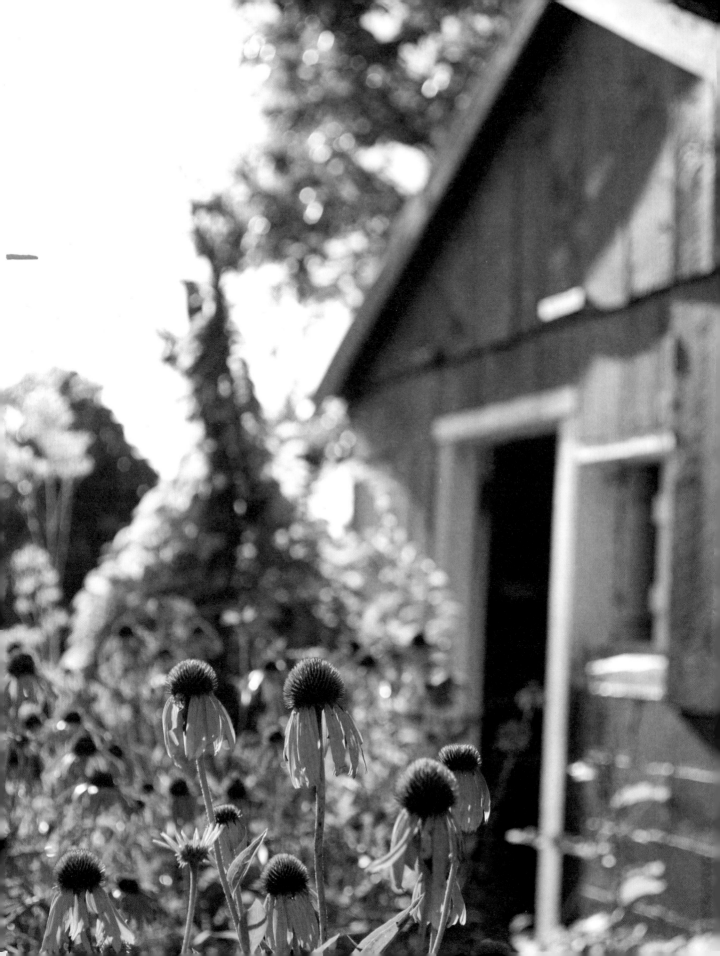

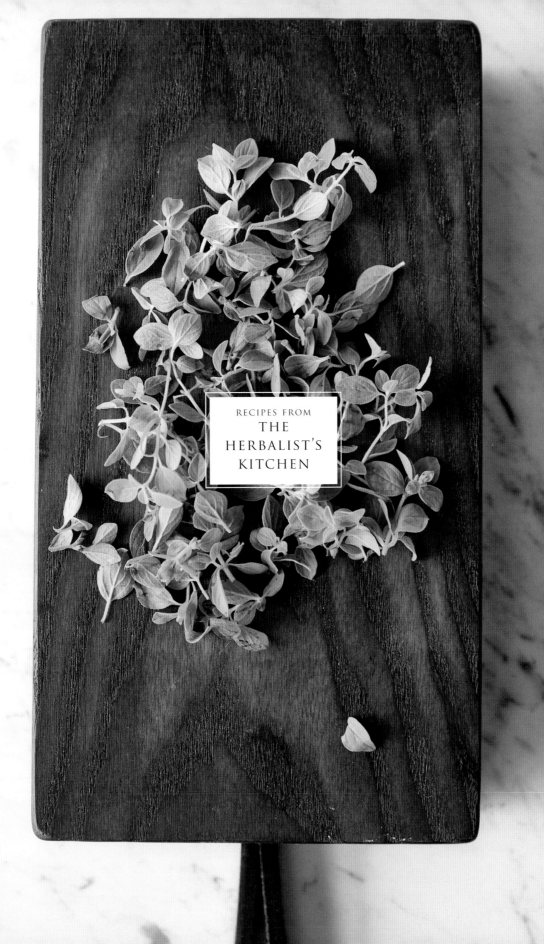

RECIPES FROM
THE
HERBALIST'S
KITCHEN

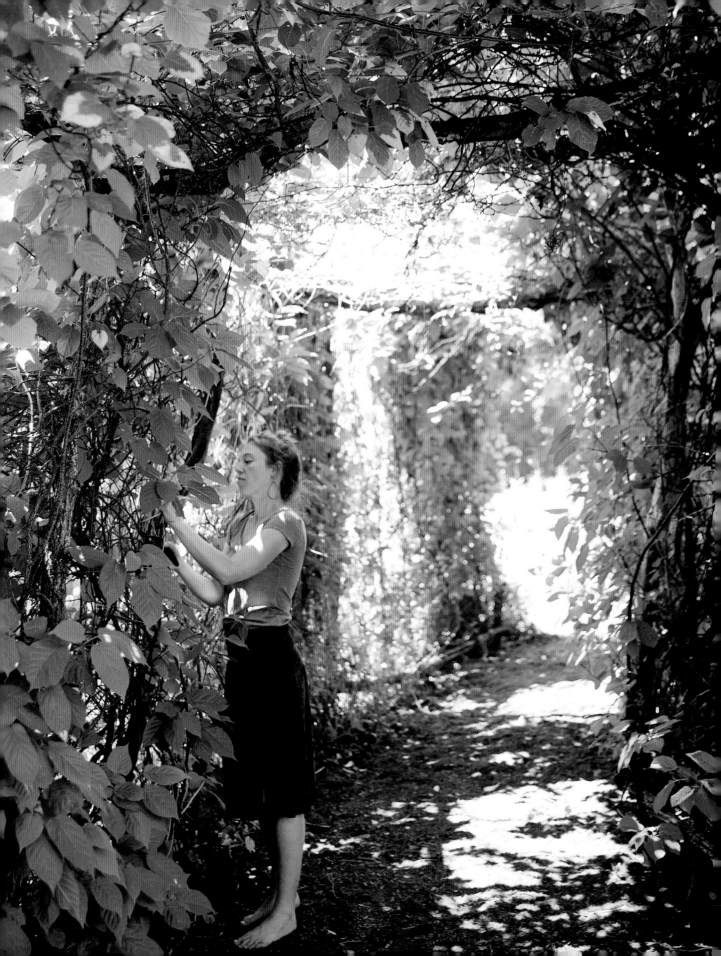

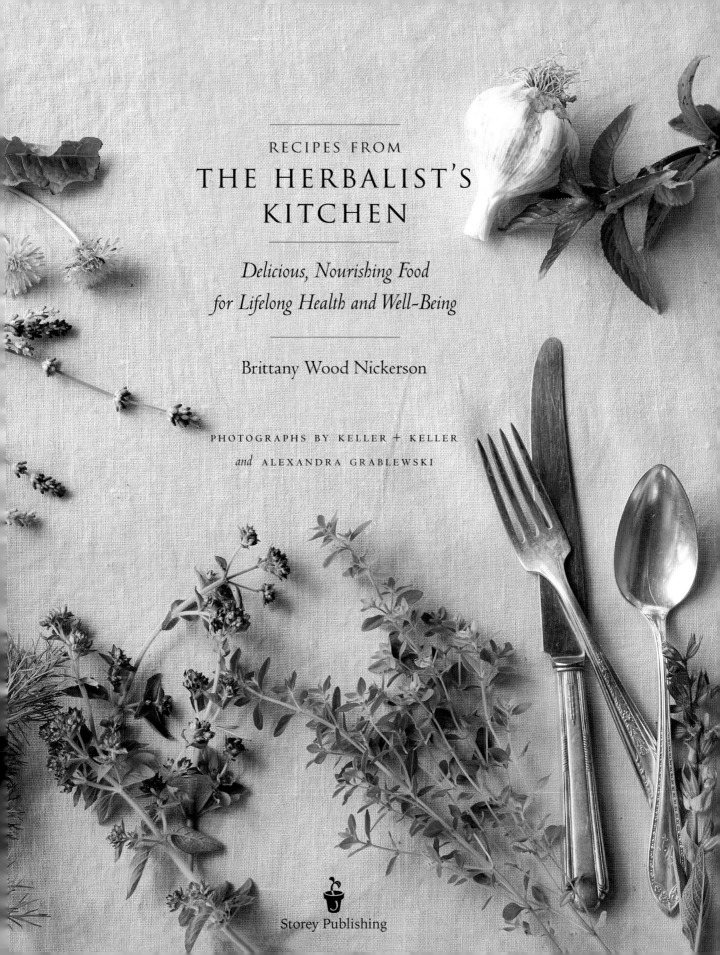

RECIPES FROM

THE HERBALIST'S KITCHEN

Delicious, Nourishing Food
for Lifelong Health and Well-Being

Brittany Wood Nickerson

PHOTOGRAPHS BY KELLER + KELLER
and ALEXANDRA GRABLEWSKI

Storey Publishing

The mission of Storey Publishing is to serve our customers by
publishing practical information that encourages
personal independence in harmony with the environment.

EDITED BY Nancy Ringer and Michal Lumsden
ART DIRECTION AND BOOK DESIGN BY Carolyn Eckert
TEXT PRODUCTION BY Slavica A. Walzl
INDEXED BY Christine R. Lindemer, Boston Road Communications

COVER PHOTOGRAPHY BY © Keller + Keller Photography

INTERIOR PHOTOGRAPHY BY © Keller + Keller Photography, back end pages, i–iii, v, viii, 1–4, 6 (t.r & b.r.), 7–9, 11, 24, 26, 35, 36 (left), 41 (t.r.), 44, 46, 49 (left), 51, 60, 61, 63, 66, 68, 70, 71, 73, 74, 76, 78, 82, 84–86, 90 (except b.l.), 92, 100, 102, 103, 109, 110, 113, 114, 117 (left), 119, 121, 125, 127, 132, 133, 137, 141, 142, 145, 149, 150, 152, 154, 159–161, 163, 164, 168, 174, 179, 181, 185, 188, 190, 191, 193, 211, 214, 215, 216 (right), 217, 221, 222, 225, 226, 229, 231 (right), 234, 242–244, 247, 250, 252–254, 261, 266–267, 269, 271, 277, 278, 282, 284, 285, 287 (b.l.), 291, 292, 295, 297, 304;

© Alexandra Grablewski, front end page (cone flowers), vi-vii, 6 (t.l. & b.l.), 10, 14, 16, 18, 20, 22, 23, 25, 28–32, 34, 36 (right), 38, 41 (except t.r.), 42, 43, 45, 47, 49 (right), 52–56, 59, 65, 67, 89, 90 (b.l.), 93, 94, 99, 101, 105, 106, 117 (right), 122, 128, 131, 139, 147, 157, 158, 166–167, 171, 177, 182–183, 187, 199, 200, 205, 208, 209, 213, 216 (left), 218, 230, 231 (left), 233, 238, 241, 265, 287 (except b.l.), 289, 294, 305; Carolyn Eckert, front end pages (purple meadow), 13

FOOD STYLING BY Sally Staub, with assistance by Ginger Heafey

Storey Publishing
210 MASS MoCA Way
North Adams, MA 01247
storey.com

Printed in China by R.R. Donnelley
10 9 8 7 6 5 4 3 2 1

Library of Congress Cataloging-in-Publication Data

Names: Nickerson, Brittany Wood, author.
Title: Recipes from the herbalist's kitchen /
by Brittany Wood Nickerson.
Description: North Adams, MA : Storey Publishing,
[2017] | Includes index.
Identifiers: LCCN 2016059760 (print) |
LCCN 2017003910 (ebook) |
ISBN 9781612126906 (hardcover : alk. paper) |
ISBN 9781612126913 (ebook)
Subjects: LCSH: Cooking (Herbs). | Nutrition. |
LCGFT: Cookbooks.
Classification: LCC TX819.H4 N53 2017 (print) |
LCC TX819.H4 (ebook) | DDC
   641.6/57—dc23
LC record available at https://lccn.loc
.gov/2016059760

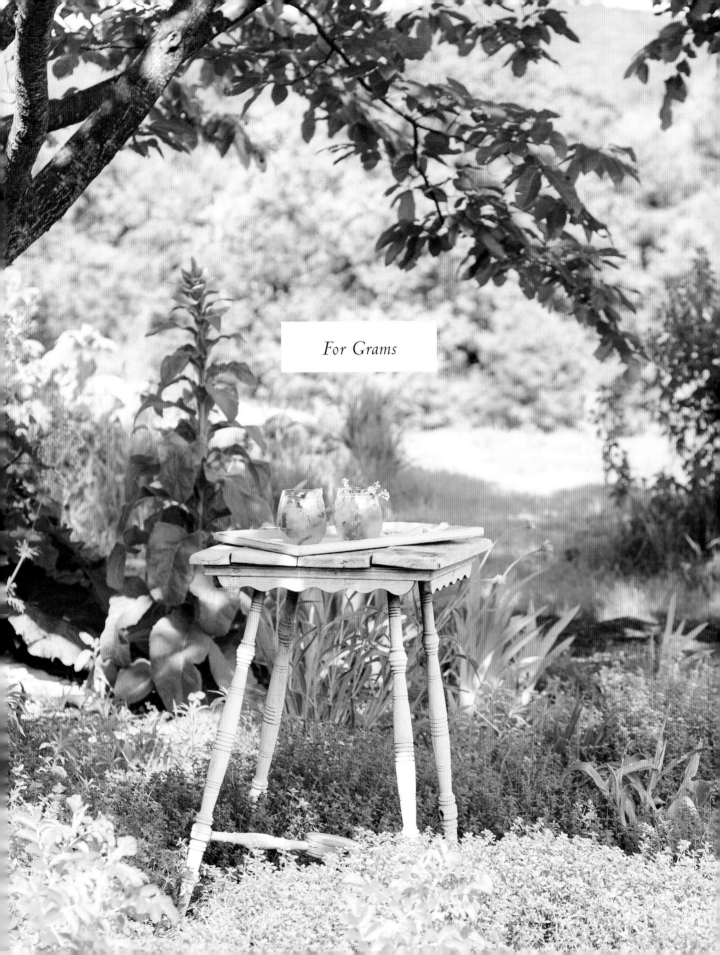

For Grams

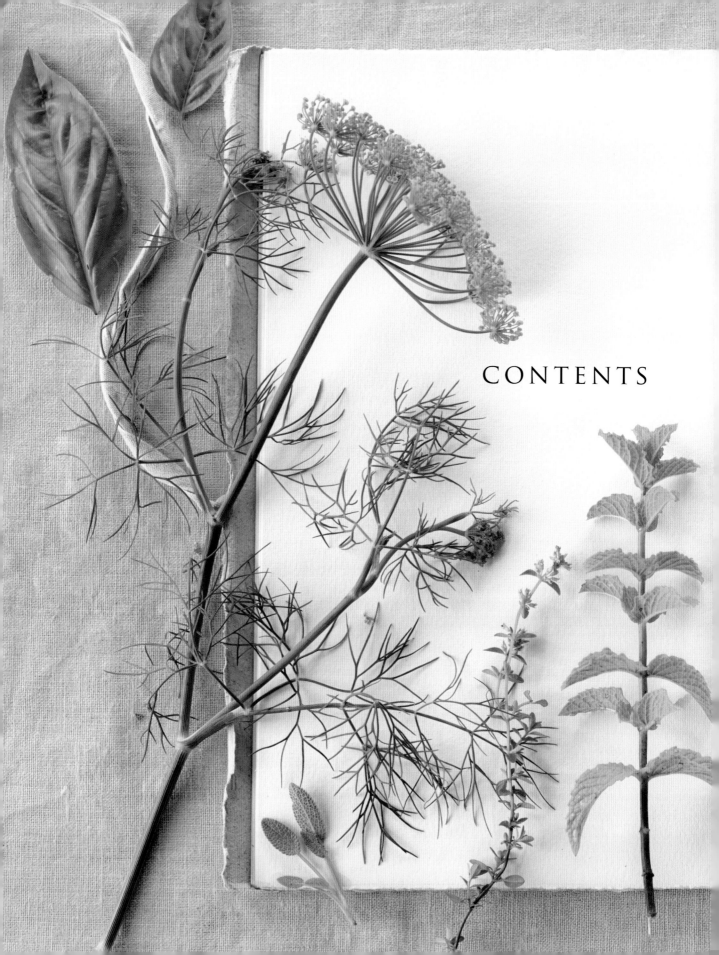

CONTENTS

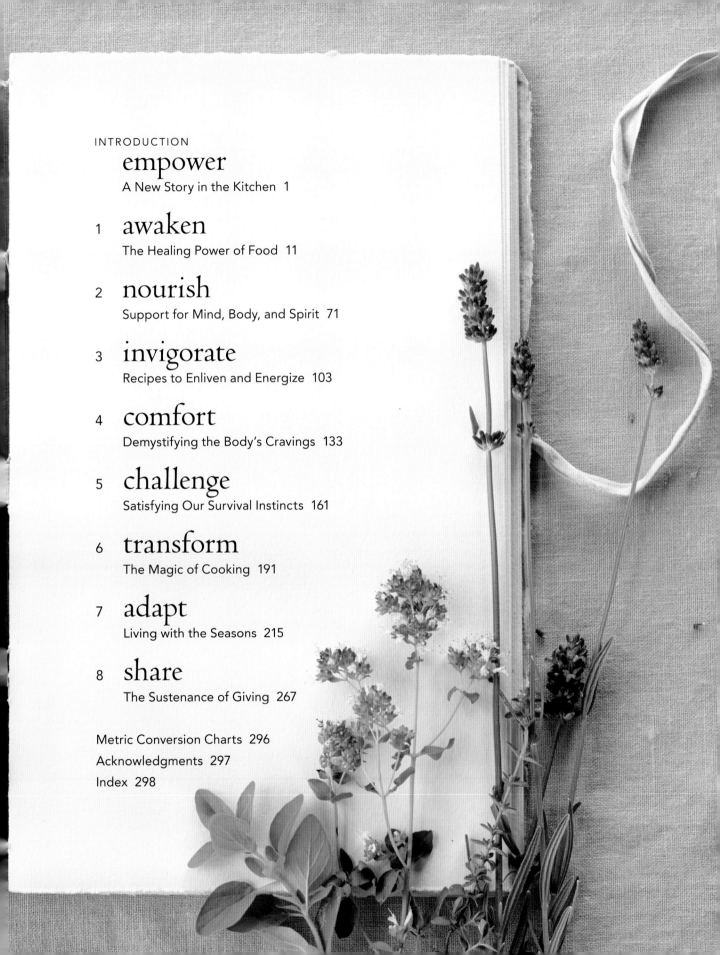

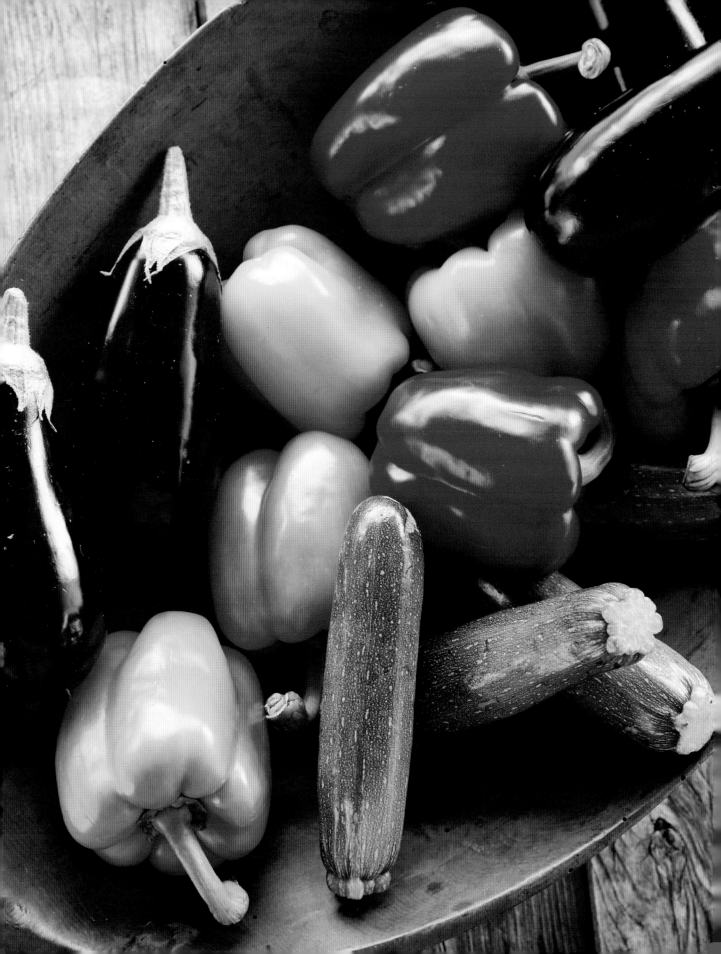

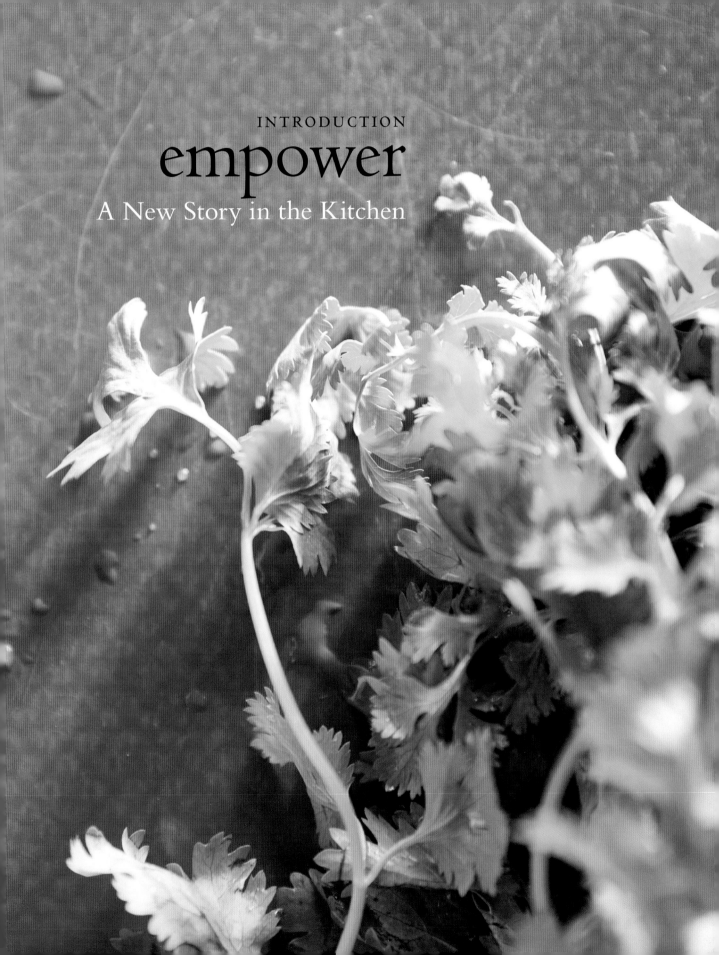

empower

A New Story in the Kitchen

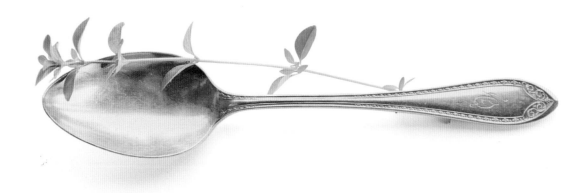

EVERY GREAT STORY HAS A HERO, that awe-inspiring figure who overcomes all manner of obstacles to meet a challenge head-on and triumph over it. In our current medical system the hero is the doctor, the scientist, the surgeon, the specialist, the expert who rushes in to diagnose the problem and tell us how to fix it. In the culinary world the hero is the food writer, the celebrity chef, the fitness trainer, the health guru, the expert who tells us exactly what to eat and how to prepare it. In fact, as a general principle we have developed a cultural habit of outsourcing heroism, finding it anywhere but inside ourselves. That mind-set — that habit of depending on outside experts to "save" us by telling us how to live well — may be one of the biggest factors holding us back from true, deep, vibrant well-being.

It's as if society is selling us a dream, a fantastical story in which our happiness and contentment are guaranteed if only we follow the advice of the right experts, eat the right foods, exercise the right amount, have the right stuff in our homes, live the right way. But does this expert "prescription" for a good life really feel good to us? Or is it actually an obstacle between us and an open, intimate, authentic experience of our world?

Empowerment through Herbalism

Herbal medicine is a time-tested system of healing, practiced around the world for thousands of years, and modern science has now confirmed its efficacy for a wide range of health concerns. However, herbalism doesn't just put forth a prescription of what herbs to take to be healthy. When applied holistically, herbalism offers us an opportunity not just to *feel well* but to *live well* — to engage intimately and authentically with our own health and our world in ways that feel fulfilling and meaningful.

At its most basic level, the work of making and using herbal medicine at home connects us to our individual needs: what sort of ailments we tend to experience, and which remedies work best for us. On a broader scale, home herbalism teaches us that each of us has different needs, that self-care requires self-knowledge, and that balance is the root of wellness. It asks us to walk the path of empowerment and self-discovery, and in this way, it positions us as the heroes of our own story.

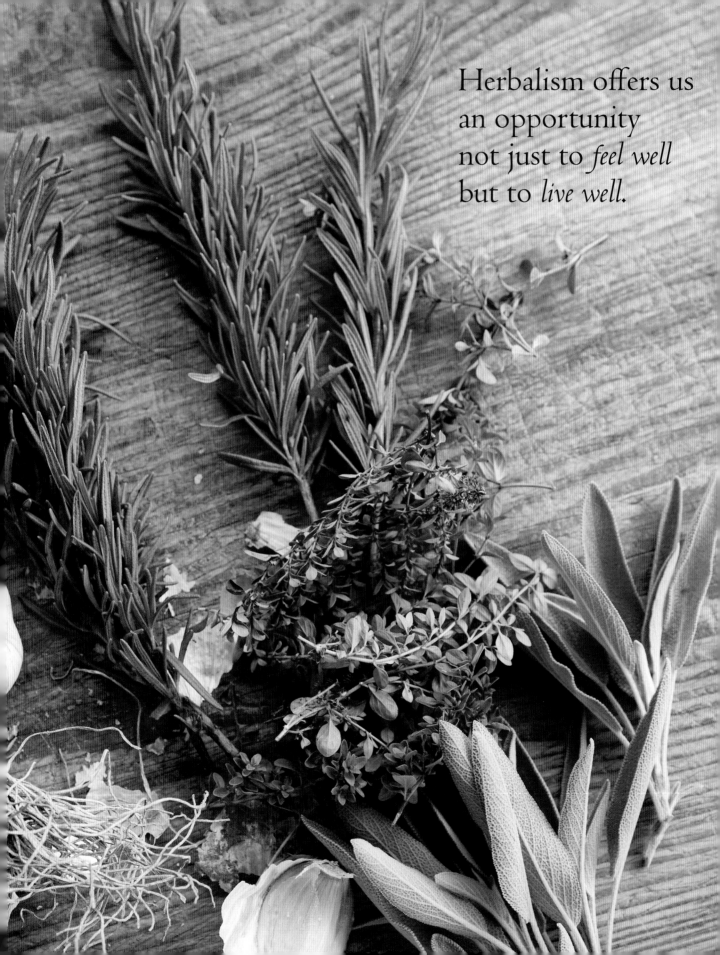

Herbalism offers us
an opportunity
not just to *feel well*
but to *live well*.

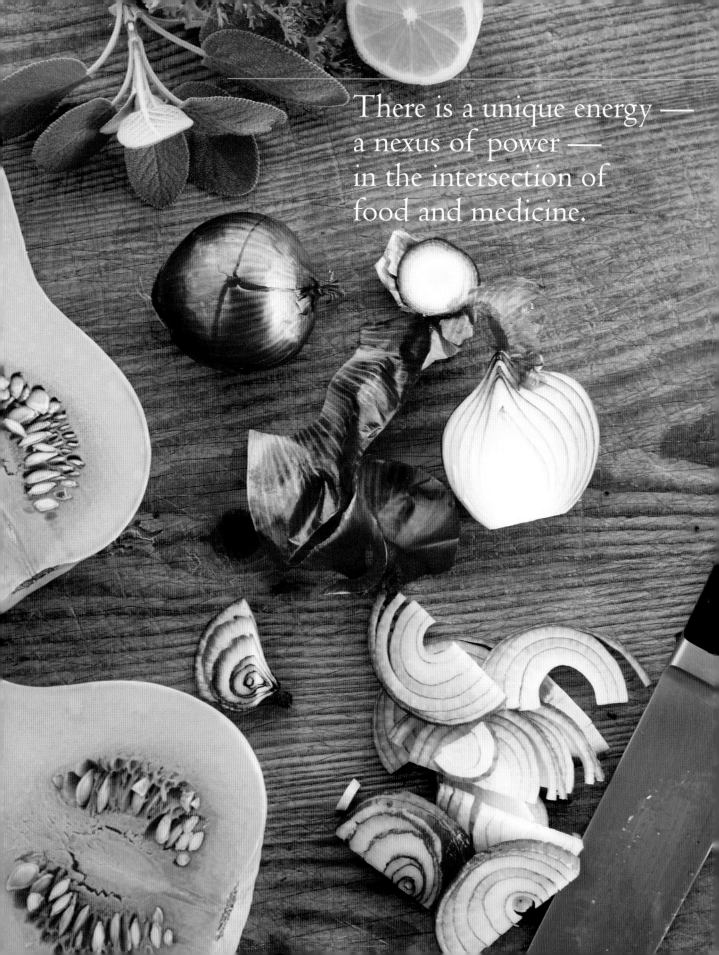

There is a unique energy —
a nexus of power —
in the intersection of
food and medicine.

Awakening to Connections

I have always loved both cooking and plants, and as a kid, I spent a lot of time in the kitchen, in the woods, and in the garden, soaking up everything I could. I began formally studying herbal medicine when I was in college in northern California. At the same time I started cooking, privately and professionally, all over the Bay Area. Eventually I started a business, Thyme Herbal, teaching cooking classes that emphasized the use of herbs and simple, good food prepared in ways that maximized their benefit to the body.

When I first started teaching classes, I realized that my students were looking at me as the expert. They wanted me to tell them what they needed to know and do to live well. I felt uncomfortable, and a little perplexed. Who was I to decide what was best for others? After all, each of us is a unique organism, and what makes us healthy is as diverse as our taste in clothing and our preferences in books and music. Being healthy is just that: a state of *being*, a subjective experience that varies from person to person.

This awareness helps us recognize that health and healing are acts of *connection*. To be healthy requires us to connect with our body — its processes and inclinations — and also with our families, our communities, our home and work environments, our food systems, and the natural world. Every aspect of our lives contributes to our physical and emotional nourishment. We all possess the inherent wisdom to nurture and heal ourselves by getting to know our own rhythms, embedded as they are in the larger picture of our lives and the patterns of the earth. We simply need to learn to listen to and connect with ourselves.

As an herbalist and healer, my role is to empower people, rather than telling them what to do. I want to help people cultivate their own skills and tune in to their own intuitive wisdom. This view of health operates outside the experts' paradigm of "right answers" and "cures." It allows for the possibility that we can know ourselves, and it recognizes that the process of self-knowing in itself is a large part of our well-being. It requires us to appreciate that health can be different things for different people, that each person's healing path is unique, and that our desire to be well and to live in balance with our body and our world is our most powerful, important medicine. These concepts have become the cornerstones of my philosophies about health and healing.

Kitchen Medicine

There is a unique energy — a nexus of power — in the intersection of food and medicine. We are taught that each has its own place: food nourishes the body; medicine cures the body. But what if we recognized that food and medicine can be one and the same? When we learn to make use of the power of food and herbs to heal and support the body we celebrate and utilize the potent medicine found in some of our most basic ingredients.

Take herbs as an example. Our traditional culinary herbs and spices, like basil, black pepper, cilantro, and parsley, have formidable medicinal abilities. They support everything from digestion and metabolism to immune function, circulation, and the nervous system. If you've ever used herbs and spices in your cooking — and most of us have — you've

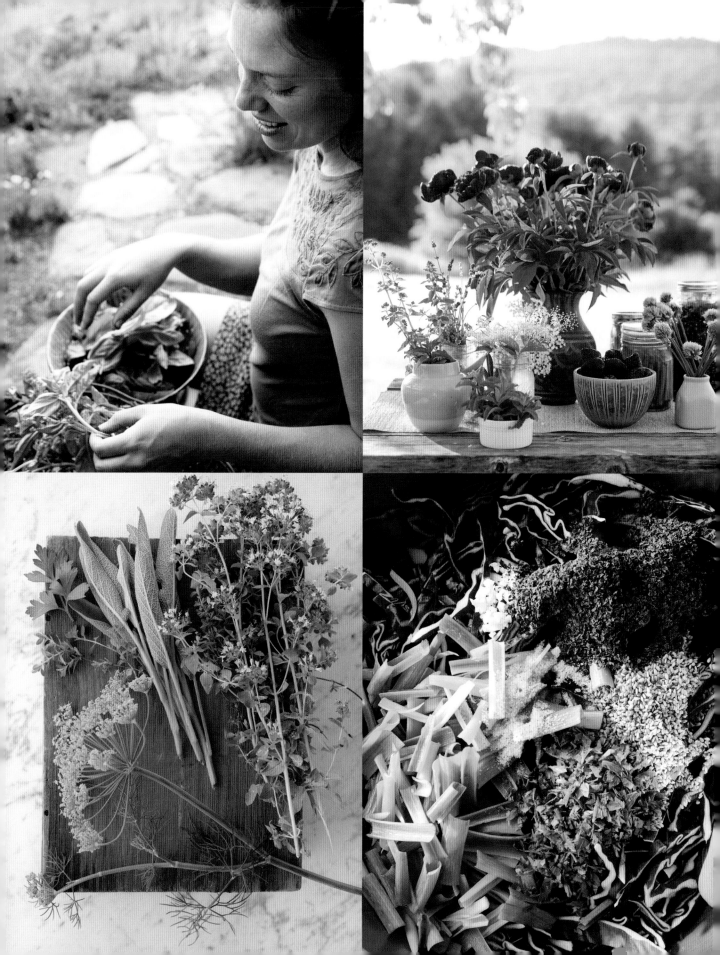

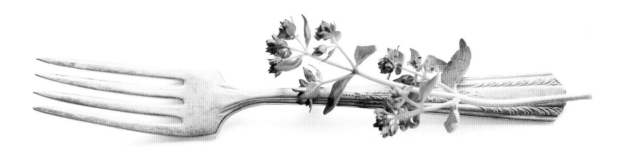

been practicing herbal medicine. Right at home. With no help from the "experts."

Herbs are not miracle cures. They don't work like heroic medicine: instead of curing a problem *for* you, they almost always help you better heal yourself. A spoonful of sage honey boosts the immune system and helps the body fight off a cold. A cup of hot peppermint tea encourages the body to sweat and helps break a fever. Offer someone a cup of basil tea, and you help them relax so they can sort through their anxiety with greater ease. Put a dollop of herb pesto alongside a heavy meal, and you help the body digest fats and ease indigestion. The list goes on and on.

We can think of food in general, as well as the very act of cooking, in a similar vein. Good, fresh, wholesome ingredients have tremendous capacity to support the body and all its systems. Preparing those foods in ways that bring out their best — that make them more nourishing for the body and a feast for the senses — is a powerful form of medicine that cultivates the health of the body, mind, and spirit.

Cooking and eating are sensual and evocative experiences. Reconnecting with these aspects of food has nothing to do with experts — it is about an intimacy of experience that is born through relationship. The kitchen is a place where we can develop this relationship and unleash our own power by unlocking all of our senses. In preparing food and medicine, we can experience beauty, get our hands dirty, savor smells, appreciate flavors, connect with ourselves and others, and nourish our physical, spiritual, and emotional world. This deep intimacy of experience is the medicine of our future. It is also the medicine of the kitchen.

The Herbalist's Kitchen

In my vision for the world, we all practice home herbalism, and our kitchens are places of meaningful ritual. The medicine and food we make are alike infused with intention and love, nourished by human hands, the use of herbs, and prepared in accord with age-old wisdom passed down from our ancestors. When you begin to use herbal medicine at home, making and concocting home remedies becomes an extension of other kitchen work. Making a tincture or infusing herbs into honey comes as naturally as frying an egg, and putting oregano in spaghetti sauce or basil with mozzarella is as instinctual as hunger. The line between our food and our medicine becomes blurry, as does the line between the healing power of food and medicine and the healing that is inherently wrapped up in our experience of the world. In the herbalist's kitchen, how we live — our participation and

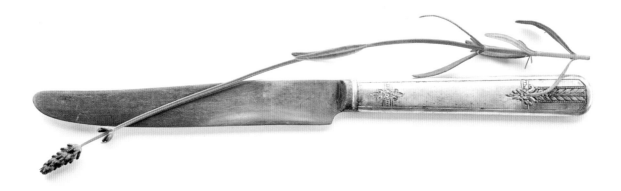

awareness — is as important, if not more so, as any recipe we follow or any ingredients we use.

As you move through the pages of this book, you will learn why, over the vast span of culinary history, we have come to cook with herbs the way we do — why we use certain herbs (and spices) in certain dishes, and why we pair certain flavors with others. Our food traditions have evolved to optimize flavor, nutrition, and digestion. When you come to understand the concepts behind these traditions, then you will be able to cook like an herbalist: you will be able to look at the ingredients you have and pick the right herbs for the season, the situation, and the ingredients. Learning skills and tools that cultivate intuition builds a deep, satisfying sense of empowerment.

It is my hope that this book can help guide you in finding your own deep, meaningful, intimate relationship with herbs, cooking, medicine, and health. There are simple principles that underpin this work. True to the tenets of holistic herbalism, they are embedded in larger life processes, they are flexible and adaptable, and they encourage empowerment.

These guiding principles for the herbalist's kitchen are as follows:

- To revitalize rituals around homemade food and medicine, including cooking and eating together

- To cultivate and nourish herbal medicine as an empowering, intrinsic component of home health care

- To make cooking and eating nutritionally dense foods a daily practice

- To slow down and enjoy the process of growing, preparing, and eating and to embrace food as our sustenance

- To realize that, as individuals, we are the stewards of our own health, and we must learn the patterns and nature of our own body to heal

Food provides an invitation to connect and reconnect, to nourish and be nourished, to invigorate and challenge, to adapt and transform, to comfort and share. May your healing herbal kitchen embody these principles in a truly unique and empowered way. And as the story of your herbal kitchen unfolds and becomes, may you be the hero.

What if we recognized
that food and medicine
can be one and the same?

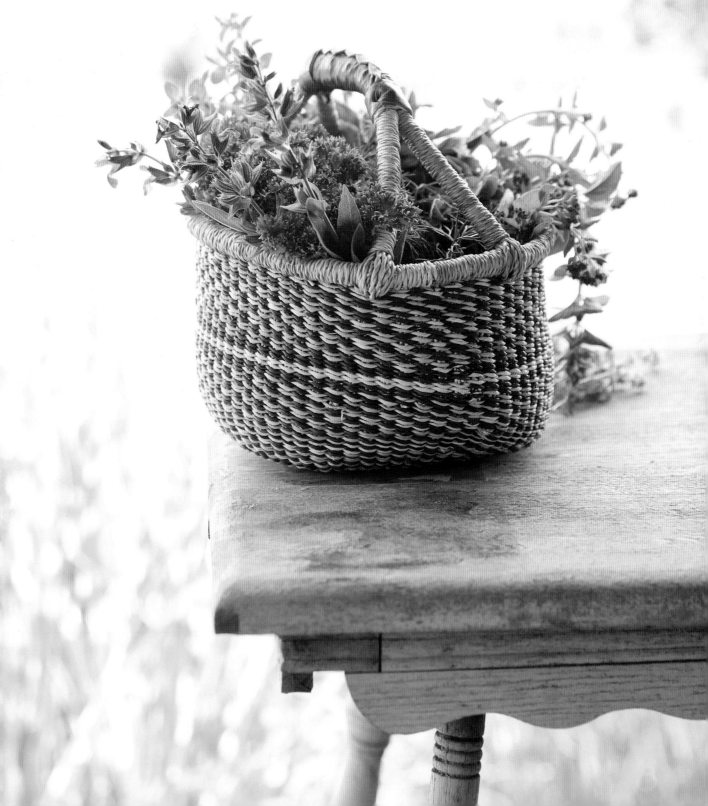

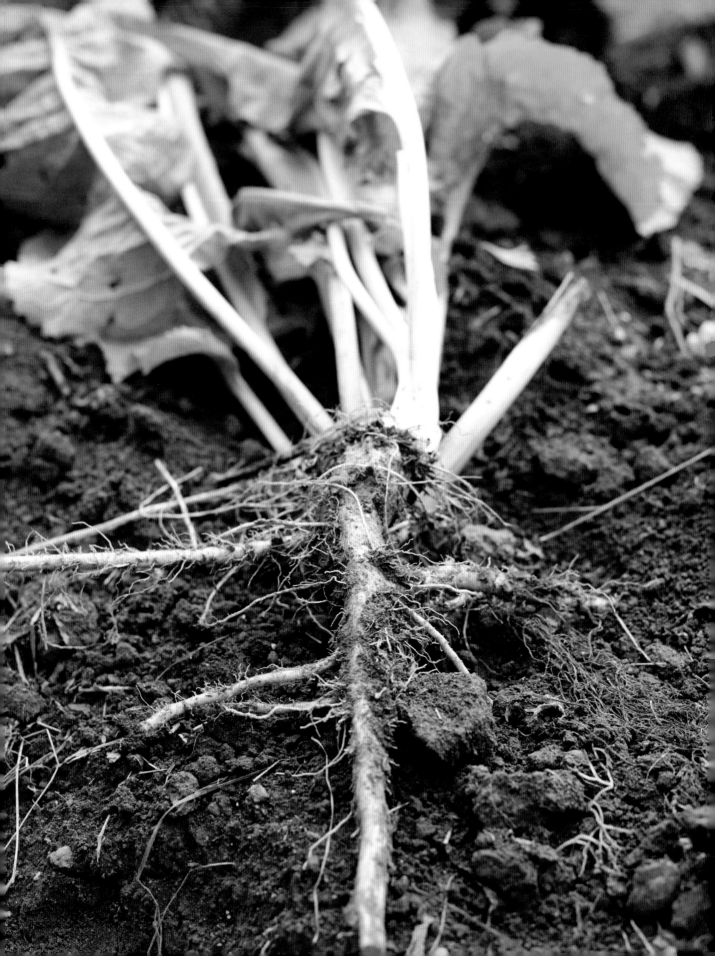

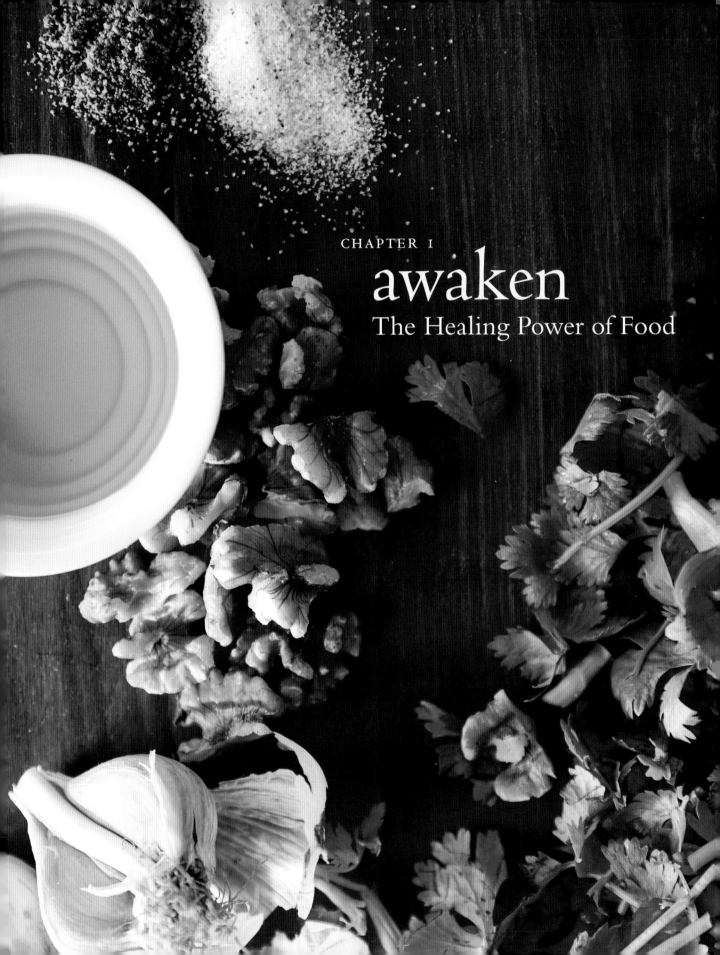

CHAPTER I

awaken

The Healing Power of Food

Most of us live disembodied lives — that is, we are out of touch with our body. We are not taught how to listen to our body or how to decipher and make meaning of how we feel when our body is trying to speak to us. Awakening to that communication — to how our body speaks to us — is an essential step in the journey to health.

Herbs, whether traditionally used in culinary or medicinal preparations, have tremendous power to influence the body and its systems. We can use herbs (and all food) to support our health and well-being, but before we can truly benefit from them, we have to learn how our body reacts to them. The interplay between herbs, the body, and healing has its own language. Learn to speak that language and you will be able to communicate, problem-solve, and create better harmony within your body. Just memorizing a list of herbs and their uses is like memorizing vocabulary words: it will give you tools to use while speaking, but it won't help you learn how to communicate. We learn to speak a language when it becomes embedded in us, natural, a part of our senses and our understandings, when we really feel comfortable in it and begin to live it. When it comes to learning the language of the body and how we can nourish and comfort it with food, medicine, experiences, relationships, and all the other factors that contribute to our well-being, personal experience is the most powerful teacher. This means that collecting ingredients, dreaming up what we want to eat, poring over recipe books, chopping, smelling, tasting, and enjoying are all experiences that help us learn to communicate and build a deep and intimate relationship with our own bodies. Personal connection to our body and our own experience is foundational for health and well-being.

Taste as Medicine

For thousands of years, medical systems from around the world — traditional Chinese medicine, Ayurveda, Native American healing practices, and other folk and herbal traditions — have focused on the body's response to taste as a means of understanding and applying herbal therapeutics and the ways in which diet supports health. Modern science has come to support this time-tested wisdom, providing evidence of two important points: first, that the taste of an herb can serve as an indicator of its constituents, and second, that stimulation of the taste buds by the different flavors initiates specific physiological responses. In other words, the *taste* of an herb both indicates and initiates an effect on the body.

Our sense of taste, then, can allow us to build a more empowered relationship with food, plant medicine, and our own body. Once you understand the medicinal actions that the different tastes have on physiology, you can begin to build a new relationship with your palate and with the herbs, foods, and drinks that you ingest. Rather than memorizing the benefits of a food or herb, you can learn to let your taste buds reveal information about its applications. You can learn to trust yourself in determining whether a particular food or herb is helpful for your particular needs. You can also begin to understand more generally which situations and contexts call for which flavors and draw conclusions about foods and herbs that may be useful.

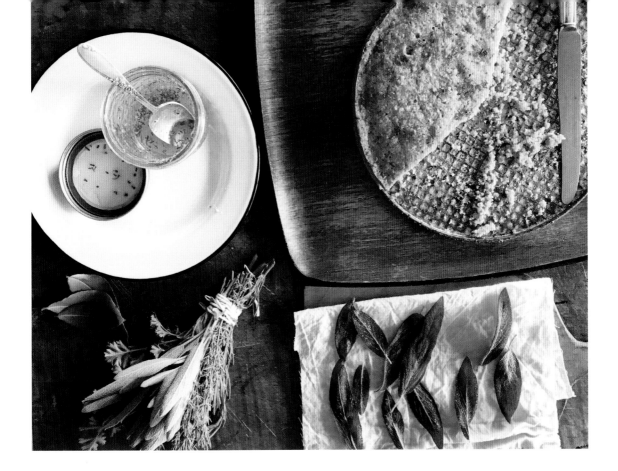

In general, tastes can be broken down into five categories: sweet, salty, sour, pungent, and bitter. Every meal you eat should include all five flavors. You don't need a lot; in some cases a condiment-size portion is fine. (And you'll find lots of condiment recipes in this book, because having them made up in advance makes it easier to balance your plate!) Another important thing to remember is that herbs and foods can have more than one taste. A carrot, for example, might be mostly sweet, but with a hint of bitterness. A green apple might taste both sour and sweet. And produce can vary depending on the variety, the time of year, the crop, or the part of the plant used.

As you gain experience with using taste as a guide, you will begin to trust your instincts; you will learn to better understand the language of your body. Your experience will help you learn to balance your diet in a very direct and personal manner, rather than simply trying to get on your plate everything that you have heard is "good for you." This awakening of your sense of taste can help guide you in the kitchen and at the table, allowing you to enjoy your meals and make food choices with a more empowered appreciation for the ways in which they nourish you.

NOTE: Every healing system that uses tastes and flavors as indicators of medicinal action on the body is unique, and in many cases there are large differences between how they are understood and their applications. The descriptions that follow are informed by my study of traditional healing systems and my own experience as a practicing herbalist. You will find that they do not stand in perfect alignment with any one traditional system of medicine. I am grateful to all of these systems for their knowledge and wisdom.

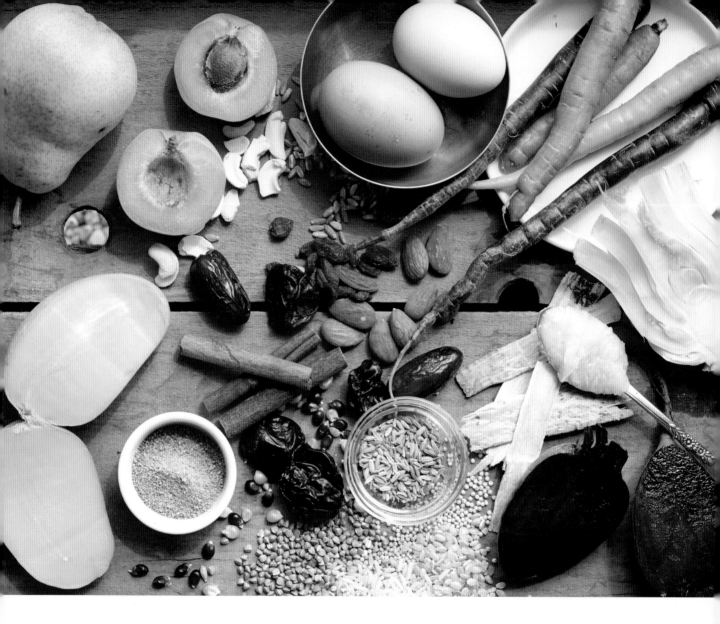

sweet/bland

The sweet taste is the most nourishing. We think of sweet as being sugary, but as a category, sweet also includes bland foods. Most of the world's staple foods, including starches and animal-based proteins, fall into this category. Most of our common culinary herbs, however, are not categorized as sweet. In fact we most often use culinary herbs to counterbalance the sweet taste of our staple nourishing foods and bring balance to the flavors of a dish.

Sweet foods are staples of the human diet for a reason: the sweet (or bland) taste indicates a high nutrient content, with fat, protein, carbohydrates, and often good quantities of vitamins and minerals. In other words, sweet/bland foods are high-calorie foods — they provide short- and long-term energy for the body. They are nutritive and regenerative; they provide all the building blocks for growth and help the body build, repair, and sustain energy. They supply nutrients that strengthen muscles, bones, nerves, and connective tissues and build body fluids including blood, semen, and milk. They are mostly demulcent, emollient, moistening, softening, and soothing, having a gentle and nourishing effect on the system.

Too much sweet food in the diet can cause dampness in the system, leading to sluggish digestion, poor absorption of nutrients, reduced appetite, bloating, stagnant circulation and elimination, increased mucus production, low energy, and difficulty focusing. Refined carbohydrates and foods sweetened with refined sugars are most likely to aggravate the body and cause such symptoms.

When you find yourself craving sugar, turn to high-quality unrefined carbohydrates and naturally sweet foods like fruit, and balance them with protein-rich foods. The combination will satiate the craving, provide the body with sustained energy, and help reduce sugar cravings overall.

In addition to being the most nourishing, sweet foods are the heaviest. You may be able to sense that fact by the list of symptoms that occur when you eat too much; slow and sluggish seems to be the theme. That heaviness also means that sweet foods are grounding and comforting; they help the body relax and are great for people who often feel cold, dry, nervous, and restless. After all, what could be more comforting than feeling nourished?

Since these foods are the most nourishing, they should comprise a significant portion of most people's diet — but make sure you're getting good-quality, unprocessed sweet/bland foods. Because sweet foods are heavier and can be more difficult to digest, it is important to dress them up with herbs, spices, and other flavorful accompaniments that are more stimulating and help improve their digestibility. In other words, sweet foods alone or in excess can have negative consequences, but when combined with all the other wonderful flavors that are more stimulating to the system, they become more nutritious and easier for the body to process.

SWEET/BLAND FOODS

- Animal fats
- Eggs
- Fruit juices
- Fruits (pears, figs, dates, apricots, mangoes, bananas, prunes, peaches)
- Grains (wheat, oats, barley, rice, corn, quinoa, millet)
- Meat and fish
- Milk and cream
- Milk substitutes (except soy)
- Nuts and seeds
- Root crops (sweet potatoes, beets, parsnips, carrots)
- Sweeteners (cane sugar, honey, maple syrup)
- Winter squashes

SWEET/BLAND HERBS

- Astragalus
- Cinnamon
- Codonopsis
- Fennel
- Goji berry
- Licorice
- Marshmallow
- Shatavari

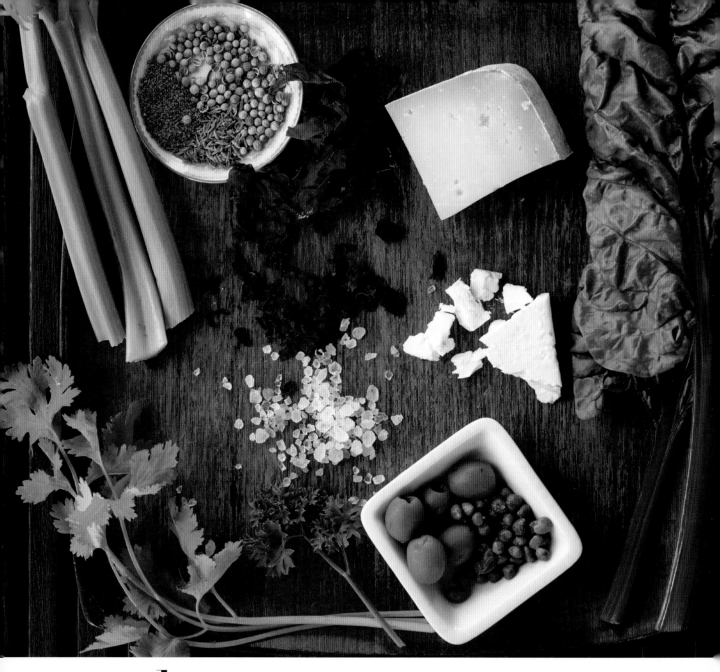

salty

The salty taste is heavy, grounding, moistening, soothing, and warming. In moderation the salty taste promotes digestion and appetite and improves our absorption of nutrients. But too much can overstimulate digestion and irritate acid reflux, heartburn, and indigestion. It can also irritate other symptoms of heat in the body, including inflammation, tissue irritation, nerve irritation, and skin rashes. Too much salty food can even make some people feel irritable and agitated.

Salt causes the body to retain fluids. Healthy fluid levels are necesary to hydrate the cells, dilute phlegm, and soften hard and dense materials that can clog the body's channels and cause stagnation. It helps move fluids, cleanse, moisten, and detoxify; it can help dissolve fatty or fluid-filled cysts and can be useful for cleansing the blood, lymph, liver, and kidneys. Too much salt, however, can lead to excessive water retention, edema, swelling, stagnant blood, and increased blood pressure.

Salt increases and enhances our taste buds' experiences of other flavors, which makes it a valuable asset in cooking — and also explains its overuse in fast food and processed, packaged foods. Because the salty taste is grounding, salty foods in moderation can be beneficial for people who have a lightness of being that leads to ungroundedness, anxiety, or feeling flustered. It is good for nervous people or people who are prone to dryness, including dry skin, hair, or nails. It may also be good for those with weak digestion or low appetite. It is important for detoxification protocols, hydration, and general good health.

There are different kinds of salt, and the quality is important. Unrefined, unprocessed salt is the best, most nourishing salt for the body. Rather than just sodium chloride, unrefined salt contains minerals and trace minerals that are nutritionally important. The minerals tend to give unrefined salts a bit of color, ranging from gray to pink, green, or any shade in between. The body metabolizes and utilizes this salt better than refined, simplified sodium chloride. Unrefined salt can be sourced from either land or sea. Both forms are wonderful — it's the unrefined quality that's important.

While the saltiest flavor comes from true salt, whether refined or unrefined, many foods and herbs have a naturally salty flavor to them. Foods that taste naturally salty generally have high levels of minerals. Sea vegetables are a great example because they have both true salt and mineral salt flavors. The first taste will be salty from ocean water, but once that subsides you will taste the salty taste of minerals. Celery, Swiss chard, and spinach are other examples of naturally salty, high-mineral vegetables.

Foods that display the mineral salt flavor are deeply nourishing to the musculoskeletal system, including the bones, muscles, and ligaments, as well as the blood and nervous system tissues. These tissues need sodium, potassium, calcium, and magnesium for proper functioning — minerals that these herbs and foods often contain in high amounts.

SALTY FOODS

- Anchovies
- Celery
- Hard cheeses
- Nettles
- Olives
- Sea vegetables (kelp, alaria, dulse, wakame)
- Smoked meats and fish
- Spinach
- Swiss chard

SALTY HERBS

- Celery seed
- Cilantro
- Coriander seed
- Cumin seed
- Dill seed
- Lovage
- Parsley

sour

The sour flavor is toning, contracting, cooling, and moistening. It causes contraction of tissues and strengthens and tones mucous membranes. This has an astringing effect that prevents leakage of fluids and energy and helps firm up tissue integrity. It can tonify and build up the tissues of the GI tract, urinary tract, lungs, and liver. It has a refreshing effect, stimulating the mind, enhancing metabolism, and stimulating the liver and gallbladder. It increases the flow of saliva and other digestive juices, which stimulates the appetite, improves digestion and absorption, and regulates peristalsis. It is particularly helpful in the digestion of fats, oils, and protein-rich foods. It also works to break up and improve assimilation of minerals; this may be the reason, in part, that traditional preparations of mineral-rich dark, leafy greens — think of kale and collards — so often include citrus or vinegar.

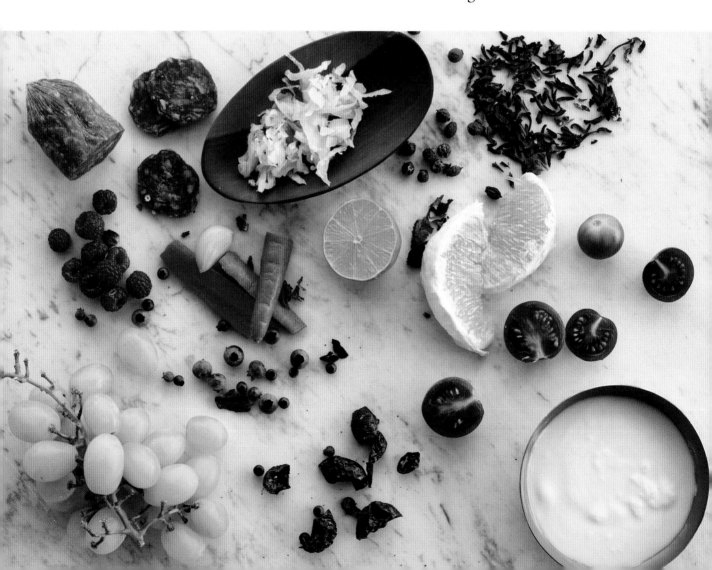

The sour flavor comes from a variety of acids, including citric acid, tannic acid, and ascorbic acid. Fermented foods, with their acetic and lactic acids, are also sour, as are many kinds of fruits, from grapes to citrus. Of course, sour foods can have other flavors as well, as is the case with many fermented foods, which are also salty, or many fruits, which are also sweet.

While the sour flavor is cooling in small amounts, large amounts, whether consumed all at once or over time, can cause heat, aggravating excessive acidity in the upper GI tract (acid reflux, heartburn, indigestion). In folks with an already fast metabolism, it can spur hunger and symptoms of low blood sugar, possibly leading to irritation and agitation. Too much sour can also lead to skin issues, including acne, boils, eczema, and psoriasis, and it can aggravate arthritic conditions and cause oversensitivity of the teeth.

According to Chinese medicine, the sour flavor is said to promote balance between the heart and the mind, steadying a scattered mind and emotions. In Ayurveda the sour flavor is said to lead to the desire for more — more food, more thoughts, and more inquisitiveness, for example. In people who lack motivation or have undirected energy, the sour taste may provide some inspiration and focus. Too much can lead to overanalysis of thoughts and emotions, jealousy, competitiveness, and envy.

Sour foods are great in spring because they stimulate the release of bile from the liver and gallbladder, which has a detoxifying and stimulating effect on overall liver metabolism. They're also helpful in fall; because they have a contracting nature that pulls energy inward, sour foods encourage the body's natural turn inward and help the body preserve heat in preparation for the colder months.

With their digestion-enhancing effects, sour foods are great complements to fatty foods, proteins, and mineral-rich vegetables. I like to include a sour condiment, often a fermented one, at each meal. Condiment-size portions are enough to introduce the health benefits of the flavor — and to introduce the probiotic bacteria in the case of the fermented foods — without overdoing it, which could cause irritation or aggravation.

SOUR FOODS

- Berries (raspberries, blackberries, blueberries, strawberries)
- Citrus (oranges, grapefruits, lemons, limes, pomelos)
- Fermented dairy (yogurt, sour cream, kefir, aged cheese)
- Fermented sausages (salami, linguiça, chorizo, prosciutto)
- Some fruits (green apples, green grapes, plums)
- Kombucha
- Miso
- Pickled and fermented vegetables
- Pomegranates
- Tomatoes
- Vinegar
- Wine

SOUR HERBS

- Hawthorn berry
- Hibiscus
- Rose hips
- Rose petals
- Schizandra berry
- Sorrel

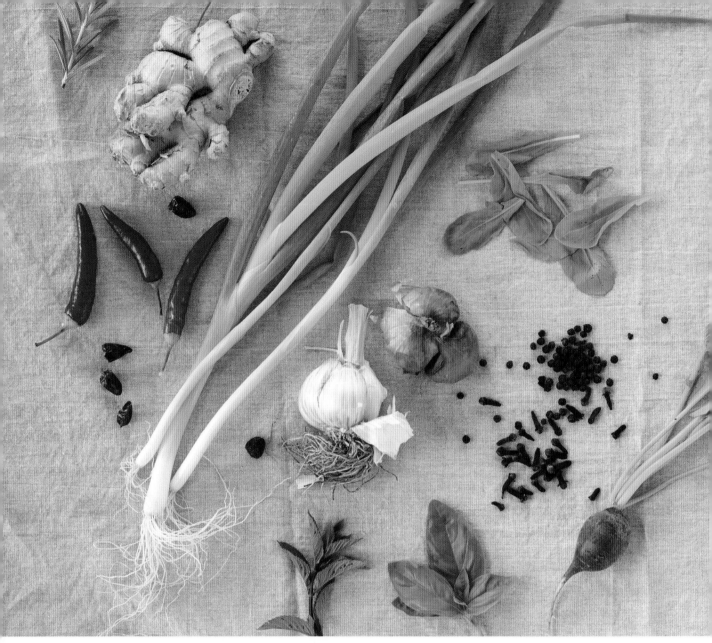

pungent

The pungent category includes spicy, acrid, and aromatic flavors. Pungent herbs and foods are warming, drying, light, and dispersive. They are stimulating, and like sour and bitter herbs and foods, they are used in cooking for balancing heavier flavors like sweet and salty. Consider, as examples, Indian curries with meats and cheeses, cinnamon added to applesauce, ginger in cake, sage or rosemary with roasted meats, or hot peppers in chili and other bean dishes.

The warming nature of pungent herbs and foods stimulates digestion and assimilation. Those pungent herbs that are also aromatic, like most culinary herbs (think of black pepper, ginger, and sage), help relax the GI tract and relieve gas and bloating. This makes them especially helpful in digesting more astringent-tasting foods that are often gas forming, like beans and brassicas.

Spicy, pungent foods and herbs warm and thin body fluids, stimulating their movement — particularly the circulation of blood and lymphatic fluids. They move blood from the core to the periphery of the body, opening the pores and promoting a sweat. While they warm the body by stimulating metabolic actions and encouraging circulation, sweating can create a cooling sensation because as sweat evaporates, it cools.

The pungent flavor helps reduce mucus production, making it beneficial for those who often find themselves stuffy-nosed or who often have mucus in their throat or lungs. They also help thin and make it easier to expectorate mucus from the sinuses and lungs and will often make the nose and eyes run. Though they are helpful for mucousy, damp conditions, they are less appropriate for hot or dry conditions, like dry coughs, since they are themselves hot and dry.

Most pungent herbs are antimicrobial, with some spectrum of antibacterial, antiviral, or even antifungal activity. By stimulating circulation of blood and lymph, many of them also improve the body's immune response.

Pungent and spicy flavors give clarity to the senses and are associated with excitement and stimulation. Too much can tax us emotionally, leading to overstimulation, overintensity, irritability, and exhaustion. Too much will do the same thing to the tissues of the body, overstimulating muscle, nerve, and mucous membrane tissues and creating a dried-out environment. An abundance of spicy, pungent food at any one sitting or over time will also aggravate acidic stomach conditions such as acid reflux, heartburn, and indigestion.

The pungent category includes all the classic spicy foods, like hot peppers and ginger. In some foods, pungency is transformed through cooking — raw onions are pungent, for example, but cooked onions are sweet, and the same is true of radishes and cabbage.

PUNGENT FOODS

- Arugula
- Cabbage
- Coffee
- Horseradish
- Hot peppers
- Mustard greens
- Radishes
- Raw onions, raw leeks, raw garlic
- Watercress

PUNGENT HERBS

- Basil
- Black pepper
- Cayenne
- Cinnamon
- Clove
- Cumin
- Ginger
- Mint
- Nutmeg
- Rosemary
- Sage
- Thyme
- Turmeric

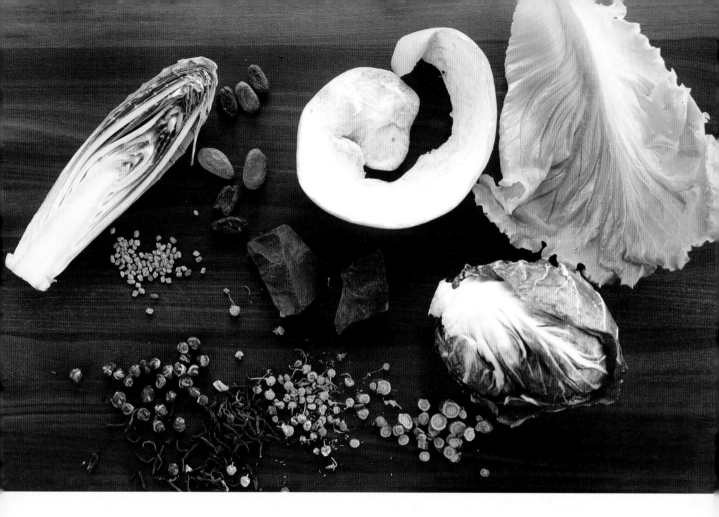

bitter

The most metabolically active of the five flavors, bitter is, unfortunately, the flavor most absent in the modern Western diet. It is cooling, drying, detoxifying, and anti-inflammatory. The bitter flavor stimulates the entire digestive process through a reflex via the taste buds. The bitter taste on your tongue activates those taste buds, and they, in turn, stimulate the enteric nervous system, which orchestrates the digestive process. Specifically, the bitter taste stimulates the secretion of hydrochloric acid, pepsin, and digestive enzymes in the stomach, the release of bile from the liver and gallbladder, the release of pancreatic juices and enzymes, and peristalsis (the muscular action that moves food through the digestive system). It is a powerful metabolic stimulant: it improves sluggish digestion, supports a healthy appetite, and helps with weight management and blood sugar balance.

THE ASTRINGENT FLAVOR

In Ayurveda the astringent flavor is separated out as its own category, while in many other traditions it is included in the sour category. While both flavors tonify tissues, astringent foods are lighter than sour foods and can be more drying. Astringent foods will usually cause the mouth to pucker, reduce saliva, stop diarrhea, and reduce bleeding. They have a similar healing effect on mucous membranes, reducing irritation, inflammation, and infection and promoting healthy tissues. Examples of astringent foods include green and black tea, dry red wine, green banana, pomegranate, rose, beans and legumes, brassicas (including cabbage, broccoli, Brussels sprouts, and cauliflower), cranberry, and sunchokes.

The astringent flavor has more of the air element than the sour flavor and is therefore lighter. This lightness makes astringent foods more gas forming, hence the status of brassicas, sunchokes, and beans as promoting gassiness.

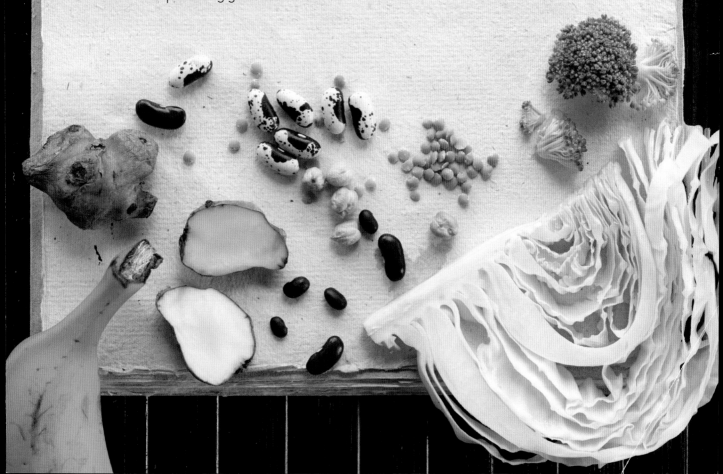

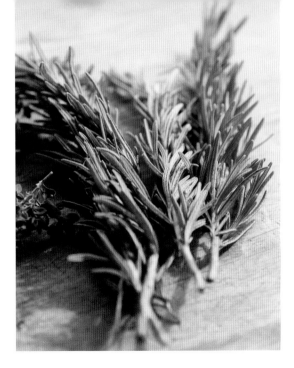
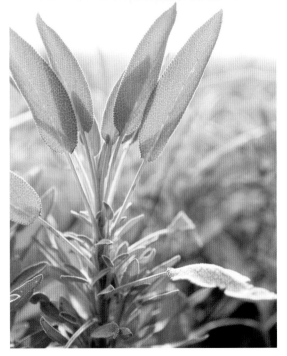

Because the bitter flavor supports the entire digestive process, bitter foods and herbs can be of help with many types of digestive issues. They are a great remedy for upper GI irritations, including acid reflux, heartburn, and indigestion. They improve our digestion, especially of fats, and our absorption of nutrients. And when taken as a predigestive, before meals, they can reduce nausea, cramping, bloating, and other discomforts sometimes associated with eating.

The bitter flavor stimulates metabolic function in the liver, promoting detoxification, nutrient metabolism, and hormone regulation. It is also excellent for the heart, clearing heat and blockages in the cardiovascular system, reducing cholesterol levels, and supporting cholesterol utilization. It reduces inflammation of the GI tract, musculoskeletal system, and skin (including skin rashes and acne), supports healthy tissue integrity for the skin, and reduces water retention. With its cooling effect, bitterness also helps clear hot emotions like anger, frustration, and irritation.

The bitter taste tends to diminish cravings by helping to balance the tastes and our desires for them. It is particularly good at helping to address sugar cravings, which many people experience strongly, by improving metabolism and helping the liver balance blood sugar levels, which are often the root cause of those cravings.

Incorporating the bitter flavor into the diet is so important for health, but that doesn't mean you have to consume large quantities. Bitter foods and herbs are rarely meant to be consumed in large amounts; they are great as side dishes, condiments, sauces, garnishes, and so on. Many common culinary herbs have bitterness to them, so just cooking with herbs introduces this important medicine to the diet. The light, cooling, stimulating bitter flavor improves the digestibility of starches, proteins, and fats, boosting nutrient absorption and utilization. This is the wisdom of traditional

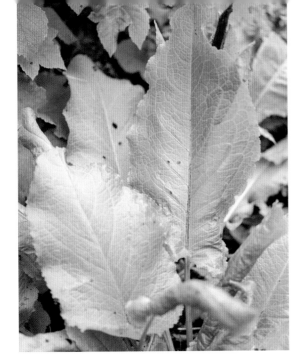
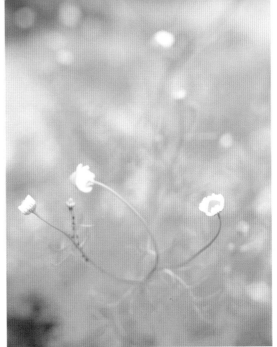

BITTER FOODS

- Artichoke
- Bitter lettuces and salad greens (radicchio, endive, frisée)
- Cocktail bitters
- Coffee, black and green tea
- Dark chocolate
- Dark leafy greens (kale, collards, dandelion greens)

BITTER HERBS

- Burdock root
- Caraway seed
- Chamomile
- Coriander seed
- Dandelion root
- Fenugreek seed
- Orange peel
- Rosemary
- Sage
- Thyme
- Yellow dock

cookery and why so many of our classic culinary herbs have strong bitter flavors. Many of the recipes in this book call on this wisdom of using bitter herbs to make sweeter, nutrient-rich foods more digestible. You can also serve a salad or other side dish of bitter herbs to incorporate this important flavor into a meal.

Like all the flavors, bitter can be overdone, especially in those who already have a fast metabolism. People who are cold, dry, nervous, deficient, or weak may find the bitter taste to be irritating. They should focus on bitter foods and herbs that are also sweet, like a salad of bitter greens with herbal balsamic vinaigrette (page 239), for example, or just a small taste of a bitter condiment alongside heavier, more grounding foods. In addition to incorporating bitter foods and herbs into the diet, you can also introduce the flavor through herbal bitters; see the recipe for basil bitters (page 184) for one that focuses on culinary herbs.

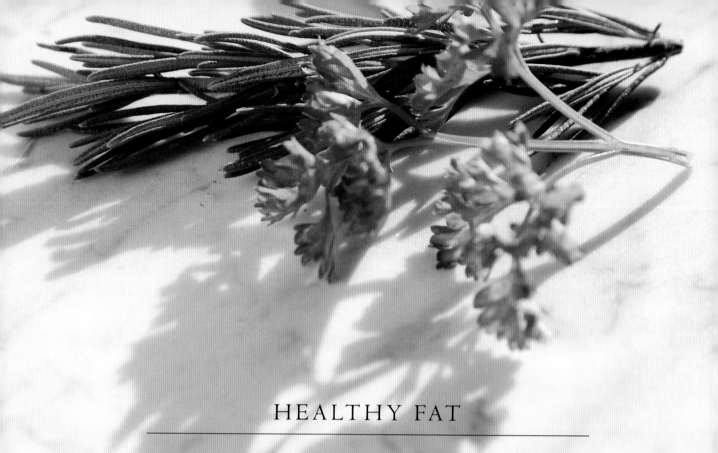

HEALTHY FAT

In the last 50 years, our culture has spent a great deal of time focusing on avoiding fat, forgetting that fat is healthful and nourishing and has historically been a very important part of the human diet. In fact, many traditional cultures prized fat as the most nutritious food available. It is incredibly nutrient dense and a rich source of fat-soluble vitamins and other compounds essential for tissue, joint, brain, and endocrine health. Though we should avoid some fats, like hydrogenated oils and corn and soy oils, plant-based fats from sources such as nuts and seed, olives, and coconut as well as animal fats from healthy pastured animals are all wonderful for the body.

Fat is heavy, dense, and sweet. While these qualities tell us that fat contains a huge amount of nourishment, they also indicate that fat can prove hard to digest. When we eat fat with herbs and spices that support digestion and assimilation, the body can access and process its vital nutrition more effectively and efficiently. Put some rosemary on your chicken or thyme on your beef, sprinkle cardamom and cinnamon on your milk or over your yogurt — these simple, and delicious, additions make the fats and proteins easier to digest and all the more nourishing. Certain cooking techniques can improve the bioavailability of the fats and proteins found in meats; braising, stewing, and roasting are all examples. You can also improve the digestibility of fat-rich nuts and seeds by soaking and roasting them, and you'll see these techniques often in my recipes.

Culinary Herbs as Medicine

Herbs have been a central component of culinary traditions around the world for hundreds and thousands of years. While many of us may cook with herbs simply because they taste good or because that's what the recipe or the tradition calls for, herbs have actually become culinary superstars for important health reasons. In fact, culinary herbs tend to be among the most useful of medicinal herbs. If you have ever cooked with an herb or spice, even just cinnamon or black pepper, you have engaged in the practice of using herbs medicinally. When we cook with diverse flavors and use herbs and spices, our goal may be to make our food taste good, but that simple intention makes our food easier to digest and assimilate and therefore more nutritious.

This realization can be liberating, helping us to learn that we can indulge in and truly enjoy food and still have it be healthy — that eating right and taking care of ourselves does not require deprivation or boring food choices. This knowledge can help us find deeper meaning in our relationship with food: letting our senses guide us, learning to listen to our body — desires, tastes, smells, and more. Ideally this can make our food choices come from a place of excitement, empowerment, and self-assurance rather than guilt and worry. Spending your time wondering what you *should* buy or eat, or what is good for you or not, is stressful and one of the worst things you can do for your health.

Once we learn to tune in to our body and speak its language, we can use food and herbs — with their nutrients, flavors, energies, and healing qualities — as tools to respond and help our body get what it needs. Communicating with the body in this way is easy and intuitive. We just need to learn to listen. With this communication in place, your kitchen can be a place of confidence, joy, and true nourishment. Health is a process, a language, and an experience that largely follows your own attitude and disposition. Give yourself the chance to tap into this wisdom and craft a few kitchen creations, or at least to just follow the recipes and know why they are the way they are!

Though each herb has its own particular flavor, its own long list of bioactive constituents, and its own unique effect on the body, most culinary herbs have in common three main medicinal categories of action:

- **Support for digestion and assimilation.** Food is only as good for us as our ability to digest it. Even the healthiest, most nutrient-dense foods are of little use to the body if we cannot absorb their nutrients. By providing diverse, complex, and stimulating flavor profiles, all culinary herbs improve digestion and the absorption of nutrients.

- **Antispasmodic properties.** Culinary herbs are almost always aromatic. Aromatic herbs help open up the nervous system, relax smooth muscle tissues, stimulate blood flow, and relieve tension. In the GI tract, this can alleviate gas, bloating, and cramping. In the rest of the body, it soothes tight muscles and may ease such conditions as anxiety, restlessness, and headaches.

- **Antimicrobial action.** Before refrigeration and modern food-processing techniques, food preservation and safe storage was a big deal. Cooking with antimicrobial herbs and spices helped to preserve food by preventing the growth of organisms that cause food to spoil or that cause food-borne illnesses. Antimicrobial herbs also kill harmful organisms in the GI tract, helping to balance gut flora and support the health of the microbiome. They can help the body combat bacterial or viral infection as well, making them great allies for common ailments such as cold and flu.

You may wonder how much of an herb you have to eat for it to have a medicinal effect. As we discussed earlier in this chapter, flavor is a powerful force driving physiological reactions. So as long as you can taste an herb, it is having a medicinal effect.

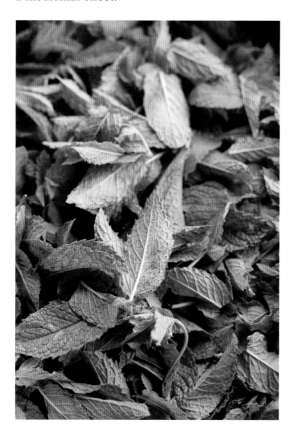

That being said, if you want to use rosemary to improve circulation or cilantro to help detoxify your body of heavy metals or mint to clear the sinuses or thyme to prevent a lung infection or parsley as a diuretic — if you want an herb to have a deep impact on your body — you will need to use more than just a taste. In these cases you will need a larger amount, or what I refer to in the descriptions that follow as a "medicinal dose." This does not mean that small amounts of an herb in food are not medicinal or that they do not influence the body; it just means that the ability of that herb to act specifically and significantly on the system is limited with smaller doses. So, for example, cooking with thyme is great for stimulating digestion, but it won't act as a lung tonic unless you are eating a tablespoon or so of thyme three times a day. And it would likely be even more effective as a tea than it would be if you just ate it plain — the hot water activates the volatile oils and accentuates the medicinal properties of the herb.

You might ask yourself, why culinary herbs? Why not just write a book about cooking with any and all herbs? Culinary herbs are powerful because they have an embedded history in our culture that is already part of a common language. Most people are familiar with culinary herbs and may have them in their kitchen already; they are widespread and accessible. As we learn to understand the uses of these herbs and apply them in the home kitchen/pharmacy, we are adding to and participating in a shared history. When we bring our own experiences to that history, we feed our common heritage and renew our connections with age-old cherished traditions.

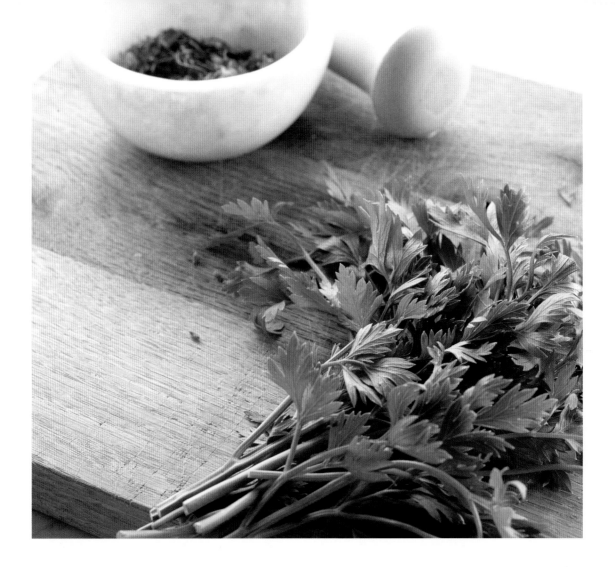

COOKING FOR A MEDICINAL DOSE

If you're looking to get a medicinal dose of an herb through your food, you have some good options. Pestos are one of the best ways to incorporate a large amount of herbs into your diet, and you can make pesto from any fresh herb, not just basil — try recipes using parsley (page 45), oregano (page 43), or cilantro (page 32), or just experiment on your own. Using fresh herbs and other ingredients (like citrus, berries, and other fruit) in blended beverages can provide a medicinal dose of an herb; cilantro lemonade (page 129) is a good example. These medicinal beverage blends are refreshing, delicious, and potently supportive of health and well-being.

You can also use culinary herbs to make teas, syrups, tinctures, and infused oils for home remedies. You'll find instructions for making these classic forms of herbal medicines later in this chapter. With these simple remedies at your disposal, you can use your culinary herbs as so much more than just food, bringing them to your bathing and self-care rituals, your first aid remedies, and your home medicine chest.

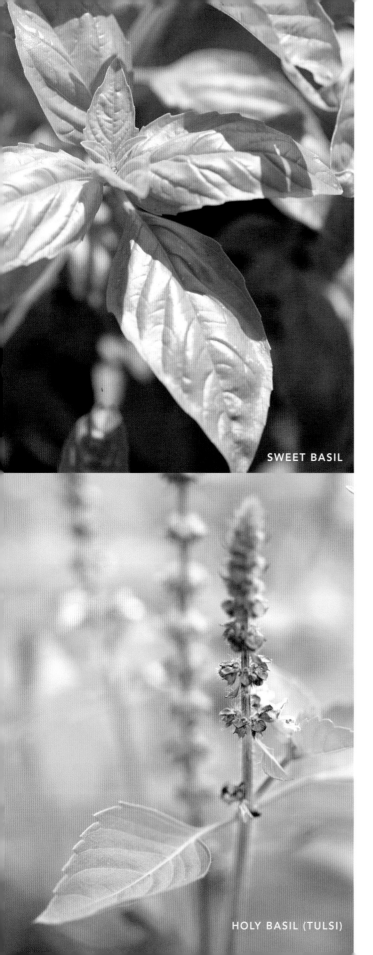

SWEET BASIL

HOLY BASIL (TULSI)

basil

Ocimum basilicum

FLAVORS: Pungent, bitter

Basil has high levels of volatile oils, which make it very aromatic, and as is the case with many culinary herbs, these oils are responsible for many of its medicinal properties.

When taken hot, basil is an effective diaphoretic (makes you sweat) and can help fight off bacterial or viral infection and purge toxins from the system through the skin. For these reasons, it can be an important herb for promoting detoxification and stimulating the release of heat and tension in the body. These diverse actions make basil both warming and cooling. Its stimulating function creates an initial warming effect, yet in many cases this improvement to metabolic function can clear heat and blockages, resulting in a cooling effect.

Basil is an important and often overlooked rejuvenating tonic that supports the mind, body, and spirit. It helps relieve fatigue and exhaustion and restore energy in cases of deep depletion. Basil seems to first stimulate and then relax the nervous system, making it a great herb for promoting mental clarity and cognitive function while helping you to stay focused, grounded, and calm. Long revered as an antidepressant, basil lifts the spirits and lightens the load on the heart. Simply smelling fresh basil can bring a sense of calm and peace. A cup of basil tea or a few drops of tincture can trigger the same sunny effect.

As is often the case with aromatic herbs, basil opens up the nervous system, dissolves tension, and thus stimulates the circulation of blood and other fluids. It can provide relief from mild headaches, especially tension headaches.

Relieving tension not only helps the musculoskeletal system and our state of mind but is excellent for the digestive system. Basil is a carminative: it eases intestinal cramping, gas, and bloating. It also warms the "digestive fire," which promotes the breakdown of food into absorbable nutrients and improves the absorption of those nutrients. It can help relieve nausea and vomiting.

Basil is also good for respiratory conditions, helping to expel mucus and relax the lung tissues, easing bronchial spasms and coughing. It has strong antimicrobial properties and is a wonderful herb to use to both prevent and nurse the symptoms of cold and flu. A hot tea will open up the pores, promote a sweat, and stimulate the immune system. In a steam, basil provides great support for the lungs (helping to expel mucus and ease other symptoms) and helps disinfect the mucous membranes of the eyes, nose, throat, and lungs.

Basil-infused oil can be applied externally to the back and chest to support the lungs during times of congestion, infection, spasms, and stress- or panic-induced shortness of breath. A strong tea can be used as a disinfectant wash or added to the bath to relieve muscle tension and cramping and promote relaxation and spiritual clarity.

USE IN THE KITCHEN

Basil, both fresh and dried, should be used freely in cooking to support digestion. Basil generally tastes strongest and is most potent when it is fresh, rather than dried or cooked. Add it at the end of cooking to preserve its volatile oils and flavor.

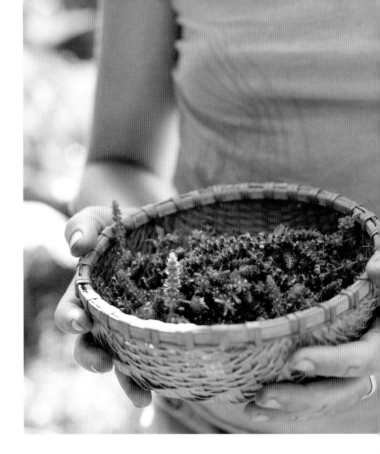

Notice the use of basil in large quantities in rich, heavy dishes like pasta, pizza, cream sauce, and meat. The basil helps us digest the starches, fats, and proteins found in these dishes. Large doses of basil in pesto, salads, teas, or other preparations not only support digestion but also have calming and soothing effects on the nervous system.

Basil is an important example of how our culinary herbs can be powerful tools for healing yet are often reserved for sprinkling on pizza. Today, an Ayurvedic variety of basil called tulsi (or holy basil) receives a lot of attention for its health benefits and tonic properties. While tulsi is undoubtedly a very special herb, in my opinion it should in no way outshine the magic of our everyday garden-variety basil. I suggest we take basil's common nature as a sign of its longstanding wisdom.

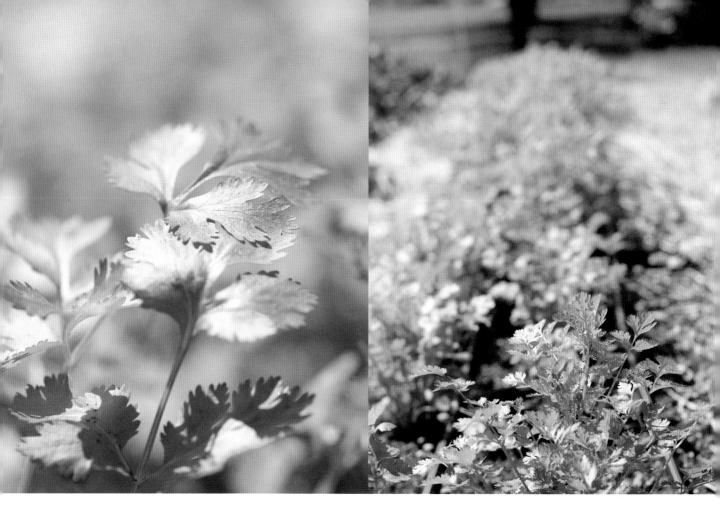

cilantro

Coriandrum sativum

FLAVOR: Sweet, bitter, astringent, pungent

Cilantro has an overall detoxifying, cooling, and grounding effect. Like many common culinary herbs, it has been used for thousands of years as a digestive aid. Cilantro increases the secretion of gastric juices, stimulates the appetite, and alleviates nausea. As a carminative, cilantro improves digestion and assimilation and helps relieve gas and bloating. It is great for easing indigestion and diarrhea.

This herb has also been shown to help the body process and utilize cholesterol, reducing cholesterol and triglyceride levels and increasing levels of high-density lipoproteins, which help transport fats like cholesterol and triglycerides. These benefits are most likely due to cilantro's effects on the liver: cilantro supports liver function and stimulates the secretion of bile, which the body uses to break down and digest fats and oils.

Cilantro is an excellent anti-inflammatory, particularly when inflammation is accompanied by heat. Medicinal doses of cilantro can ease inflammation and heat associated with hives, rashes, flushed or red skin, and excess sweating. It can also help balance inflammatory emotions of a hot nature, like rage, frustration, anger, or irritation. Cilantro can also be used externally as a poultice to reduce heat (redness and inflammation) on the surface of the skin, such as sunburn, rash, or acne. Internally or externally, it can be used acutely to address a specific situation or consistently as a tonic for people who have a "hot" constitution (perhaps they are hot to the touch, they always feel hot, or they are prone to inflammatory reactions).

Cilantro and its seed, coriander, are both mild diuretics. Medicinal doses can increase urination and relieve burning sensations associated with cystitis or urinary tract infections (UTIs). (Note that cilantro is not a strong enough antiseptic to treat a UTI and will not replace the need for medical attention, but it can reduce symptoms. It can also help prevent recurrence of chronic UTIs.)

Extracts of cilantro leaf have been shown to help balance blood sugar levels, and the herb may be of benefit in preventing metabolic syndrome and type 2 diabetes. Cilantro increases the amount of insulin released from cells and has insulin-like qualities, which both work to remove excessive amounts of glucose from the blood. Cilantro also aids the liver in converting glucose (available in high amounts when blood sugar is high) into glycogen, a storable energy source that the body can convert back into glucose as needed. Adequate stores of glycogen allow the body to balance its own blood sugar, helping to reduce sugar cravings. If you can't quite seem to kick the sugar habit, consider adding cilantro into your diet as a support.

Last, but certainly not least, cilantro can be used as an effective natural chelator. Chelators are substances that bind with heavy metals in the body so they can be carried out. One study showed that cilantro reduced lead counts in mice, and I suspect that it is effective in reducing levels of other heavy metals, such as mercury and cadmium, as well. When you eat seafood, consider also eating a medicinal dose of cilantro in a salad, pesto, or herbal drink to ensure that any heavy metals deposited in the seafood from polluted ocean waters do not get stored in your body.

USE IN THE KITCHEN

The volatile oils and aromas that give cilantro much of its unique, refreshing flavor dissipate once the plant is heated, dried, or frozen. For this reason, it is often used as a garnish or served raw in salsas, chutneys, sauces, and salads. When I want to put cilantro in a stew or other slow-cooked dish, I add the fresh leaves at the very end or save them for a garnish on top. Or I use the root — it imparts an unusual earthy and cilantro-rich flavor, holds up better to cooking, and offers many of the same benefits as the leaf.

You may have noticed that cilantro is commonly used with spicy foods, like salsa and chili. Cilantro has an overall cooling effect, helping to relieve heat in the body, which makes it a nice complement for dishes with heat. It is also used heavily in cuisines from hot climates. The next time you need a refreshing drink at the end of a long, hot day, try a glass of cilantro lemonade (page 129)!

Coriander seed is also popular in the kitchen and shares many of the same medicinal properties as cilantro.

dill

Anethum graveolens

FLAVOR: Pungent, bitter

The feathery dill leaves most commonly used in cooking are sometimes called dill weed. The seeds are the strongest part of the plant (flavorwise and medicinally) and can be used in cooking and home remedies. I also like to use dill flower and the immature seeds as well as the pollen. The pollen can be collected during the flowering stage by tapping the flower umbel inside a brown bag or over a bowl. The pollen makes a lovely flavorful garnish.

Dill is an all-around fabulous digestive remedy, carminative, and digestive stimulant. It's great for gas, bloating, and indigestion, and it eases nausea, vomiting, and diarrhea. It has long been revered as a remedy for halitosis (bad breath), which makes sense given that dill

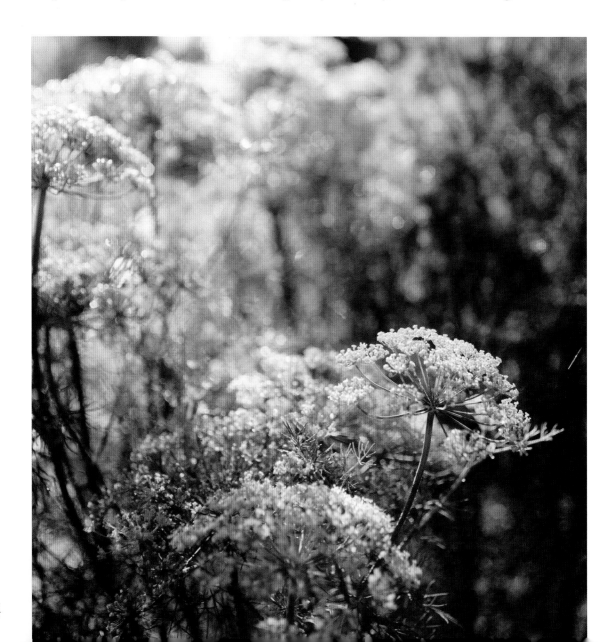

supports proper digestion and metabolism. It is also excellent for soothing fever from bacterial or viral infection.

This gentle herb lends itself well to use with children. Dill is a famous old European remedy for colic, often administered to infant children in a weak tea called dill water. Like its cousin fennel, dill is a galactogogue, meaning that it helps increase the flow of breast milk. One of the best ways to administer herbs to infants is through the breast milk of the nursing mother. So while dill water is appropriate for infants, it can also be given to those who nurse them, infusing their milk with anti-colicky compounds!

Dill-infused vinegar is another common European remedy. Dill is rich in minerals, and because vinegar is an excellent solvent of minerals, dill vinegar makes a great tonic for both digestion and the structures of the body, like the hair, nails, bones, and nerves. This remedy is delicious!

USE IN THE KITCHEN

Dill's complex flavor profile gives rise to mixed feelings for many. If you love dill, fabulous, enjoy it! If you're less enamored, start with small bits — a little goes a long way. Dill is in the same family as anise and fennel and shares some of their flavoring. Combining dill with sweet flavors helps bring out that anise- and fennel-like character. In fact, dill is a traditional flavoring in French cakes and pastries. It pairs well with citrus, cream, and yogurt, which all bring out similar subtle notes of anise and fennel. In addition, I love dill with boiled eggs, in salads, on potatoes, and with fish.

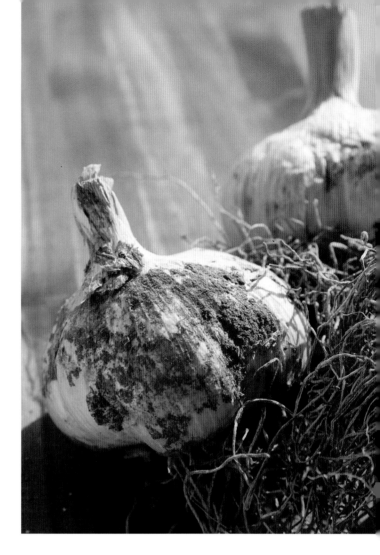

garlic

Allium sativum

FLAVOR: Pungent (when raw), sweet (when cooked)

Garlic contains highly medicinal sulfur compounds, including alliin, which, when acted upon by an enzyme called alliinase, is converted into allicin. A powerful antioxidant, allicin has attracted a lot of attention from researchers because of its potent antibacterial, antiviral, antifungal, antiprotozoal, and anticancer activity. Garlic just happens to contain

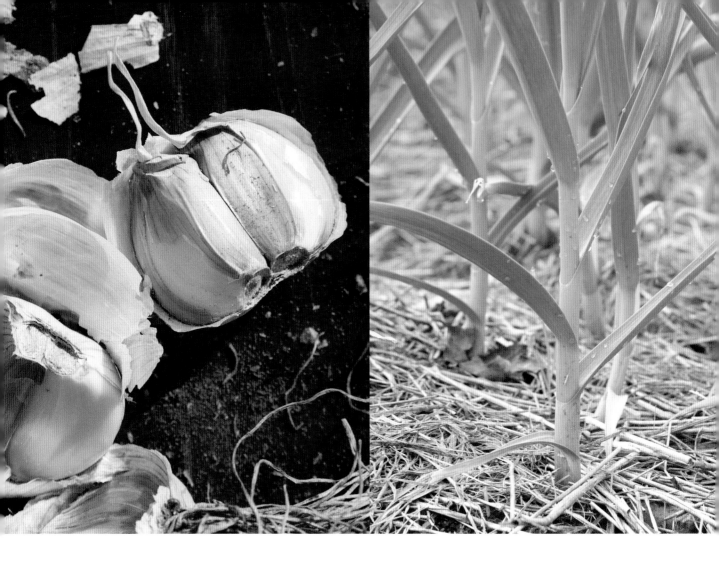

both alliin and alliinase; they are stored in different parts of the bulb, kept apart from one another by cell membranes. When you cut, crush, or juice garlic, these compounds come together and produce allicin. This is just one more reminder of why using whole plants for medicine, rather than isolated constituents, is so powerful; garlic teaches us that the medicine is locked up in the ecosystem of the plant in its whole form. Because the enzymatic reaction that forms allicin takes time, it is best to let freshly chopped or pressed garlic sit for 5 to 10 minutes before using it.

As a vasodilator, bronchodilator, and decongestant, garlic has long been used as a remedy for asthma and other respiratory issues. Garlic infused in vinegar with honey is a classic and effective tonic for upper respiratory congestion, asthma, and seasonal allergies. If you find the garlic too harsh for the stomach, try adding fennel seed to this remedy to soothe and soften that pungent flavor.

Garlic offers incredible tonic properties to the cardiovascular system as well. It thins the blood, reducing blood pressure and preventing blood clots. It supports elasticity of the arteries and blood vessels, preventing and addressing hardening of the arteries (arteriosclerosis). It can have a beneficial effect on cholesterol levels, helping the body better synthesize and utilize cholesterol compounds.

The sulfur compounds in garlic, notably allicin, are immune stimulants that work to raise white blood cell counts. And its powerful antimicrobial compounds act on mucous membrane tissues and can be of assistance in cases of everything from intestinal bugs and parasites to cold, flu, and sore throat. Garlic has even been shown to fight off some strains of antibiotic-resistant bacteria. It can be effective against fungal infections as well, including candidiasis and oral thrush.

As an antiseptic and circulatory stimulant, garlic disinfects the blood throughout the body, including in the brain. When there is no infection to deal with, this has an effect of blood cleansing, making garlic an effective alterative (blood purifier) and anti-inflammatory. It can be used to reduce inflammation of the joints and improve joint mobility.

Chopped or crushed garlic can be preserved in oil, which keeps it isolated from oxygen and seems to preserve the active compounds. Externally, the infused oil, water-based infusion, or fresh plant poultice can be used on fungal or bacterial infections of the skin or nails, inflammatory conditions such as aches, sprains, and bruises, and mild skin irritations. A drop of warm garlic-infused oil in the ear can prevent and treat infection.

While garlic oil is considered a delicacy that people make and enjoy all the time in their cooking, I feel obliged to at least mention that the food safety field warns of the risk of botulism from garlic oil. I don't worry about this too much myself, but you should know the word on that side of the street.

USE IN THE KITCHEN

Both cooked and raw garlic should be used freely in the diet. While cooked garlic contains many wonderful health benefits, raw or lightly cooked garlic contains more, particularly those antimicrobial and immune-stimulating compounds. Raw garlic is lovely in salad dressings and other condiments; if you want to use it in a cooked dish, add it at or near the very end of cooking to preserve its volatile constituents. Adding garlic in the early stages of cooking a dish will develop deeper flavor profiles, so often I add it at both the beginning and the end.

Many folks find raw garlic to be harsh on their stomach but still want to incorporate it into their diet. Consider garlic-infused honey or garlic-infused vinegar with honey; the honey mellows and softens the harsh, pungent compounds. Eating lightly cooked garlic alongside carminative culinary herbs is also helpful. And fermented garlic in kraut or kimchi has all the same health benefits of raw garlic, with a more mellow flavor and energy. Pickled garlic, like that left over at the bottom of your Thyme and Jalapeño Pickled Carrots (page 109) or Lactofermented Dilly Beans (page 196), is also often mild enough for those with a sensitive stomach. If raw garlic continues to bother you, just eat it cooked!

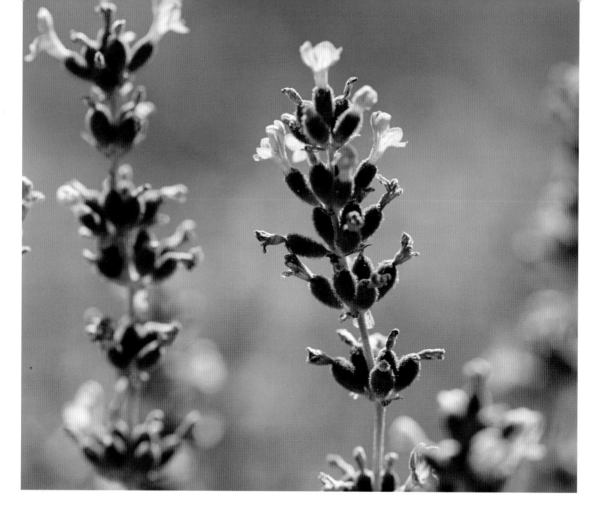

lavender

Lavandula spp.

FLAVOR: Pungent, bitter

Of the many varieties of lavender that exist, all are highly aromatic, intoxicating to the senses, relaxing, as well as clarifying, and prized as medicinals.

The flowers are the part generally called for in medicine, cosmetics, and perfumery, but the leaves contain just as many of the magical volatile oils that make lavender famous. I use the fresh leaves and flowers interchangeably in medicine and cooking. Once dried, the flowers do seem to maintain a more potent aroma and have higher oil content than the leaves, but again, both can be used.

Lavender is a powerful nervine (affects the nervous system). Its bitter, pungent flavors and aromatics are grounding and calming. It is a great ally for depression, anxiety, fear, nervousness, hysteria, obsession, negative thoughts, and panic. It helps dissolve tension and can relieve headaches, promote sleep, and reduce feelings of fatigue. It is an uplifting heart remedy — lavender helps put us back into our body and into our heart when our mind has run away from us.

Because so much of lavender's medicine lies in its volatile oils, the effects can be experienced well through aromatherapy. Lavender hydrosol or diluted tincture in a spray bottle can be sprayed around the room. The spray can also be used as an antimicrobial wash — say goodbye to antibacterial hand wipes and sanitizer. A pot of lavender tea left to simmer, uncovered, on the stovetop or woodstove will fill your house with aromatic magic too. Consider a small pillow stuffed with dried lavender beside the bed to help you relax and promote sweet dreams; I love to use lavender massage oil before bed to promote deep, restful sleep.

Lavender can also be a good herb for helping to relieve pain. Externally, in the bath or as a massage oil, it can ease tight and sore muscles, muscle spasms, and pain in the tissues and joints. Internally, it can soothe just enough to take the edge off pain.

As an antibacterial herb, lavender makes a great wash for cuts, scrapes, and other maladies and a nice addition to healing salves, natural cleaning products, and anything else you can think of. In the winter, I like to use lavender in steams for the respiratory system. The aromatic oils prevent and help clear up infections of the mucous membrane tissues and open up congestion. Some studies have shown that the oils in lavender can fight the bacteria associated with strep throat and pneumonia.

Like other bitter, pungent, and aromatic culinary herbs, lavender is a good digestive aid. Small amounts can ease indigestion and relieve intestinal cramping. It stimulates the digestive fire and improves the digestion and absorption of nutrients.

USE IN THE KITCHEN

I recommend lavender every which way — including at least one fresh plant in your life. If you don't have a garden, consider lavender in a pot on the windowsill.

In remedies and cooking, it is often the aromatic oils we are after, and they are released quickly when exposed to heat. They are easily extracted with hot water, as a tea; just make sure to cover the steeping tea to trap the oils. A longer-steeped tea will turn bitter, while a short-steeped tea will be pleasantly aromatic. In cooking, you will notice that recipes usually call for only a small amount; the lavender aroma permeates thoroughly, making a little go a long way.

POWDERING LAVENDER

Some of the recipes in this book call for powdering dried lavender blossoms. You can easily powder them in a coffee or spice grinder, or by hand with a mortar and pestle, but you can also use a blender. Just put the blossoms in the blender and turn it on. With one hand beneath the motor base and the other on the blender lid, gently lift the blender and tilt it to one side. Running the blender while it's tilted allows the blossoms to move inside the blender in a circular motion, with better access to the blade. You can use this method to powder any dried herb.

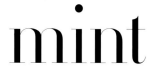

mint

Mentha spp.

FLAVOR: Pungent

There are hundreds of types of mint, from peppermint to spearmint to chocolate mint and beyond. While each has its own special attributes, they all possess that aromatic magic that gives them their medicine, and they can be used interchangeably — although keep in mind that the oils of some may be stronger than the oils of others.

Both stimulating and cooling, mint's main actions are its ability to refresh and decongest. When taken hot, it is a diaphoretic, opening the pores and promoting sweating; it stimulates stagnant fluids of the blood and lymph and helps clear heat from inside the body. An antispasmodic, it relaxes smooth muscle tissues and stimulates metabolic function, acting as a digestive and circulatory stimulant while simultaneously dissolving tension. With this diverse range of actions, mint has many uses.

Mint has a refreshing effect on the senses, rejuvenating the mind and clearing cobwebs out of both the thoughts and the sinuses. It is an excellent decongestant when taken internally or inhaled through a steam or bath. Mint also refreshes stagnant thoughts and emotions, increases vitality, and promotes energy, including sexual vitality. It is a great herb to improve concentration; mint was my favorite study herb in college. Like many members of the mint family, including lavender, basil, and rosemary, mint both stimulates and relaxes, relieving tension and helping to dissolve fear, anxiety, and restlessness, especially when they are held in the body.

In addition to being diaphoretic, mint oils are strong antimicrobials, making this herb a good choice for cold, flu, fever, intestinal illnesses, and ear and other infections. Because it stimulates circulation and clears heat, it is excellent both internally and externally for skin eruptions and infections, including hives, acne, eczema, and psoriasis. Externally, as a poultice, mint cools and soothes, relieving itching, redness, and topical inflammation.

These same qualities that move and relieve stagnancy can have great pain-relieving effects for the musculoskeletal system. Taken internally or applied externally, mint often provides relief for rheumatic pains, leg cramps, and general fatigue.

Mint also has a balancing effect on menstruation. It can help return an absent period and promote balance in the cycle. As a tonic it helps prevent painful periods and can likewise be used to alleviate symptoms of menstruation, including cramping, bloating, nausea, and fatigue.

Mint is a highly valued carminative and general digestive aid. It stimulates the digestive fire, including the secretion of bile and digestive enzymes. It promotes the appetite and is excellent for people suffering from lack of appetite or wasting conditions. While some people find that mint's cooling and soothing properties help prevent and relieve the symptoms of heartburn and acid reflux, others find that it aggravates symptoms. It makes a good after-dinner tea to counteract an overfull stomach or indigestion. Like most carminatives, it relaxes the muscles of the GI tract and helps expel gas and relieve intestinal cramping.

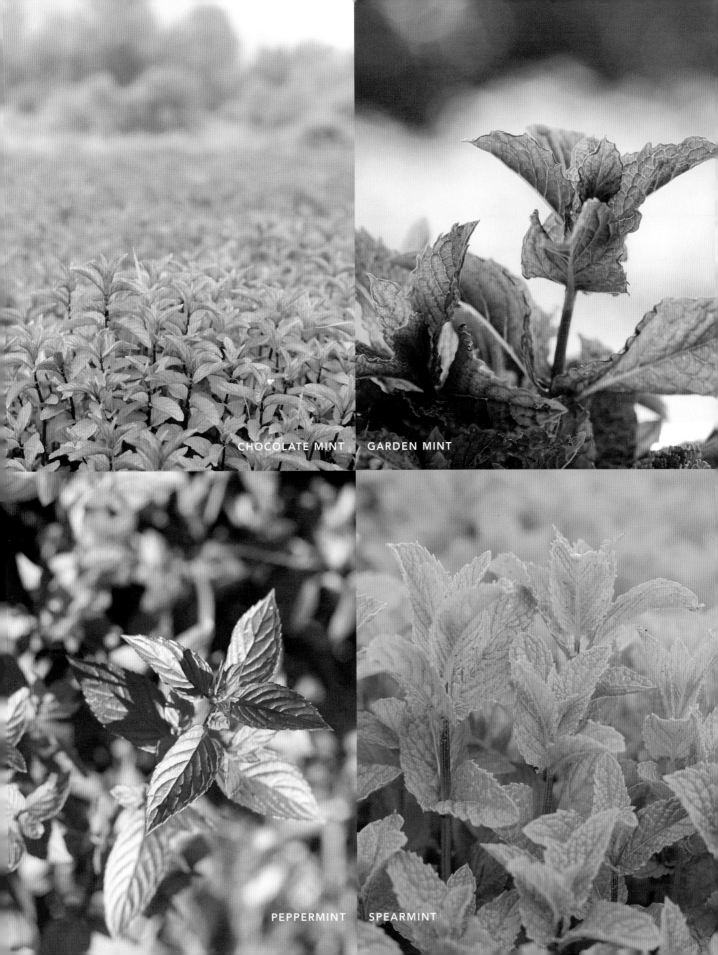

CHOCOLATE MINT | GARDEN MINT

PEPPERMINT | SPEARMINT

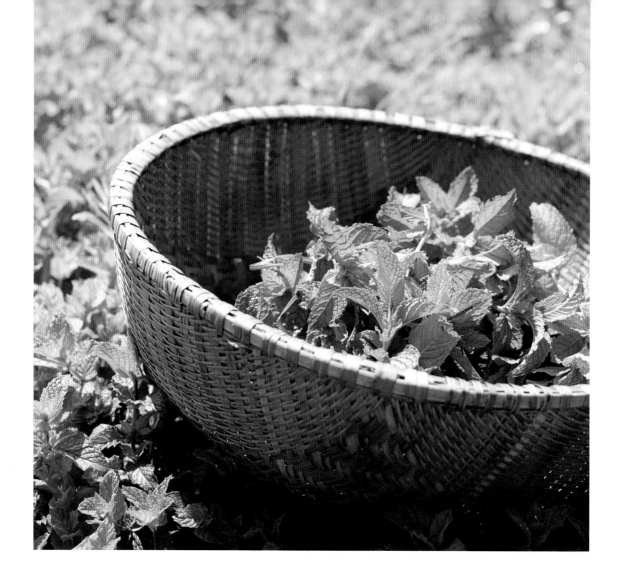

A tonic for the digestive system, mint helps relieve constipation and balance loose stools and diarrhea. Its antinausea effect should not be overlooked; it can ease the nausea associated with motion sickness, morning sickness, intestinal illness, menstruation, or migraine. Its antibacterial oils work to reduce infection or parasitic overgrowths, and its relaxing, anti-inflammatory, and antimicrobial qualities band together and make it excellent for inflammatory conditions of the digestive system, including Crohn's disease, colitis and irritable bowel syndrome.

USE IN THE KITCHEN

Like cilantro, mint's cooling nature lends itself well to spicy dishes, offering a refreshing respite from the heat. It also pairs well with other cooling foods like yogurt and cucumber that might end up as condiments and side dishes for spicy meals.

I love using mint to enliven summer drinks. Even just a few fresh sprigs in a water bottle feels uplifting on a hot day. While I make tea from both fresh and dried mint, I prefer to use fresh mint in my cooking, especially in summer, as a cooling counterpoint to the heat.

oregano

Origanum spp.

FLAVOR: Pungent, bitter

There are many varieties of oregano, including the popular marjoram, *Origanum majorana*, all of which share much in common with the common oregano, *O. vulgare*. You can use them medicinally interchangeably, remembering, as is the case for mint, that some oregano species will be stronger, with a more bitter, pungent flavor and more oils, while others (like marjoram) are more sweet. Grow a variety you love and adapt in recipes as you feel appropriate, using more of a milder variety and less of a stronger variety. It is all truly delicious and highly medicinal.

Pungent, aromatic, and warming, oregano is a stimulating diaphoretic (stimulates sweating) useful in cases of fever with chills. It helps expel cold from the body, especially when a cold invasion leads to cold, flu, or fever. As a bronchodilator and expectorant, it has traditionally been used to treat coughs and whooping cough. And as a strong antimicrobial, antifungal, and rubefacient (something that stimulates blood flow to any skin surface it comes into contact with), it can be used to relieve sore throat and infections of the mouth; just swish with a strong tea of oregano or ¼ teaspoon of the tincture diluted in an ounce of water.

Oregano contains thymol, which is a potent antifungal, making this herb a good choice for use in an oil, poultice, compress, or wash to treat fungal infections of the skin. As a rubefacient and stimulant, it can also be applied

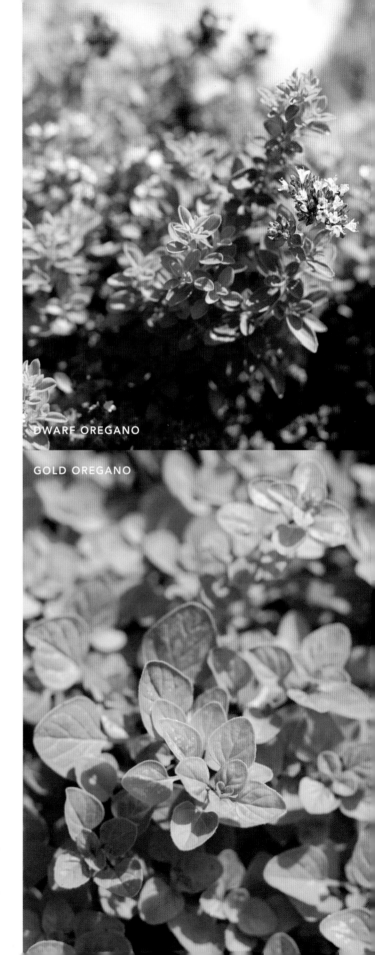

DWARF OREGANO

GOLD OREGANO

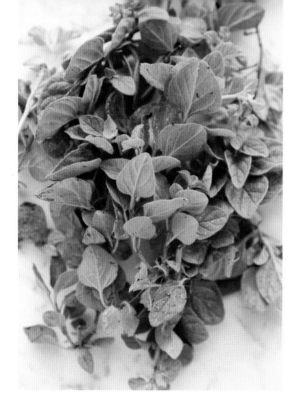

externally to soothe rheumatic pains and other stagnancies of the musculoskeletal system.

Oregano's excellent antifungal properties set it apart from other digestive aids. It helps expel toxins from the gut and fights *Candida* and other unwanted micro-organisms (a condition often referred to as gut dysbiosis). It is excellent for addressing symptoms of halitosis, putrid digestion (fermentation and stagnancy in the upper digestive tract), bloating and abdominal distension, and belching. While the essential oil is often used to treat excess *Candida* and other GI issues, I feel strongly that a tea or tincture does the job fine, and either will be easier to make at home and easier for the body to process.

This herb improves memory and concentration and is a great tonic for old age. Like its mint family cousins, it helps relieve tension. It is excellent for the high-strung "overdoer" who can't seem to relax and is particularly supportive alongside other nervines when this "overdoing" becomes part of a person's identity but is not serving him or her well. It is also useful for relieving tension headache; try a poultice of the fresh leaves right on the forehead or temples. I learned this technique from a Venezuelan nurse, Señora Carmen, who gave me a juicy and highly aromatic variety of oregano called *orégano orejón*, or "big-eared" oregano, which I still cherish.

Beyond relieving tension, oregano is an antidepressant. It calms nervousness, fear, irritability, and bad dreams.

Oregano is also an emmenagogue (meaning it stimulates menstrual bleeding). It can be used to bring on the menses or ease congestion-related menstrual pain.

USE IN THE KITCHEN

The Latin genus name, *Origanum*, is derived from two Greek words: *oros*, meaning "mountain," and *ganos*, meaning "joy." The herb grows wild on hillsides throughout the Mediterranean, where there is a long history of cooking with wild greens. With this in mind, it makes perfect sense that oregano would make its way into traditional dishes such as spanakopita (see the recipe on page 153). It is delicious on meats and with eggs and a not-to-be missed ingredient in tomato sauce!

The aromatic oils of oregano hold up well to drying, and I sometimes find the dried herb even more potent than the fresh leaves in my cooking. I use oregano fresh whenever it is in the garden and enjoy the dried herb in my cooking and in teas throughout the winter months.

parsley

Petroselinum crispum

FLAVOR: Pungent, bitter, salty

All parts of the parsley plant are incredibly nutritive, from the leaf to the root, stem, and seed. Both the curly and flat-leaf varieties of parsley are common, though each has a slightly different flavor. In my opinion the flat-leaf variety is slightly saltier, but they can be used interchangeably. I find fresh parsley from the garden to be more tender, with a subtler and more delicious flavor. If you can, grow your own; if not, be grateful for what you can buy, picking out the most tender-looking bunch as you shop.

Parsley is a valuable nutritive tonic. It is a rich source of vitamin C — pound for pound parsley has more vitamin C than an orange, and without the sugar. It also contains notable amounts of calcium, phosphorus, potassium, and iron, making it a great remedy for iron-deficiency anemia and fatigue.

Like most culinary herbs, parsley is a carminative, easing gas and bloating, and it stimulates digestion and absorption. It is a

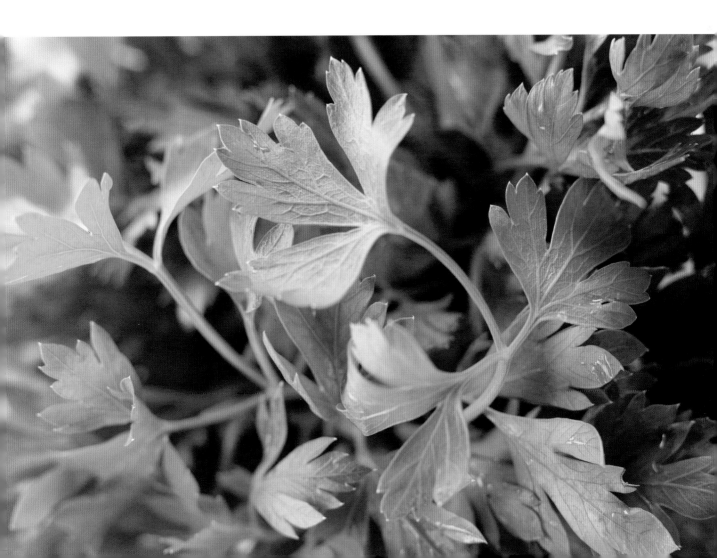

good remedy for bad breath, and is perhaps most famously known for neutralizing garlic breath! It has been used historically to expel worms and ease constipation.

This herb is an important diuretic and urinary tonic. Because it actually contains potassium, as most herbal diuretics do, it does not deplete the body of potassium, as most pharmaceutical diuretics do. It is a urinary antiseptic and demulcent and can be used for urinary stones and urinary tract infections. It is an important addition to the diet for those who suffer chronic or reoccurring urinary tract infections or for those who are recovering from one. In fact, parsley is excellent for helping to stimulate movement of fluids of all kind, working to break up the stagnancy of edema and reduce general water retention, including that associated with premenstruation.

Parsley is a valuable metabolic stimulator, promoting detoxification through the kidneys and liver. This makes it a great remedy for seasonal allergies, all manner of premenstrual difficulties, hot flashes, headaches, night sweats, and arthritis. Parsley also improves thyroid function and helps address secondary symptoms of diabetes, particularly those of the kidneys. Compounds in parsley have been found to prevent the growth of tumor cells, making parsley an anticancer herb as well. It is also a uterine tonic, and as an emmenagogue, it can help bring on menses and relieve congestion-related menstrual cramping.

Externally, a poultice of the leaves or grated root works to relieve swelling, stagnation, heat, and infection associated with mastitis and other infections.

USE IN THE KITCHEN

I use fresh parsley freely as a green in my cooking. I add it to salads or eat it as a salad green on its own, use it in soups and sautés, and throw it into pestos and other sauces. You can dry it to use as a seasoning or to make tea, but you will find that dried parsley is not nearly as flavorful as fresh when it comes to cooking.

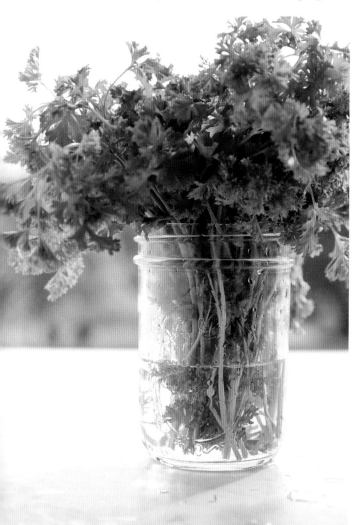

rosemary

Rosmarinus officinalis
FLAVOR: Pungent, bitter

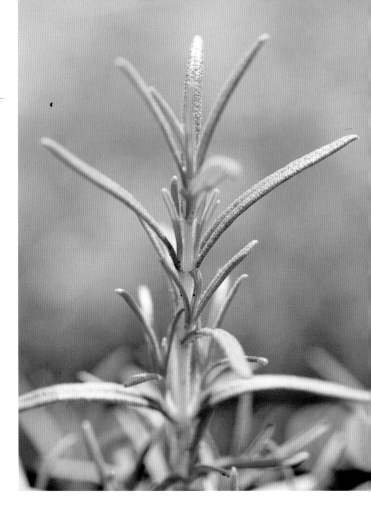

Rosemary is a wonderful tonic herb. When used over time, its effects on the metabolic system build on themselves and create lasting positive effects. To begin, rosemary stimulates the metabolism; its bitter taste stimulates liver and gallbladder function and it also supports kidney function. It also regulates the function of smooth muscle tissue through parasympathetic nervous system pathways (the so-called "rest and digest" part of the nervous system, which primarily encourages relaxation, rest, and rejuvenation), toning the arteries, digestive system, heart, and lungs. Throughout the body this herb has a warming, clearing, and oxygenating effect on blood, tissues, and organs. These properties contribute to most of its effects on the nervous system, digestive system, and cardiovascular system.

An excellent carminative and bitter, rosemary stimulates healthy peristalsis and liver function, supports the digestion and assimilation of fats and oils, and eases gas, bloating, and intestinal cramping and colic. As an antimicrobial, it kills intestinal parasites and bacteria. Because it operates through parasympathetic pathways, it helps relax smooth muscle tissue spasms and is good for an upset or nervous stomach. Rosemary also works to delay the uptake of carbohydrates in the system, leading to a slower increase in blood sugar levels.

As a tonic for the nervous system, rosemary can relieve headaches and calm nervousness and anxiety. I often use a bit of rosemary in tea or tincture blends to support people with anxiety. As a warming and stimulating tonic, rosemary activates other calming sedative herbs, opening the nervous system and stimulating a sense of purpose in the body and thus in the spirit. Rosemary is both mentally uplifting and clarifying; it is excellent for depression and for uplifting the heart.

Rosemary is a great tonic for the heart and cardiovascular system. It strengthens the heart muscle, helps regulate blood pressure, stimulates circulation, and tonifies blood vessels.

An excellent tonic for the brain, rosemary helps strengthen memory, clear foggy thinking, and even improve vision. It has long been cited as an herb of remembrance — it is associated with love and friendship and the bond of such connections.

One compound found in rosemary, carnosic acid (which is also found in sage), is an antioxidant that prevents food spoiling. It seems to be particularly good at preventing fats from going rancid, making rosemary a first choice for preserving meats — hence much of our culinary associations of rosemary with roasts of all kinds. This high antioxidant activity is thought to contribute to some of this herb's benefits to the brain, circulatory system, and nervous system and to reduce the growth of cancer and tumors.

In addition to antioxidants, rosemary contains acetylcholinesterase inhibitors, which slow the breakdown of acetylcholine in the brain. (This breakdown has been linked to Alzheimer's and other memory issues.) To benefit from these properties, you should use rosemary as a tonic to build and strengthen memory and metabolism over time.

Rosemary is an antispasmodic (which means it reduces spasms of smooth muscle tissues), which, as we have seen, has a positive effect on digestion and circulation. It also has an affinity for the female reproductive system and is helpful for reducing spasm-related menstrual cramps (the kinds of cramps that begin at the onset of bleeding). As a warming, circulation-stimulating decongestant, rosemary also lends itself well to congestive menstrual cramping (the kinds of cramps that begin before you bleed and are often greatly relieved at the onset of menstruation). A hot rosemary tea or the tincture in hot water is excellent for either type of cramping.

Externally, rosemary is a rubefacient and can be applied topically as an infused oil, compress, or poultice — or used in a bath — to ease congestion and pain in the musculoskeletal system, including symptoms of gout and bruising, as well as the pain of menstruation or stomachache. A rosemary bath or footbath, perhaps with a touch of lavender, is a marvelous way to unwind at the end of the day.

USE IN THE KITCHEN

Rosemary has a deep earthy flavor that lends itself particularly well to all types of meat, from chicken to beef to lamb, as well as potatoes and other root vegetables. The aromatics infuse wonderfully into breads and other baked goods, and I find the herb lovely in sweet treats and desserts. Because of its potent rubefacient and disinfectant properties, it also works well in body-care preparations, including hair rinses, shampoos, infused oils, baths, and facial and body scrubs.

Rosemary's strong flavor holds up well to cooking and to drying. I use both fresh and dried rosemary in my cooking.

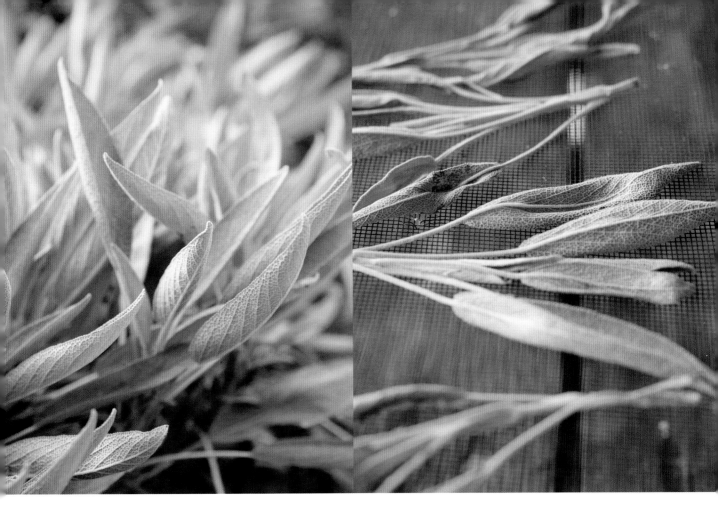

sage

Salvia officinalis

FLAVOR: Pungent, bitter, astringent

There are many kinds of sage, each with diverse medicinal and ceremonial applications. While they all share similarities in flavor and constituents, we will focus on the garden variety, *Salvia officinalis*. It is an active healer with a wide range of uses.

Sage is astringent, pungent, oily, aromatic, bitter, and mildly warming. It is an excellent carminative and digestive bitter, stimulating the liver and gallbladder. It aids with the digestion of fats and oils and stimulates peristalsis. As a carminative it eases all manner of general digestive upsets, including indigestion, gas, bloating, lack of appetite, discomfort after eating, and poor nutrient absorption. Sage's astringent properties make it a great remedy for overly loose stools and diarrhea; for this application, it is best to take the tea cold.

Sage supports the body's utilization of lipids and cholesterol, from the digestive system all the way to the cellular level. This promotes healthy cell membranes and reduces dryness in the cells, tendons, and skin. Because sex hormones and other steroid-based hormones use fat and cholesterol as precursors, sage seems to help the body better produce these hormones

(I thank herbalist Matthew Wood for this insight and have found it to be effective in my practice). Alongside this action, sage has been credited with estrogenic effects (it interacts with estrogen receptors in the body), and it does help regulate the hormonal cycle — making it good for relieving premenstrual issues, hot flashes, and symptoms of menopause.

As the wisdom in its name implies, sage promotes longevity, working to strengthen and rejuvenate at a cellular level. It is excellent for restoring vitality during and after periods of illness or general debility.

An outstanding herb for the nervous system, sage can help relieve tension. It is a great remedy for what I call "split ends of the nerves" — a characteristic of people who are quick to jump or shout, reactive, and easily agitated, frustrated, or made angry, nervous, or upset by a disruption to their routine. It is a good choice for the strung-out and overstressed person who has been exhausted for so long that the body adapts to this state of stress and has a hard time relaxing because of it. In cases such as this, including exhaustion and insomnia, sage is wonderful alongside other nervines as a short-term tonic.

Sage encourages clarity and peace of mind. It has a long history of being burned to clear energy, uplift the senses, and promote mental alertness, relaxation, and protection. While white sage is most commonly used for burning, the culinary variety can also be used.

A powerful antimicrobial, sage contains potent oils, similar to those found in other culinary herbs, that disinfect and support the health of mucous membranes. It also contains carnosic acid, the antioxidant that has been found particularly helpful in preserving meats;

it is no wonder that sage, like rosemary, is often reserved for seasoning meats.

Sage has a well-earned reputation for remedying sore throat and infection of the mouth and throat, including gum infections and irritations, strep, laryngitis, and tonsillitis. For this purpose you can use room-temperature tea or diluted tincture or glycerin as a gargle; I add a bit of salt to my gargle. You could also apply any of these preparations as a spray to the throat or gums. I use sage as an ingredient in my homemade herbal tooth and gum rinse; I make a tincture with some combination of other excellent herbs for oral health, such as calendula, echinacea, thyme, mint, cinnamon, or clove, which I then dilute (20 drops to a mouthful of water) and swish for 30 to 60 seconds.

Externally, as a poultice, compress, wash, or infused oil, sage supports the healing of wounds. It helps move stagnant blood, making it a superb remedy for poor circulation, bruises, hard swellings, and infection. Internally, the tea or tincture can be used to help reduce blood clots and blood stagnation; it's especially supportive for those who bruise easily or who have varicose and spider veins. This is an important use of this herb and one that provides valuable support in old age as well as in cases of poor circulation and blood stagnation. It is no wonder sage is prized as a rejuvenative — increasing circulation and clearing blockages opens up space for more mental and physical energy.

A note about administration: When served hot, sage is a diaphoretic, stimulating sweating, detoxification, and fluid loss through the pores of the skin. In this instance it has a warming effect on metabolism, and it can also have a cooling effect overall, since sweat cools as it dries. When served cold, sage is a much more powerful astringent, drying up and eliminating fluids, including sweat and other discharges (this is why you drink cold tea to help relieve loose stools and diarrhea). Along these lines, it is famous for helping to dry up breast milk production.

USE IN THE KITCHEN

With its strong oils and pungent flavor, sage lends itself to cooking. It holds up to heat and readily infuses into meats and other dishes. It is classically used on poultry and in bread stuffing, and I also love it with onions, hard squashes, and sweet root vegetables. It is hardy enough to hold up to crisping and is famously browned in butter or oil, giving it a lovely texture and deep, earthy flavor. I love to add crispy sage to grain, bean, and pasta dishes (see Crispy Sage and Roasted Garlic Risotto, page 144).

I love using sage in tea for its strong yet simple flavor, lovely aromatics, and rich medicine. It makes a great after-dinner tea to clear the palate and support digestion, and it even helps the body fight colds and flu.

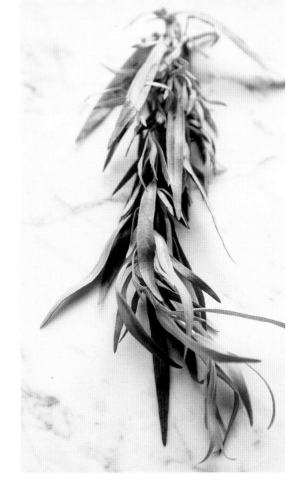

tarragon

Artemisia dracunculus

FLAVOR: Bitter, pungent

Like all culinary herbs, tarragon is richly aromatic. It holds notes of anise in its smell and taste, along with a little bit of bitterness. One of its volatile aromatic constituents, estragole, is also found in anise, fennel, bay, basil, and other culinary herbs, which might explain why tarragon's flavor has some likeness to the flavor of these other herbs. The aromatics transfer well during cooking, which gives tarragon a notable place in cuisine. Tarragon also contains compounds that can make the tongue tingle or feel slightly numb, so don't be alarmed if tarragon-heavy recipes leave a slight tingling sensation on the tongue. This effect is benign and perhaps even mildly entertaining.

Tarragon is a member of the artemisia family, related to mugwort, wormwood, and sweet Annie — a truly magical lineage with a long history of use in shifting and transitioning consciousness. In fact, tarragon is an old folk remedy for insomnia and hyperactivity. It soothes the nervous system and promotes the shift in consciousness that helps us to enter dreamtime. While its cousin mugwort may help us remember our dreams, tarragon encourages us to settle into a restful place and get to the kind of deep sleep where dreams happen!

Tarragon supports the digestive system by stimulating the release of bile and other digestive juices. It is a great aid for relieving gas and indigestion and is excellent following a large meal (think Thanksgiving). It relieves discomfort associated with the digestion of fat as well as complicated food combinations.

Tarragon is an appetite stimulant — it is probably one of my favorite culinary herbs for improving the appetite and restoring a desire for food. I find this particularly helpful in two situations: The first is for people in high-stress or high-anxiety crisis, when the appetite wanes or the stomach is tied in knots and food just doesn't sound good. It may be normal to feel like your stomach is tied in knots for a short time before a particular event, but when that feeling lasts for days or weeks, weight loss and weakness can result. Tarragon is your friend here, as it both soothes the nerves and stimulates the appetite. The second situation is for someone with appetite loss due to illness or debility; here tarragon boosts the appetite by improving metabolism.

Tarragon also can revive sluggish kidneys, flushing the system, including the bladder, and relieving symptoms of gout and rheumatism.

USE IN THE KITCHEN

Tarragon's complex flavor lends itself well to both sweet and savory dishes. It is commonly found in egg dishes and dairy-based sauces and can also be a nice accompaniment to white fish or aioli. When paired with fruit, pastry, cakes, or other sweet foods, its anise- and fennel-like flavors shine.

While I prefer to use fresh tarragon when I have the option, the dried leaves can hold their own in a recipe. When using dried tarragon make sure it still looks, smells, and tastes vibrant — it has a tendency to lose its potency more quickly than many other dried culinary herbs.

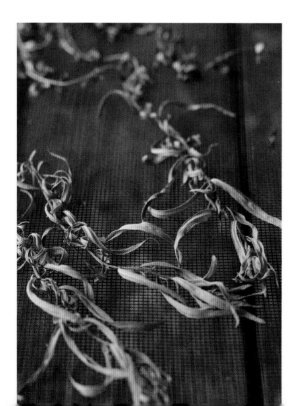

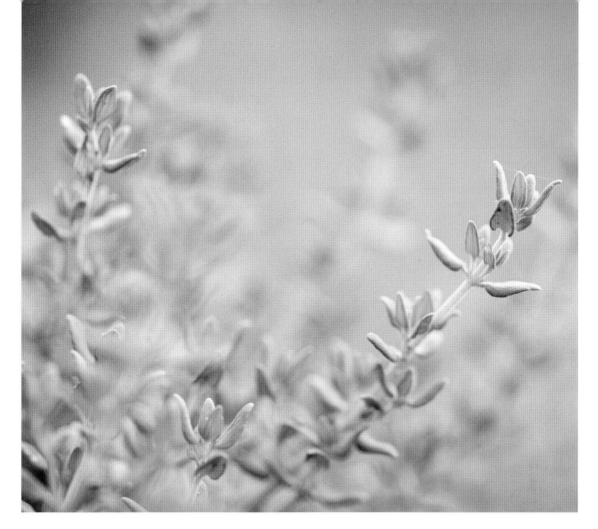

thyme

Thymus vulgaris

FLAVOR: Bitter, pungent

There are many varieties of culinary and ornamental thyme. While some have stronger oils than others, they can be used medicinally interchangeably.

Thyme is a strong antimicrobial and anti-fungal, with two notable active constituents: thymol (often found in pharmaceutical anti-fungal medications) and carvacol.(Both are also found in oregano.) It can be used internally and externally as an antiseptic, antiviral, and antifungal for a range of ailments, including colds and flu, intestinal parasites and worms, gut dysbiosis, eczema, oral thrush, vaginal yeast, athlete's foot, and fungal infections of the skin or nails.

Thyme is an antispasmodic, relaxing smooth muscle tissue throughout the body. In the GI tract, like most carminatives, it relaxes sphinc-ter muscles and relieves gas, bloating, and indigestion. In the respiratory system, it relaxes the muscles and provides relief for spasming coughs. In the circulatory system,

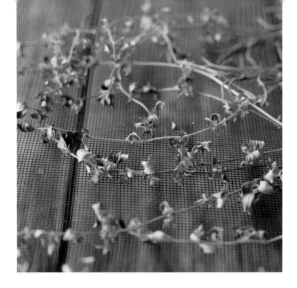

it eases tension and promotes circulation at the level of the capillaries, which can provide relief from headaches, pain, and cold extremities. In the reproductive system, it eases tension and cramping associated with menstruation.

As a stimulating rubefacient and antispasmodic, thyme relaxes tight blood vessels and relieves tension when applied externally as well. My preferred applications for external use include the infused oil and strong tea; the tea can be added to a bath, hot compresses, or respiratory steams. Applied topically to the abdomen, thyme will help relieve menstrual cramping; on the chest and back, it will reduce congestion and ease a cough (good for asthma and bronchitis as well); on the back of the neck, it will relieve tension and soothe a headache or head cold; and on sore muscles or cold-aggravated arthritic conditions, it will warm, comfort, and ease pain. Consider it as a massage oil or in the bath for fever with chills or for preventing colds or flu. As a wash, in a compress, or in the bath, it can also offer general support to ease red, flaky, dry skin (including on the scalp) as well as curb fungal and other infections as mentioned earlier.

When taken internally, thyme's antimicrobial constituents are released through the lungs, which makes it excellent for preventing or relieving lung infections (including bronchitis, whooping cough, croup, and asthma). Its warming, stimulating energy helps improve the expectoration of mucus. I find it very useful alongside peppermint to open up the sinuses and relieve congestion of the upper and lower respiratory systems. For best results for the respiratory system, drink the hot tea or use a hot steam.

Thyme's potent antimicrobial oils lend themselves well to oral hygiene routines. I include thyme in my tooth rinse tincture, swishing with about 20 drops of the tincture in a mouthful of water for 30 to 60 seconds after brushing. You could also swish with room-temperature tea. A gargle of the diluted tincture or tea is also excellent for sore throat and or throat infection, including tonsillitis, laryngitis, and strep.

The pungent and bitter tastes working together are the most stimulating and detoxifying combination. Thyme possesses this powerful flavor profile and stimulates liver metabolism, increases secretion of bile, and improves the breakdown and absorption of fats and oils. It helps balance cholesterol levels and improve cholesterol utilization. By warming the digestive fire and improving the breakdown of food and proper absorption of nutrients, it reduces the production of phlegm.

USE IN THE KITCHEN

Thyme goes well with with almost any type of food. It pairs well with a variety of other spice flavors ranging from oregano, sage, and parsley to cinnamon, paprika, and coriander. I find it a very versatile herb in the kitchen and use it liberally both fresh and dried. All aromatic varieties of thyme can be used in cooking.

MEDICINAL CONSIDERATIONS

Culinary herbs are generally considered to be very safe. After all, we've cooked with these herbs for generations. Although it's always possible for someone to have an idiosyncratic reaction to an herb — in the same way any one of us might be allergic to a particular food — cooking with culinary herbs is considered a safe practice.

When you get into using larger, medicinal doses of herbs, there are some safety considerations. The first is to recognize that those idiosyncratic reactions are possible, even with those herbs that are considered perfectly safe. If you don't think an herb is sitting well with you — if it makes you feel sick to your stomach or causes skin irritation, headache, or other symptoms — trust yourself and stop using it. It doesn't matter if all the books say that herb is safe and no one else in history has ever had that reaction before; you still need to honor your body's unique and individual relationship to that herb.

Pregnancy and breastfeeding are times to be cautious. Cooking with culinary herbs is considered safe during pregnancy and while breastfeeding, but some herbs, such as lavender, are too strong to be taken in large doses during pregnancy and should be used in moderation while breastfeeding. Other herbs, such as parsley and oregano, have an emmenagogue action; while you can use them in cooking, they are not considered safe in large doses during pregnancy. While breastfeeding, herbs such as dill are incredibly helpful to increase milk production and help ease symptoms of colic, while herbs such as sage decrease milk production. It is important to know the medicinal effects of the herbs you are using so that you can make informed choices.

Another important consideration is the interaction of herbs with pharmaceutical medications, including oral contraceptives. In regard to culinary herbs, be cautious with large doses of herbs that stimulate liver metabolism, such as rosemary. They may increase the rate at which the body processes medications, potentially reducing the drugs' efficacy. Other herbs may affect the same systems that the medications affect, reducing or increasing the drugs' efficacy.

Such precautions are most important when you are taking medicinal doses of an herb consistently over time (we will consider "consistently over time" to be medicinal doses taken every day or multiple times a day); they are not a concern when you are cooking with herbs. If in doubt, consult an herb-knowledgeable practitioner.

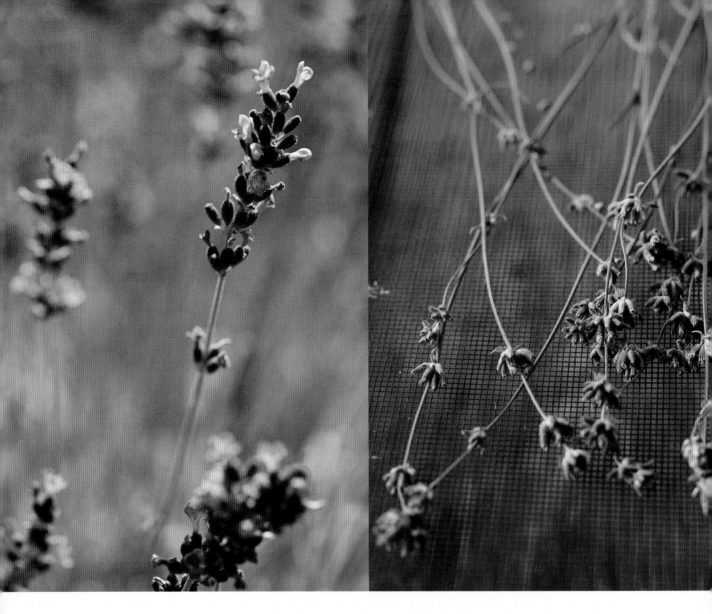

FRESH VS. DRIED

When a plant is dried, it loses volume due to the loss of water, so it becomes a more concentrated form of the plant. Thus, while you can generally use fresh and dried herbs interchangeably, you may want to adjust quantities. If a recipe calls for fresh herbs and all you have is dried, use about one-half to two-thirds the amount called for in the recipe.

As you cook with herbs, you will learn that some are just better fresh. Mint, cilantro, basil, and parsley are examples. While you can certainly use dried parsley, it doesn't have nearly the same rich flavor as fresh parsley. You will also learn that there are differences in flavor between fresh and dried herbs, and over time you will come to know when to use fresh versus dried to get the flavor you desire.

Throughout the book I give specifications for using fresh or dried herbs in recipes. If only one is mentioned, it means that the recipe is best made with that form of the herb.

Kitchen Medicine:
Techniques for Working with Herbs

When you learn the medicinal uses of the herbs in your pantry, they become so much more than seasonings. In fact, you will probably want at least twice as much of all your favorite herbs around! Crafting home remedies and using them for everyday ailments is an age-old tradition. Once you get the hang of medicine making, it can become an extension of other kitchen projects. It becomes something you do while you prep for dinner, and that "medicine" may even be a part of your meal, like an infused oil that you add to your salad dressing or an herb pesto you serve with chicken, for example. In the kitchen, the line between food and medicine can become blurry, as it should be.

The following preparation techniques are designed to help introduce the ideas of making medicine and open up some of the many possible ways in which you can use culinary herbs as both food and medicine, helping you to build a diverse, extensive, and accessible home pharmacy.

STORING HERBS

While the freshest-tasting herbs might be those you can pick from the garden or windowbox just before you use them, that isn't always the way things work out. Of course if you have access, pick your herbs fresh and use them right away. For those of us who do not grow our own herbs, properly storing herbs, whether fresh or dried, allows us to keep them on hand and preserve their culinary and medicinal constituents.

STORING FRESH HERBS

Fresh herbs store best when they are kept dry in a plastic bag in the refrigerator. Wet herbs will be more likely to rot around the edges and spoil more quickly. However, it can be convenient to wash a bunch of herbs all at once; in this case, pat or spin them dry as thoroughly as possible and put a paper towel or dishcloth in the bag with the herbs to absorb the extra water. Stored this way, herbs can last up to a week. Unless they are very dirty or have been handled a lot, I don't usually wash highly aromatic herbs such as basil, thyme, and oregano; washing them also washes off the volatile oils that are responsible for much of their unique flavor.

Some herbs do well when kept in water on the countertop; basil and mint in particular can store well this way for 4 to 6 days.

DRYING HERBS

You may find that there are times when you prefer to use dried herbs in cooking and in medicine making. They will have different flavors, and they are very convenient to keep on hand and use. I rely on dried herbs a lot in the winter when my garden is hibernating. If you have access to fresh herbs, drying them can be a great way to save an abundant harvest for later use. You may even find that the herbs you grow and dry yourself have a stronger, richer flavor than those dried herbs you buy at the store.

The best place to dry herbs is in a hot, dry environment with good air circulation. Don't dry them in direct sunlight, as the sun will fade the plants and break down their volatile oil and other constituents. Attic spaces work well, or the upper levels of a barn. You can also dry herbs in your kitchen or pantry.

When I was in college living in San Francisco, I dried a lot of herbs in my closet!

To ensure that herbs dry without becoming moldy, you will need good airflow around the plant material. Lay the herbs flat in a single layer on a basket or screen where air can circulate around them. Or pick the herbs with stems long enough that you can bundle them and hang them to dry. Once the herbs are completely dry to the touch — they should crumble or break apart between your fingers — they are ready to store. If you dried them on the stem, you may want to separate out the woody stems before storing them; this makes the herbs more convenient to use later on. Store dried herbs in an airtight container out of direct sunlight. They will keep for 1 to 2 years.

People often ask me if the dried herbs they have on their spice shelf, which may have sat there for years, are still good. I tell people to use their senses to determine if an herb is still good to use. Does it smell fresh and aromatic, does it look vibrant and colorful, does it taste rich and flavorful? If a jar of dried herbs has lost its color, smells like dust, or tastes like unidentifiable twigs, it is probably a good time to restock the pantry.

TEAS

Tea can be made from fresh or dried herbs. Teas made from fresh herbs are light, with little color, and richly aromatic. Culinary herbs generally lend themselves well to fresh-plant teas because they have so many potent, delicious volatile oils. Those volatile oils also tend to hold up well to drying, so dried-plant teas can be equally aromatic, but they usually have a thicker, richer flavor and a darker color. Teas made from dried plants are richer in vitamins and minerals than fresh teas; the drying process breaks open the cell walls of the plant and gives the water greater access to plant constituents.

YIELD: 1 CUP

INGREDIENTS

- 2 tablespoons fresh herbs or 1 tablespoon dried
- 1 cup boiling water

PROCESS

Place the herbs in a mug, jar, or teapot. Pour the boiling water over the herbs and cover with a lid. Let steep for 5 to 15 minutes. Strain before drinking.

USE

Teas can be drunk hot or cold, but consider whether the temperature will add to the medicine. For example, if you have a head cold, hot tea will help break up congestion and expectorate mucus, whereas room-temperature or cool tea on a hot day will help you feel refreshed.

SEE THESE RECIPES:

- Centered and Focused Tea, page 157
- Lavender After-Dinner Tea, page 100
- Mint Tisane, page 211
- Garden Tea, page 239
- Sage and Orange Peel Throat Soother Tea, page 210

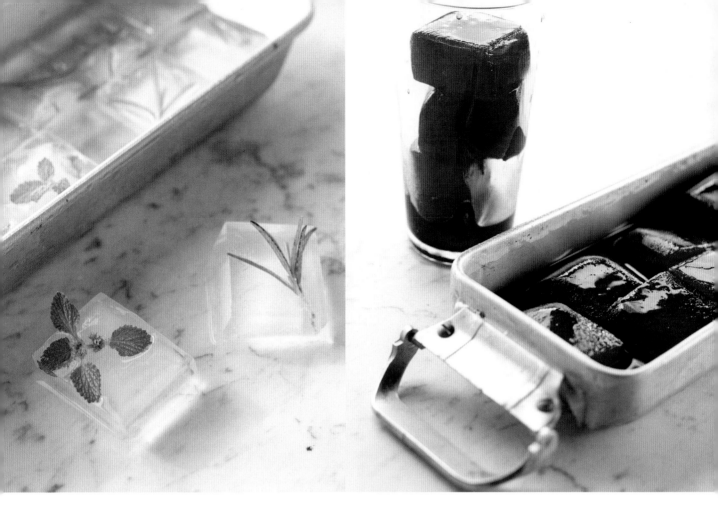

HERBAL ICE CUBES

Herbal ice cubes are a great way to incorporate herbs into everyday beverages, adding flavor and a little medicine to any occasion. I use them mostly in the summer to make refreshing drinks at the end of a long day. Depending on the color of the herb you use, they can be very exotic. Hibiscus and rose hips, for example, make a red/pink ice cube. Adding fruit juice or puréed fruit and berries to the ice cubes also adds great color and flavor.

YIELD: 1 TRAY OF ICE CUBES

INGREDIENTS

1 cup fresh herbs or ½ cup dried herbs

2 cups water

PROCESS

Prepare a strong herbal tea, following the instructions on page 58. Strain, cool, and then freeze in an ice cube tray.

USE

Herbal ice cubes can also be added to hot tea, soups, oatmeal, or anything else you might want to cool off or pump with more flavor or herbal goodness.

SEE THIS RECIPE:

• Elderflower Ice Cubes, page 293

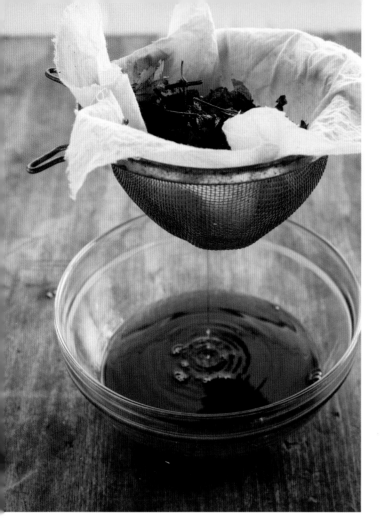

1. If you're using fresh herbs, chop them. Pack the herbs into a clean pint jar.

2. Pour enough alcohol over the herbs to cover them by several inches. Usually 1 to 1½ cups will do it.

3. Cover, label with the date and contents, and set aside to steep for 4 to 6 weeks in a cool, dark place, shaking the jar whenever you remember or are inspired. Herbs that pop up above the alcohol may discolor; this is not a problem, but push them down below the alcohol if you can, or add more alcohol to cover them if needed.

4. After 4 to 6 weeks, strain the tincture through fine cheesecloth or cotton muslin.

5. Store the tincture in a glass jar with a tight-fitting lid in a cool, dark place, where it will keep for up to 3 years. Transfer an ounce or two to a small dosage bottle with a dropper for daily use.

USE

The average adult medicinal dose for tinctures, whether alcohol or glycerin based, is 30 to 60 drops, two or three times daily. People who are more sensitive should start with less. This dosage is based on a 150-pound adult. Adjust accordingly for larger or smaller people. Children over 30 pounds can be dosed proportionately by weight.

SEE THIS RECIPE:

- Basil Bitters, page 184

TINCTURES

While tinctures can be made with a base of alcohol, vinegar, or glycerin, the most common are alcohol extracts. Alcohol is an excellent solvent, extracting a wide range of valuable medicinal constituents. Glycerin, which is made through the saponification of fats, is sweet and thick, and it is a great alcohol-free option for tincture making.

YIELD: ABOUT 1½ CUPS

INGREDIENTS

1½ cups packed fresh herbs or 1 cup dried

1–1½ cups 100-proof vodka or 80-proof brandy

HERBAL VINEGARS

Vinegar is the oldest solvent used in herbal medicine besides water. It is particularly effective at extracting vitamins and minerals. Herb-infused vinegar adds flavor and nutrition to your cooking. It is also a great way to preserve the bounty and flavor of the harvest into later seasons. Vinegar picks up subtle flavors in an herb, including aromatics as well as the nutritional properties. In addition to making infused vinegars with flavorful culinary herbs and spices, I often add high-mineral wild weeds (such as dandelion greens, cleavers, plantain leaf, violet leaf and flower, and purslane) to the mix for added nutrition.

YIELD: ABOUT 1½ CUPS

INGREDIENTS

1½ cups packed fresh herbs or 1 cup dried

1–1½ cups raw apple cider vinegar

PROCESS

1. If you're using fresh herbs, chop them. Pack the herbs into a clean pint jar.

2. Pour enough vinegar over the herbs to cover them by 1 to 2 inches. Usually about 1½ cups will do it.

3. Cover, label with the date and contents, and set aside to steep for 3 to 4 weeks in a cool, dark place, shaking the jar when you remember or are inspired. Herbs that pop up above the vinegar may discolor; this is not a problem, but push them down below the vinegar if you can or add more vinegar to cover them if needed.

4. After 3 to 4 weeks, strain the vinegar through fine cheesecloth or cotton muslin.

5. Store the infused vinegar in a glass jar with a tight-fitting lid in the refrigerator, where it will keep for at least a year.

NOTE: Vinegar erodes metal. To cover a jar of vinegar, use a glass, plastic, or cork lid or put a layer of waxed paper between the vinegar and a metal lid.

USE

Use herbal vinegars freely in cooking. Raw apple cider vinegar itself is a great digestive aid, rich in biologically active enzymes and cultures; add herbs to it and you get even more health benefits. To support healthy digestion or to take herbal vinegars as a dietary supplement, dilute 1 teaspoon to 1 tablespoon of herbal vinegar in a few ounces of water and sip before meals. Those with acid reflux, indigestion, heartburn, and other upper GI irritations may find vinegar irritating, but others find it helpful — start with small amounts well diluted.

SEE THESE RECIPES:

- Turmeric Fire Cider, page 185
- Nourishing Rosemary Hair Rinse, page 101
- Tarragon-Infused Vinegar, page 186

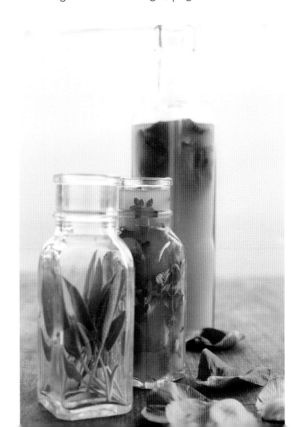

HERB BUTTER

Herb butters turn even the simplest of dishes into a delicacy. Butter is rich in the fat-soluble vitamins A, D, E, and K, nutrients that are important to every system of the body, from the brain and nervous system to the musculoskeletal, endocrine, immune, and reproductive systems. These vitamins can also be important for the assimilation of other nutrients. Vitamin A is necessary for protein assimilation and the absorption of calcium, while vitamin D increases our absorption and utilization of both calcium and phosphorus.

For this reason, butter and other fats rich in the fat-soluble vitamins are seen as important carriers — they assist in the uptake and utilization of nutrition throughout the body. This is yet another reminder of the brilliant synergy of cooking: vegetables and proteins should always be consumed with fat to help maximize their nutritional value.

YIELD: ½ CUP

INGREDIENTS

½ cup (1 stick) unsalted butter, softened

2–6 tablespoons fresh or dried herbs, finely chopped or ground

¼–½ teaspoon salt

PROCESS

Combine the butter, herbs, and salt in a bowl. Mix until thoroughly combined.

USE

You can use herb butters just like plain butter, cooking with them or just slathering them on steamed vegetables, grains, grilled meats, fish — the possibilities are endless.

Herb butters will keep for 7 to 10 days in an airtight container or glass jar in the refrigerator, or in the freezer for 3 to 6 months. To freeze the butter, you'll want to wrap it up first: Scoop the butter onto a piece of waxed paper or parchment paper. Use the paper to shape the butter into a round log, pushing out air as you do. Roll the butter log tightly in the paper and pinch and twist the edges to seal off any air.

SEE THESE RECIPES:

- White Fish with Herb Butter, page 249
- Roasted Onions with Sage Butter, page 136

HERB BUTTER COMBINATIONS

Be as creative as you like with your herb combinations. In addition to herbs, you can use cheeses, nuts, and dried fruits in your butters. A few of my favorite combinations not used in recipes elsewhere in the book include:

- Tarragon with orange zest

- Toasted oregano and pine nuts

- Paprika, garlic, and thyme

- Cilantro and jalapeño

HERBAL WATERS

What I call herbal waters are like herb juice — you don't actually juice the herb, but you purée it with water and strain out the plant material, leaving a rich, flavorful, delicious beverage that captures all the qualities of the fresh herb in a refreshing form. Herbal waters taste very alive and vibrant. You can add many other wonderful flavors to them, from sweeteners to vinegars to fruits and veggies.

YIELD: 3 CUPS

INGREDIENTS

1 cup packed fresh herbs of your choice

2 cups water

PROCESS

Combine the herbs and water in a blender and purée. Strain, if desired. Store in the refrigerator, where it will keep for 2 days.

USE

Drink your herbal waters straight up or over ice. Or use them as a base for smoothies or cocktails.

SEE THIS RECIPE:

- Cilantro Lemonade, page 129

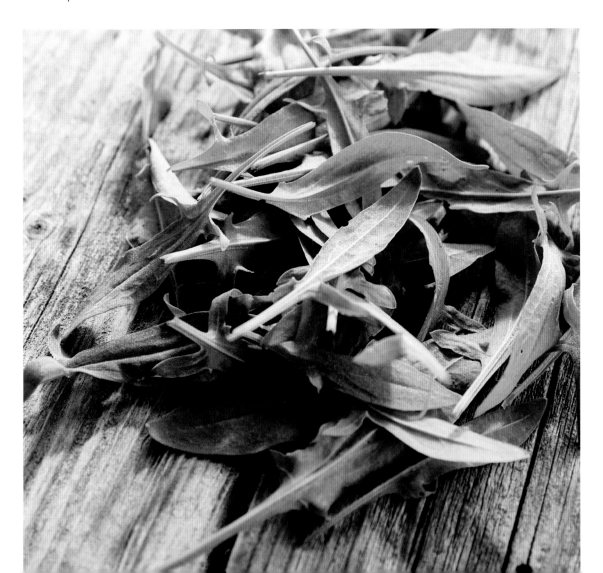

HERB-INFUSED OILS

Through long steeping or slow heating, you can infuse an oil with the aromatics and other constituents of an herb. You can use any oil as the base for your infused oils. For culinary use, choose an oil that suits your intended purpose: sautéing, salad dressing, dipping, and so on. For external medicinal use, choose whatever feels right for you and works with your skin type. I often use olive oil, which is rich with antioxidants and very nourishing. I also like sesame oil, which has a warming quality excellent for people who have a tendency to run cold. If you run hot, you might like coconut oil, which is cooling, anti-inflammatory, antiviral, and antifungal. Oils like grapeseed and almond are also favorites for the skin.

Whenever possible, use unrefined oils. The less processed the oil is, the more nutrients it will retain. If you're using an oil that is solid at room temperature, like coconut oil, follow the instructions for making a medicinal oil with dried herbs (at right).

YIELD: 1½ CUPS

INGREDIENTS

1–1½ cups oil

1½ cups packed fresh herbs or 1 cup dried

MAKING MEDICINAL OILS WITH FRESH HERBS

1. Begin with dry fresh herbs; do not wash them first or use herbs that are wet from dew or rain. Chop the herbs and pack them into a clean pint jar.

2. Pour the oil over the herbs. Use a fork or spoon to gently release any air bubbles. The oil should cover the herbs by ½ to 1 inch; add more if necessary. Push any floating herbs down under the oil; any herbs exposed to air may mold.

3. Cover, label with the date and contents, and set aside to steep for 2 to 4 weeks in a cool, dark place.

4. Check the oil on days 1 and 3. Push down any herbs that have floated up and add more oil to cover as necessary. Check again at 1 to 2 weeks.

5. After 3 to 4 weeks, strain the oil through fine cheesecloth or cotton muslin. (If there is any surface mold on the oil, scrape it off before straining.) Gently press the oil from the spent herbs — but do not press too hard or moisture from the plant material will enter the oil and decrease its shelf life.

6. Store the infused oil in a glass jar with a tight-fitting lid in a cool, dark place. Infused oils made from fresh plants will keep for 1 to 2 years.

MAKING MEDICINAL OILS WITH DRIED HERBS

1. Combine the dried herbs and oil in the top of a double boiler. Bring an inch or two of water in the lower pan to a boil, then reduce the heat to low and let the herbs and oil infuse, stirring often, for 45 to 60 minutes.

2. Let the oil cool completely, then strain through fine cheesecloth or cotton muslin. Press the oil from the spent herbs — the dried herbs you used will not have had any moisture in them, so press thoroughly.

3. Store the infused oil in a glass jar with a tight-fitting lid in a cool, dark place. Infused oils made from dried plants will keep for 1 to 3 years.

MAKING CULINARY OILS WITH FRESH OR DRIED HERBS

Culinary infused oils are made following the previously outlined methods for fresh or dried herbs, but you'll want to keep a closer eye on them to minimize the potential for mold growth. If you're working with fresh herbs, reduce the steeping time to 2 weeks and check the oil every few days during the entire steeping process to make sure the herbs are submerged beneath the oil and mold has not formed on top. If you do find mold on your infused oil, scrape it off and add more oil to thoroughly cover the herbs.

After straining, store your culinary oils in a cool, dark place. Use fresh-plant culinary herbal oils within 3 months, and use dried-plant culinary oils within 6 months.

These methods work well for making culinary oils for woodier herbs such as rosemary, thyme, sage, and oregano. Herbs with more tender leaves, such as basil, parsley, cilantro, and mint, are more flavorful when prepared using the method outlined for Basil Oil (page 274).

USE

For culinary use, infused oils make lovely dressings, dipping oils, and so on. For medicinal use, infused oils are a wonderful way to apply the healing power of herbs to the skin. The aromatics of the herbs infused into the oil affect the nervous system as you apply them, and the oil base and

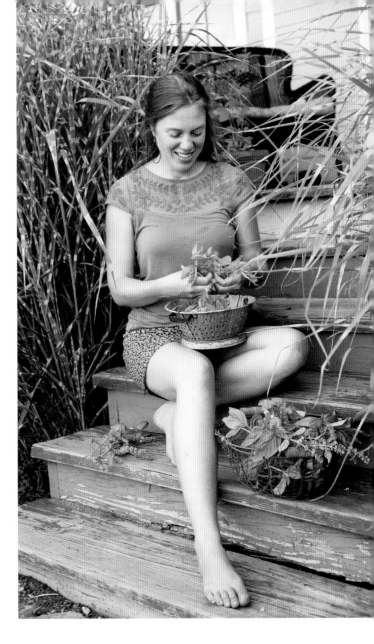

other plant constituents extracted into the oil nourish and feed the skin. Keeping the skin well oiled supports elimination of toxins and circulation of blood and lymph fluids and calms the nervous system. Regular self-massage with herb-infused oils is a great way to stay grounded, calm, and focused.

SEE THIS RECIPE:

• Basil Oil, page 274

HERB-INFUSED HONEYS

Honey is demulcent, soothing, antimicrobial, rich in enzymes, and delicious. The healing magic of this sticky, sweet substance is augmented by whatever herbs you combine it with.

YIELD: ABOUT ¾ CUP

INGREDIENTS

⅓ cup fresh herbs or ½ cup dried

¾ cup raw honey

PROCESS

1. If you're using fresh herbs, make sure they are dry. Chop them, combine them with the honey in a clean half-pint jar, and mix well. Do your best to push the herbs down into honey.

2. Cover, label with the date and contents, and set aside to steep for 3 to 4 weeks in a cool, dark place.

3. After 3 to 4 weeks, strain the honey through a fine-mesh strainer, if you like; you can also skip this step and enjoy your infused honey herbs and all. If the honey has crystallized during the steeping period, so that you can't strain it, place the jar in a pan of warm water to liquefy.

4. Store the infused honey in a glass jar with a tight-fitting lid in a cool, dark place. It will keep for at least a year. If you did not strain the fresh herbs from your infused honey, store it in the refrigerator.

NOTE: You can also make herb-infused honeys in a double boiler: Combine the herbs and honey in the top of a double boiler. Bring an inch or two of water in the lower pan to a boil, then reduce the heat to low and let the honey and herbs infuse gently for 45 to 60 minutes. Strain (or not), store, and use in the same way as the cold-infused version.

USE

Herb-infused honeys add complex flavors and good medicine to your cooking. They can be stirred into a cup of hot tea or enjoyed by the spoonful. Infused honeys can also be used topically to soothe, heal, and reduce inflammation. To apply herb-infused honey as a compress, moisten the skin with warm water, apply honey, and let sit for 10 to 15 minutes before gently washing off with warm water.

SEE THESE RECIPES:

- Hazelnut Cornmeal Cake with Rosemary Honey, page 189

- Sage Honey, page 126

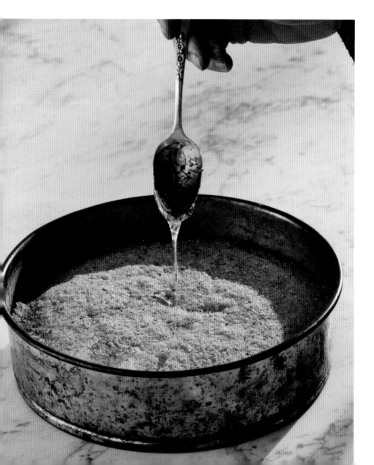

HERBAL SYRUPS

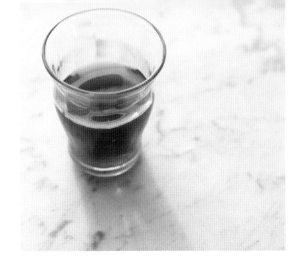

Like teas, syrups are water-based preparations, but they are more concentrated, sweetened, and longer lasting. Whereas teas will last several days in the refrigerator, a syrup will last 6 months. In addition to acting as a preservative, the sweetener makes the syrup taste great and can add its own medicinal value. If you make a syrup with honey, for example, all the medicinal properties of the honey will be present in the syrup. You can even use herb-infused honeys, for added character.

To increase the shelf life of a syrup, add a splash of brandy, apple cider vinegar, herb-infused vinegar, or alcohol-based tincture. Lemon juice also works well as a preservative, as it is high in vitamin C, and it adds great flavor.

Making syrups is an activity that children particularly enjoy. I find kids are more likely to take herbal remedies when they have a part in making them, and because syrups usually taste great, they are all the more exciting.

YIELD: 3 CUPS

INGREDIENTS

- 1½ cups fresh herbs or 1 cup dried
- 4 cups water
- 1 cup honey or other natural sweetener, such as agave, maple syrup, unrefined cane sugar, or fruit juice concentrate
- ¼ cup brandy, apple cider vinegar (plain or infused), or tincture (optional)

PROCESS

1. Combine the herbs and water in a saucepan. Bring to a boil, then reduce the heat and let simmer until the water volume has reduced by half (to about 2 cups).

2. Strain the herbs from this decoction.

3. Let the decoction cool to 100°F (38°C) or so — warm, but not steaming hot. Add the honey and mix well or shake to dissolve.

4. Let the syrup cool completely, then, if you like, add the brandy, vinegar, or tincture as a preservative.

5. Label with the date and contents and store in the refrigerator, where the syrup will keep for 6 months. If you do not add brandy, vinegar, or tincture as a preservative, mold may form on the surface of the syrup or on the edges of the jar. You can simply scrape this surface mold off, transfer the syrup to a clean jar, and continue to use it.

USE

Use herbal syrups to flavor drinks, desserts, marinades, dressings, and other creations. You can also take them as a dietary supplement, 1 tablespoon to 1 ounce once or twice daily. (Children between the ages of 3 and 10 can take 1 teaspoon to 1 tablespoon, depending on their age and weight.) Because syrups can be made ahead and stored, they are a convenient way to get herbs into your life on a daily basis.

SEE THESE RECIPES:

- Elderberry-Thyme Syrup, page 264
- Rose-merry-berry Syrup, page 212

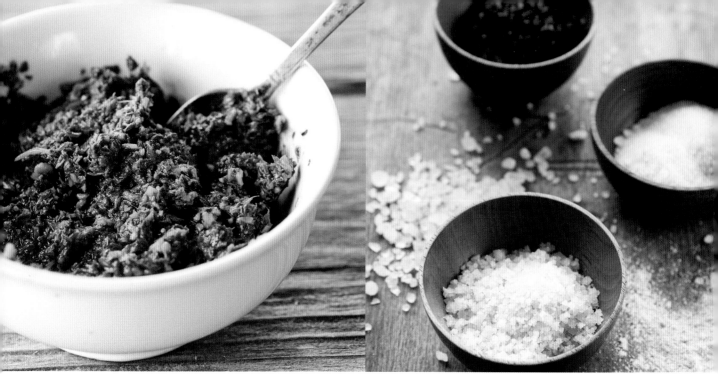

HERB PESTOS

While pesto traditionally calls for fresh basil, you can make delicious pesto using any fresh herbs or greens, alone or in combination. Experiment making different herbal pestos with single herbs or creative combinations. For greens, consider arugula, kale, or nettles. Chives, scallions, nuts, seeds, cheeses, and even citrus fruits make great additions or substitutions to traditional recipes.

YIELD: ABOUT ¾ CUP

INGREDIENTS

2–5 tablespoons nuts or seeds

2 cups packed herbs or greens

⅓–½ cup oil

2–4 tablespoons cheese (optional)

Garlic, scallions, or chives

Salt and freshly ground pepper

PROCESS

1. If you're using nuts or seeds, soak them in enough water to cover for at least 6 hours and up to overnight; strain before using. Or toast the nuts or seeds in a dry skillet over medium heat until golden brown and aromatic, 3 to 5 minutes. This makes them easier to digest and makes the flavors richer.

2. Combine all the ingredients in a food processor. Blend until smooth.

USE

Pesto is one of the best ways to get medicinal doses of herbs into your diet. Just ⅛ to ¼ cup of pesto is a healthy serving of an herb, providing nutrients, medicinal action, and digestive support. Try preparing a batch of pesto weekly to keep in the fridge; it makes it easy to incorporate herbs into your diet. In the summer months I like to make pesto to freeze so I can enjoy the flavor of fresh herbs all winter long.

SEE THESE RECIPES:

- Baked Eggs with Parsley Pesto, page 77
- Cilantro Pesto, page 169
- Oregano Pesto, page 165

HERBAL SALTS

Herb-infused salts are a great addition to the herbal pantry. They are fun to cook with, invigorating dishes with extra flavor. You can use coarse, finely ground, or flaked salt. I prefer unrefined salts, which are rich in minerals. The herbs can be fresh or dried (I use the term "herb" loosely here; you can add herbs, ground coffee, dried fruits, and so on). You can even add liquids to your salts, like vanilla or other extracts, fruit juice, wine and other alcohols, coffee, or tea. The preparation method depends on whether the ingredients are fresh, dried, or liquid.

SALTS WITH FRESH HERBS OR LIQUIDS

For salt infused with fresh herbs, I generally use a 2:1 ratio: 1 cup salt and ½ cup chopped fresh herbs per batch. With salt infused with liquid, I usually use a 1:1 ratio: 1 cup salt and 1 cup red wine, for example, or 1 cup salt, ½ cup brandy, and ½ cup black cherry juice, plus some herbs. (Note that if you're using alcohol, it will cook off in the oven!) These ratios are simply guidelines to get you started; make up your own ratios to suit your palate.

1. Preheat the oven to 200°F (95°C).

2. Combine all the ingredients and mix well. If you're using fresh herbs, chop them first, and you may want to press them into the salt with the back of a spoon to release the aromatics.

3. Spread the mixture on a baking sheet. If you start with a dry mix, bake for 15 to 20 minutes, or until any herbs are completely dried, stirring every 5 minutes or so. If you're using a liquid, bake for 20 to 30 minutes, or until the liquid has evaporated, stirring every 5 minutes or so. The salt should be crumbly when finished.

NOTE: If you're using a liquid, you can cook it down to reduce its volume before adding it to the salt; this cuts down on time in the oven.

SALTS WITH DRIED HERBS

For salt infused with dried herbs, you can use the same 2:1 ratio: 1 cup salt and ½ cup dried herbs. Combine the salt and dried herbs in a mortar and pestle or spice grinder and grind until the herbs are crushed and the mixture is well combined.

USE

You will make great discoveries and come up with dazzling new recipes as you experiment with using infused salts in your kitchen. I like to keep a bit of herb-infused salt in a small dish at the table for extra seasoning during a meal. If all that is not benefit enough, these salts make beautiful gifts.

Some of my favorite combinations for infusing salt with fresh or dried herbs:

- Rosemary and lemon zest
- Thyme, fennel seeds, and black pepper
- Garlic and chive
- Garlic and parsley
- Herbes de Provence (see page 238)
- Oregano and sage
- Mint and lavender
- Citrus medley (grapefruit, lime, and lemon zests)
- Earl Grey tea and black pepper
- Ginger and brandy
- Turmeric, garlic, and black pepper

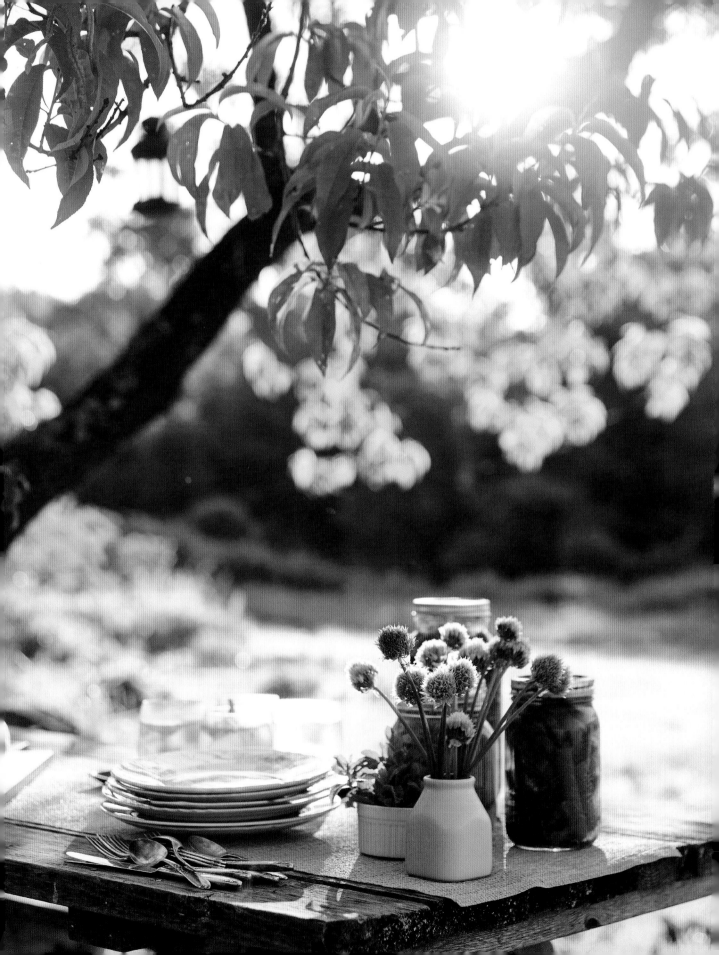

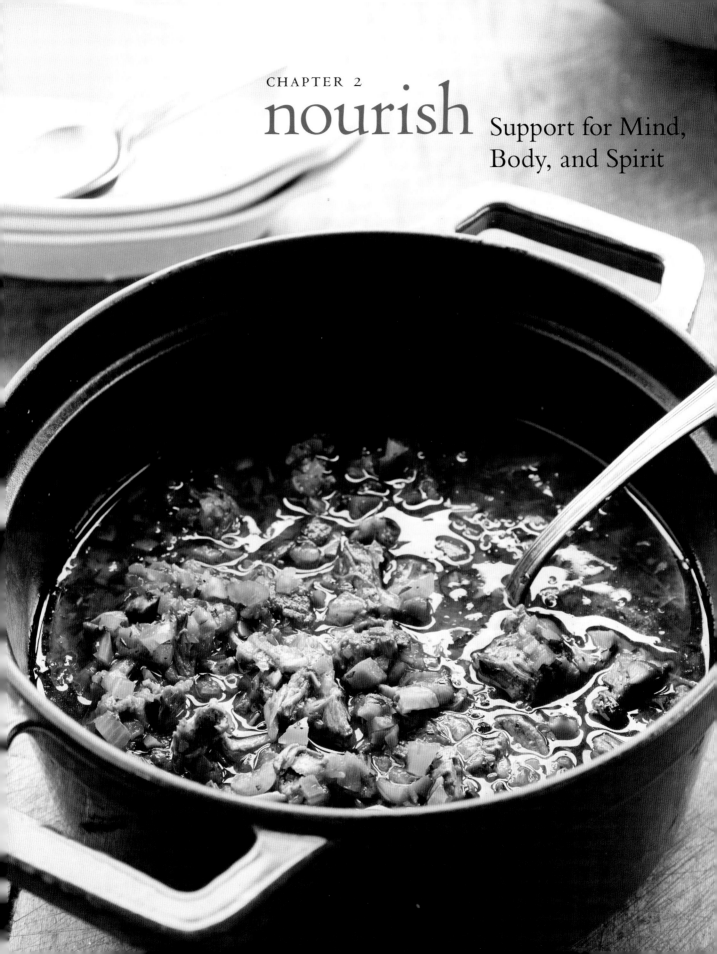

CHAPTER 2
nourish Support for Mind, Body, and Spirit

THERE ARE MANY WAYS to be nourished. The nourishment provided by food is paramount to health, well-being, and ultimately survival, yet across cultures and throughout history, food has served much more than just the physical body. Food is part of custom and celebration. It represents the fertility of land; the hands of those who grow, harvest, or prepare; and the joy, satisfaction, celebration, and thanksgiving of eating. Food feeds us, yes, but its potential to *nourish* us — deeply, on a physiological and emotional level — arises from the values, traditions, attitudes, and understandings we bring to our relationship with it.

We commonly talk about nourishment in terms of nutrition — which nutrients are present, from vitamins and minerals to antioxidants and enzymes, and how they support the body. Much of what we understand about health and diet today is framed around the concept of health foods: foods that have high levels of said nutrients and thus are acclaimed for their ability to restore and support health. While these nutrients are important for the body, this way of conceptualizing health and nutrition can overlook the importance of *process*. Not all carrots, for example, contain the same nutrients. Soil fertility, growing practices, harvesting time, and storage all influence nutrient content. Beyond that, how the carrots are cooked or prepared will influence their eventual nutrient content and the availability of those nutrients to the body. We cannot separate nourishment from larger life processes.

In the body, the process most involved with receiving nourishment is digestion.

When I was growing up, I remember hearing the phrase "You are what you eat." When I started studying herbal medicine and learning about digestion and processes of absorption, I realized, "You are what you *digest*." Food is only as nourishing as our body's ability to digest it. The most nutrient-rich health foods in the world will be of little use to the body if we are unable to digest and absorb the nutrients for which they are famed.

Good digestion is the foundation of all nourishment. Yet, like every other process, digestion does not exist in isolation but is influenced by other body systems and processes. Digestion is ruled by a branch of the autonomic nervous system called the enteric nervous system. The enteric nervous system runs the length of the digestive system and contains almost as many neurons as the brain and the spinal cord — sometimes it's called our second brain. This means that everything that affects the nervous system, from foods and medications to our emotions, attitudes, and experiences, affects our digestion and the rest of our physiology. These emotions themselves nourish us or don't, but they also affect how much nourishment we receive from our food.

Our health, then, is greatly influenced by our digestion of not just food but also experiences, thoughts, and emotions. It is influenced by our relationships with our environment, ourselves and others, and food itself. Our relationship with food can be full of enjoyment and pleasure, engaging our sense of creativity and self-expression. Or it can be wrought with tension, uncertainty, self-policing, and guilt. We digest well when we are relaxed and at ease, and digestion is compromised when

ESTABLISH BEING, PERFORM ACTION

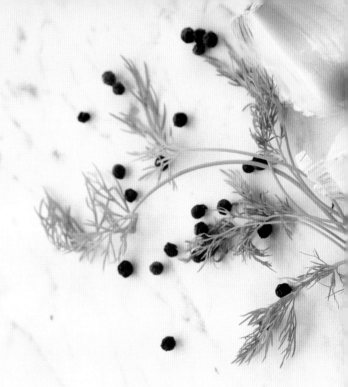

Our biological and physiological health doesn't just follow our diet, it follows our actions, our experiences, and our emotions. There is an Ayurvedic teaching that says, "Establish being, perform action." The first part of this teaching, "establish being," encourages us to settle into a place in life where we are able to be present in the moment. Learning to just *be* brings a sense of self-reflective awareness that can help us transform ingrained negative or painful patterns of behavior. The second part, "perform action," reminds us to keep moving, be proactive, and take risks. I love this teaching, because it reminds us that there are two components of making change: being (recognition, reflection, meditation, awareness) and action (doing, motivation, completion, movement). Change embodies the yin and yang of life. You cannot have one without the other. One of the secrets of health is to learn to bring the contemplative, introspective, soft, reflective nature of being to our everyday doings.

Our relationship with food gives us access to our inner landscape. There are countless moments in food production, harvesting, cooking, and eating that ask for reflection, that engage our senses, our instincts, and our relationship with our deep primal nature. Food gives us the opportunity both to establish being (think of the meditative quality that can accompany planting, weeding, harvesting, chopping, sautéing, and stirring and the being-ness of connecting to your instincts and your senses) and to perform action. This is holistic wellness at its finest, feeding both the emotional and the physical, the conceptual and the material — it provides nourishment for soul and body.

It is so important that our concepts of healing and nourishment remain reflective (being) as well as goal oriented (action). Healing gets stuck when it revolves around obstacles, wounds, and illness narratives. Because our physiology follows our emotions and spirit and our spirit and emotions follow our physiology, the same foods that challenge our system and help it work better, that nourish it and comfort it, can help us find the courage to change, relax, forgive, and let go.

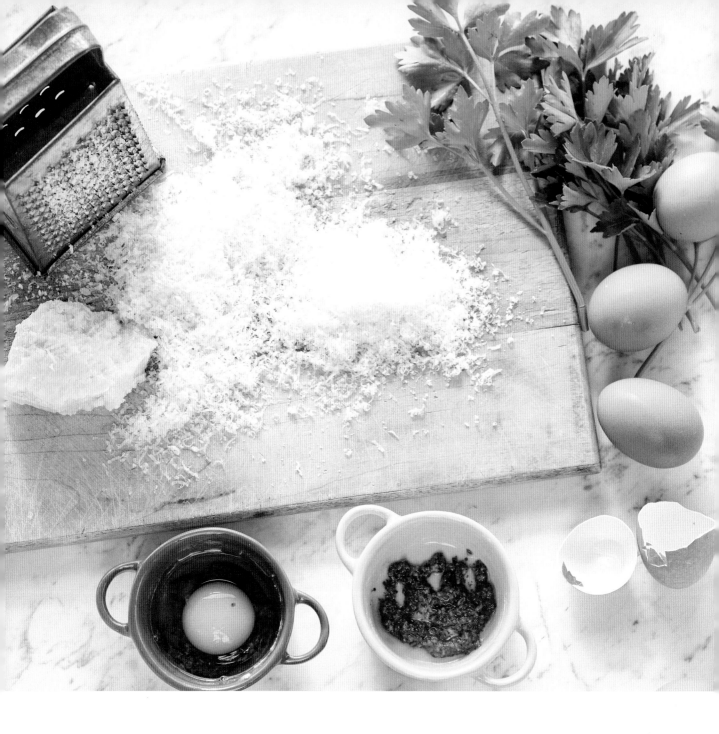

we are stressed out or anxious. Thus, stress, tension, and uncertainty surrounding our food choices will influence our ability to receive nourishment, no matter how "healthy" the food we eat is. A truly healthy diet embodies a holistic view of nourishment — one that

allows us to enjoy not just nourishing food choices but also nourishing emotions, such as joy, pleasure, satisfaction, compassion, and self-acceptance. How deeply we are nourished isn't just about food. We are nourished by love and care, by connection to others and by doing things we love. When we can integrate the many processes that influence our health and well-being, our entire life becomes a recipe for nourishment.

Food is an offering for our senses, a gift of beauty, smell, taste, *and* nourishment, and it should be enjoyed as such. If you do nothing else to nourish yourself, practice (with utter and complete compassion for the times when you fail) enjoying your food. Celebrate it, knowing that the joy you feel in each bite will nourish your whole being.

One of the most powerful things we can do to nourish ourselves and support digestion is to relax before and during meals. Make space to sit down to eat. Before you begin eating, take a few deep breaths, settle into your body, smell the food, feel your body, calm your mind, and relax your muscles. Let negative thoughts and emotions dissipate and settle. Then pull in positive associations: give thanks for the food, for your access to it, for those who grew it and prepared it. When you eat,

do your best to let go of any nagging voices or criticisms that may come up. Allow yourself to enjoy your food fully and recognize the many ways it is nourishing you.

The recipes in this chapter focus on foods that have high levels of nutrients and have been prepared in ways that make them easy to digest. The preparation methods are designed to increase the *bioavailability* of the nutrients — that is, the degree to which they are made available to our body — and often boost the nutrient content itself. Many of the recipes are slow-cooked, stewed, marinated, or fermented — connected at their very foundation to processes of hand, heat, time, and heart. These processes can be as nourishing as the foods themselves. Being in the kitchen and connecting with the culinary alchemy that feeds us is nourishing unto itself. It gives us time to focus on our self-care, to recognize the ways in which we nourish ourselves and others, and to appreciate food itself and the miracle of life.

THE ABUNDANCE MODEL

So often when we talk about our diet and our health, we talk about what not to do: what not to eat and why not, how not to be and why not, and what is wrong with the foods we eat. In these situations, our relationship with health becomes about establishing self-control and our thoughts become more focused on doubt, lack, and negativity. When we direct our energy and attention to what we want to do, what we are doing, and what we can easily and sustainably include in our life and in our diet, it is much easier to succeed because we are acknowledging ourselves for our capabilities and our accomplishments rather than our failures or limitations. With this "abundance model" in mind, over time you may find that your old attachments, self-criticisms, and "what not to do" list just sort of disappear. You will be so busy being nourished by all these great additions to your life that the things that are not serving you just naturally fall away.

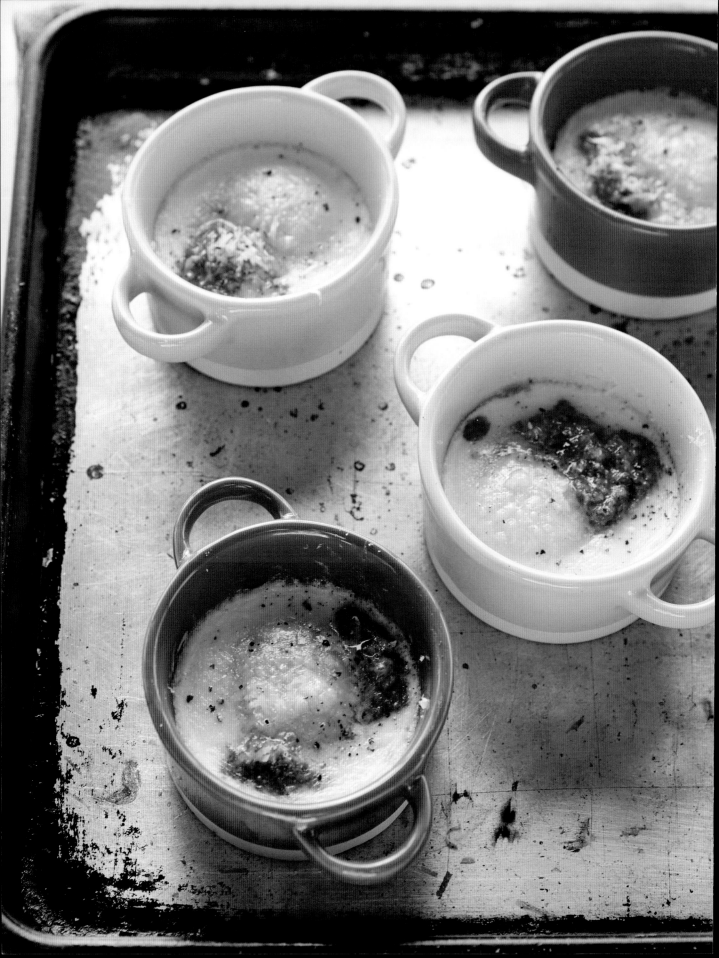

BAKED EGGS WITH PARSLEY PESTO

Eggs represent potential life, containing within themselves all the nutrients needed to get that life started. They represent new beginnings, starting points, and the kind of energy we may associate with inspiration or determination. This is the same kind of energy we need when we establish our goals and intentions for the day and set out to germinate them. Whether for a slow, leisurely morning feast or a quick breakfast before work or school, eggs are a great way way to start the day.

These eggs are excellent served with greens, roasted roots, polenta, or toast for a breakfast or brunch. They're great with parsley pesto, but you can use any kind of pesto you like. If you don't have pesto on hand or don't have time to make it, some chopped herbs and garlic in the bottom of the ramekin will be a perfectly delicious substitute.

✦ YIELD: 4 SERVINGS ✦

⅓ cup pine nuts

2 cups packed fresh flat-leaf parsley

3 garlic cloves

½ cup olive oil

¼ teaspoon salt

Freshly ground black pepper

4 tablespoons grated Parmesan cheese

8 eggs

I. Preheat the oven to 425°F (220°C). Butter eight small ramekins or four larger ramekins (you can use muffin pans if needed).

2. Toast the pine nuts in a skillet over medium heat, stirring often, until golden brown, 3 to 6 minutes. Let cool.

3. Combine the toasted pine nuts with the parsley, garlic, oil, salt, and a generous grind of pepper in a food processor. Process until smooth.

4. If you're using small ramekins, put 1 teaspoon of the parsley pesto in the bottom of each ramekin and crack one egg into each. If you're using the larger ones, put 2 teaspoons of the parsley pesto in the bottom of each ramekin and crack two eggs into each. Layer on another 1 to 2 teaspoons of the pesto and top with ½ to 1 tablespoon of the Parmesan per ramekin.

5. Place the ramekins on a baking sheet and carefully transfer to the oven. If you're using the smaller ramekins, bake for 7 to 8 minutes for an egg with a runny yolk and 10 to 12 minutes for a firm yolk. Cooking two eggs in each rame-kin takes longer, 10 to 12 minutes for a runny yolk and 14 to 16 minutes for a firm yolk. Let sit for 1 to 3 minutes before serving.

PASTURED EGGS

Eggs from chickens allowed free range on pasture, where they can eat green grass and grubs as well as grain, contain higher amounts of omega-3 fatty acids and vitamins A, D, E, K, and B_{12} than eggs from chickens raised indoors on just grain. Their yolks are darker and richer, and you can taste the difference in flavor. Beyond the health benefits, I imagine that pastured hens have a good time foraging, and they can become an important part of a small farm ecosystem.

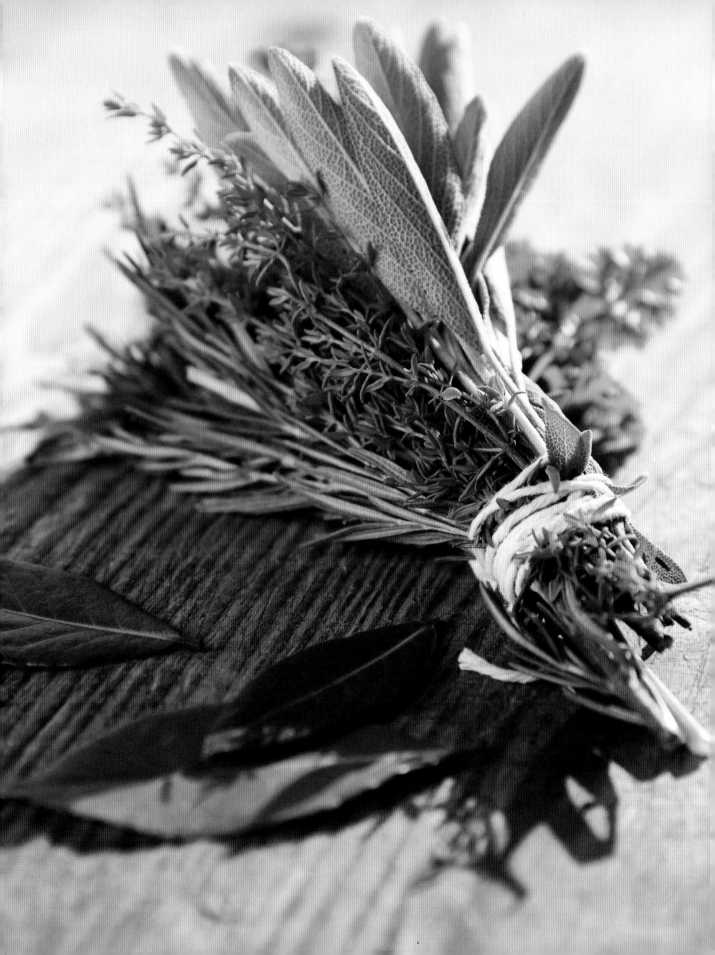

GRANDMA'S CHICKEN SOUP

Symbolic of wisdom, nurturance, and love, the grandmother figure embodies the nourishment offered by chicken soup. The slow-simmered stock breaks down the gelatin in cartilage and connective tissue and leaches minerals from bones, while taking on a rich chicken flavor. Combine that with antibacterial herbs (sage, rosemary, and thyme), immune-enhancing mushrooms, and nourishing root vegetables and you have something that supports and heals the body on all levels, helping you recover from illness, boosting immunity, and restoring energy and vitality. All food can embody the grandmother's iconic gifts, but chicken soup seems to offer powerful medicine and comforting taste in the same bite — yet another reminder that what pleases the palate can nourish the soul.

◆ YIELD: 6 SERVINGS ◆

Sprigs of fresh parsley, rosemary, sage, and thyme, for the bouquet garni

1½ pounds bone-in chicken (I use legs and thighs), with the skin

2 bay leaves

2½ quarts (10 cups) water

2 tablespoons olive oil

1 large onion, diced

1 pound potatoes, chopped into ½-inch pieces

10–12 ounces cremini or button mushrooms, sliced

3 large carrots, chopped into ¼-inch pieces (about 1½ cups)

2–3 stalks celery, chopped into ¼-inch pieces (about 1½ cups)

4–6 garlic cloves, finely chopped

2 tablespoons chopped fresh rosemary or 1 tablespoon dried

2 tablespoons chopped fresh sage or 1 tablespoon dried

2 tablespoons fresh thyme or 1 tablespoon dried

Salt and freshly ground black pepper

2 cups packed dark leafy greens (kale, collards, spinach, or Swiss chard), chopped into 1-inch pieces

1 cup chopped fresh parsley leaves

1. Fasten together the herb sprigs for the bouquet garni with kitchen twine. Put the chicken in a large pot, add the bouquet garni and bay leaves, and pour in the water. Bring to a simmer over medium heat, skim off any foam that forms on the surface, cover, and reduce the heat to low. Simmer gently for about an hour, skimming off any foam that forms as it cooks.

2. After an hour, remove the chicken from the stock and set it aside to cool. Remove and compost the herbs and set the broth aside as well.

3. Heat the oil in another large pot over medium-high heat. Add the onion and sauté until translucent, about 3 minutes. Then add the potatoes, mushrooms, carrots, celery, and half of the garlic, along with the rosemary, sage, thyme, pepper, and ½ teaspoon of salt. Sauté until the herbs become aromatic, 2 to 3 minutes.

4. Add the chicken stock to the pot and bring to a simmer. Reduce the heat to low and simmer, covered, until the vegetables are tender, 15 to 20 minutes.

5. While the soup is cooking, remove the chicken meat from the bones and shred or cut it into bite-size pieces.

6. Add the chicken meat to the soup along with the greens and cook for 2 minutes. Then add the parsley and remaining garlic. Turn off the heat and let sit, covered, for about 5 minutes to let the flavors meld. Season to taste with salt before serving.

ROASTED RED LENTIL DHAL

Red lentil dhal can vary in texture from a spoon-worthy soup to a thick stew that can be scooped and eaten with naan (see recipe, page 140) or large pieces of steamed greens, like collards or kale. Forgoing utensils and eating with your hands can seem so primal, evoking a powerful recognition that food is fundamental to our being — like breathing, eating is an instinctual skill that we practice to survive. When I engage with my food this way, I feel a great sense of appreciation for the food, for my own hands, and for the hands that grew, harvested, and prepared the meal.

◆ YIELD: 4 SERVINGS ◆

2 cups red lentils

2 tablespoons ghee (page 93) or butter

2 teaspoons whole black mustard seed

1 teaspoon ground coriander

1 teaspoon whole cumin seed

½ dried red chile, broken up, or ½ teaspoon red pepper flakes

5–6 cups water

1 teaspoon salt

¾ teaspoon ground turmeric

Half a cinnamon stick or ¼ teaspoon ground cinnamon

2 cups chopped cilantro

4–5 garlic cloves, minced

1. Set a skillet (preferably cast iron) over medium heat. Add the lentils and roast, stirring often, until just brown, 5 to 10 minutes. Keep an eye on them; you will think the lentils are not roast-ing, not roasting . . . then all of a sudden they are burning. As soon as they are done, remove the lentils from the pan and set aside to cool.

2. Heat the ghee in a small skillet over low heat. Once it is hot, add the mustard seed, coriander, cumin seed, and chile. Cook the spices, stirring often, until the mustard and cumin seeds begin to pop, about 1 minute. Turn off the heat and set aside.

3. Once they're cool, put the lentils in a colander and rinse well.

4. In a 2½- to 3-quart saucepan, combine the lentils with 5 cups of the water and the salt, turmeric, cinnamon, and ghee mixture. Bring to a simmer, then cover and let simmer over low heat until the lentils are soft and beginning to fall apart, 25 to 30 minutes. The dhal should have the consistency of a thick soup or stew. If it gets too thick before the lentils are ready, add more water, keeping in mind that the dhal will firm up as it cools.

5. When the lentils are done, stir in 1½ cups of the cilantro and the garlic. Serve garnished with the remaining ½ cup cilantro.

FRESHLY GROUND HERBS

As is the case with most herbs and spices, freshly ground coriander is wonderfully aromatic. Though you can certainly use preground coriander, the freshly ground seeds add a nice touch to this recipe. You can grind whole coriander seeds in a mortar and pestle, in a spice grinder, or in a thoroughly cleaned coffee grinder.

GREENS with GARLIC, GINGER, and TURMERIC

In recent years, eating greens seems to have become synonymous with healthy eating, and for good reason: greens provide valuable minerals and fiber and are great for the liver and digestion. They are made more digestible and their nutrients more available by the addition of herbs, spices, fats, and oils. Make sure to include a variety of different greens in your diet, and consider adding wild greens to the mix. I like to combine different varieties with diverse flavors, like the spicy mustard and the bitter collards in this recipe. Butter and coconut oil plus pungent, aromatic roots and bulbs makes for a unique combination.

◆ YIELD: 4 SERVINGS ◆

2 tablespoons butter

2 tablespoons coconut oil

1 bunch collard greens, chopped (about 4 packed cups)

1 bunch mustard greens, chopped (about 4 packed cups)

Salt and freshly ground black pepper

1–2 tablespoons chopped garlic (about 3 cloves)

1 tablespoon grated fresh ginger

1 tablespoon grated fresh turmeric root or ½ teaspoon ground dried turmeric

I. Heat the butter and oil in a large cast-iron skillet over medium heat. Add the greens and sprinkle a little salt and pepper over the top. Toss a few times in the pan, then add the garlic, ginger, and turmeric, and stir together. Reduce the heat to medium-low and cook, stirring often, until the greens are soft.

2. Season with salt and pepper to taste before serving.

TURMERIC

Turmeric is a pungent, aromatic, bitter digestive aid useful both in cooking and in medicinal preparations. It supports the breakdown of fats and oils and can reduce gas and bloating. It stimulates liver metabolism, digestive metabolism, and cellular metabolism, which helps reduce unhealthy inflammatory responses throughout the body.

Fresh turmeric root tends to have more vibrant flavor than ground dried turmeric, but by all means, use what you have. If you're using ground dried turmeric in this recipe, add it to the hot oil and sauté, stirring continuously, for 30 to 60 seconds before adding the greens; this helps bring out its flavor.

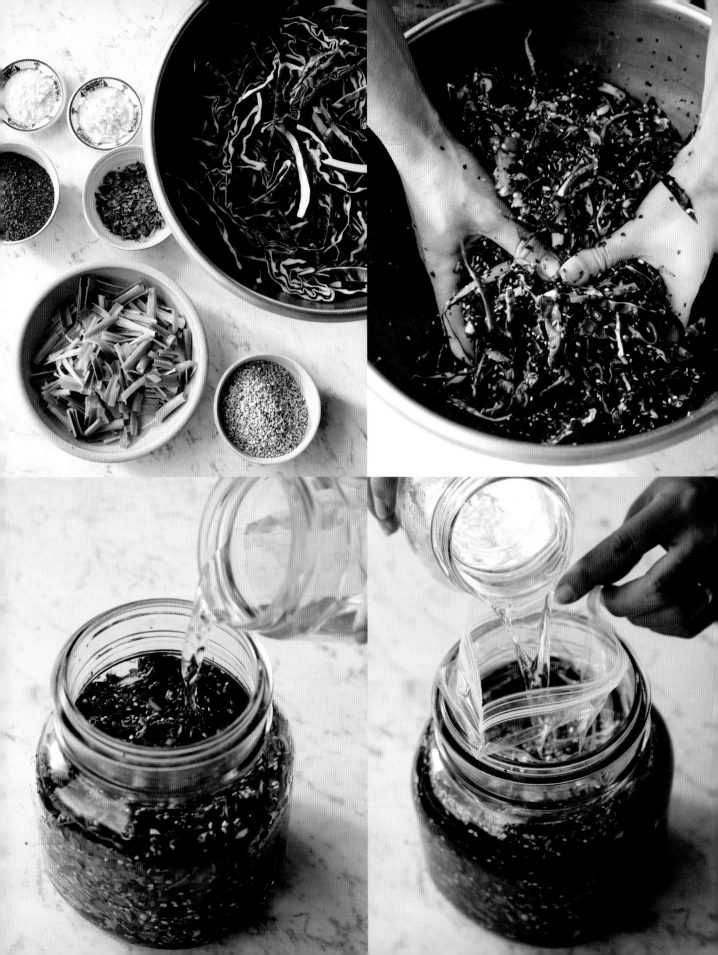

DEEP-SEA PURPLE KRAUT

Looking out over the ocean is easily one of the more mesmerizing ways to view the natural world. The constantly changing interplay of the soft gray-green foam of crashing waves, the light greens of shallow waters, and the dark blues, purples, and blacks of the deep sea is a reminder of the mutability of our perspective: it changes as we move, as the tide ebbs and flows, as what lies beneath changes.

Watching this magical kraut ferment is like watching the ocean — only the dance of change happens right on your kitchen counter. As lactic acid bacteria break down the fibers, starches, and sugars in the cabbage and seaweed, they create new nutrients (vitamins and probiotics) and new colors. Ever-changing and alive, the kraut feeds not just our body but our perspective.

Sauerkraut is excellent for digestion; the sour flavors are light and fresh and help cleanse the palate. It makes a great condiment or side dish for almost any meal.

◆ YIELD: ABOUT 6 CUPS ◆

½ cup sesame seeds

1 purple cabbage (about 3 pounds)

2 bunches scallions, sliced in half lengthwise and cut into 1-inch pieces (1½–2 cups)

½ cup packed chopped fresh parsley

½ cup finely chopped dulse or dulse flakes (about ½ ounce)

1–2 garlic cloves, finely chopped or pressed

1½ teaspoons noniodized salt

FOR THE BRINE

2 cups nonchlorinated water

1 tablespoon noniodized salt

I. Toast the sesame seeds in a skillet over medium-low heat until golden brown and aromatic, 5 to 10 minutes. Remove from the heat and set aside to cool.

2. Remove and compost the outer leaves of the cabbage. Cut the head into quarters and slice ⅛ inch thick, or as thin as you can. (You can remove the core before slicing, but I don't usually bother.) Combine the sliced cabbage in a large bowl with the toasted sesame seeds, scallions, parsley, dulse, and garlic. Sprinkle the salt over the cabbage mixture and massage with your hands by squeezing and flipping for 10 to 20 minutes. Let the cabbage rest for 10 minutes or so, then massage for another 5 to 10 minutes. By this point the cabbage should have begun to sweat, with juice collecting at the bottom of the bowl.

3. Tightly pack the cabbage mixture into a clean half-gallon mason jar or crock. Pour any juice remaining in the bowl into the jar. If that juice is enough to cover the cabbage by 1 inch, you do not need to prepare the brine.

4. Prepare the brine: Warm ¼ cup of the water, add the salt, and stir until dissolved. Stir that salty water into the rest of the water.

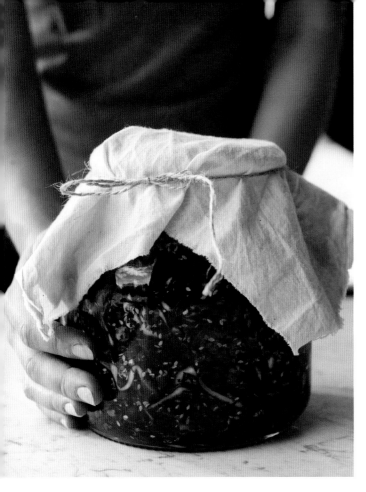

with water, so it spreads out and seals off the jar or crock. Or set a smaller glass jar filled with water as a weight on top of the cabbage. If you are using a crock rather than a jar, you can put a plate on top of the cabbage inside the crock and put a jar full of water on top of the plate to weigh it down.

6. Let the kraut ferment at room temperature until the flavor reaches your liking, 1 to 3 weeks. Check it every other day during the first week to make sure the cabbage stays submerged beneath the brine; any cabbage exposed to air may mold. Push the weight down as needed and add more brine if necessary.

7. Begin to taste the kraut after 1 week. The longer it ferments, the more sour the flavor and the softer the cabbage. The speed of fermentation will vary depending on the ambient temperature. A ferment made during a heat wave in August might take only 10 days to be as sour as you like it, whereas a ferment made in October could require 3 weeks or more.

8. When you like the taste, transfer the kraut to smaller glass jars or plastic containers and store in the refrigerator, where it will keep for 3 to 6 months. Once it is refrigerated, the kraut does not have to be submerged beneath the brine; the cold will keep it from spoiling.

PURPLE KRAUT *continued*

5. Pour enough brine over the cabbage to cover it by about 1 inch. (You should have enough brine, but make more if you need to.) To keep the cabbage submerged beneath the brine, set a ziplock bag on top of the cabbage and fill it

---

SEAWEEDS

Seaweeds are the greens of the ocean, vitamin- and mineral-rich superfoods. While there are many varieties of seaweed, each with its own unique health benefits, they all have a softening effect on the body. This is particularly noteworthy for the cardiovascular system; here, seaweed helps maintain flexibility in the blood vessels. Picture dulse, or another variety, growing on a rock, riding the waves of the sea, flexible and adaptive as wave after wave runs its course. When our arteries have become hardened by plaques and age — or our minds have become hardened by thoughts or experiences — seaweeds help us relax and soften.

Besides providing a rich array of vitamins, minerals, and trace nutrients, dulse acts as a flavor enhancer. Its presence adds an intriguing salty flavor that is sometimes hard to pinpoint.

FERMENTATION BASICS

Lactobacillus and other bacteria responsible for successful fermentation thrive in a salty environment but are harmed by chlorine and iodine. For this reason, we need to pay special attention to the ingredients we use when preparing fermented foods. Successful fermentation requires nonchlorinated water — filtered water, well or spring water, or some kinds of bottled water. Many municipal water supplies are now treated with chloramine, a more stable form of chlorine. Chloramine is harder to remove than chlorine; you may need a special filter. Call your municipality to find out how they treat your water.

It is also important to use noniodized salt. Like chlorine and chloramine, iodine disrupts the delicate balance of bacteria in your ferment and could cause it to spoil. I prefer to use unrefined salt in my cooking and for fermentation. Unrefined salt contains minerals and usually has a gray or pink color. However, any noniodized salt will work, including kosher salt and refined sea salt.

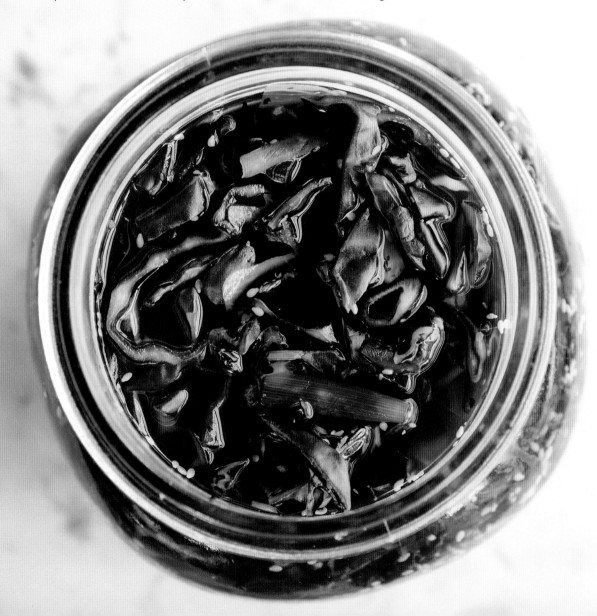

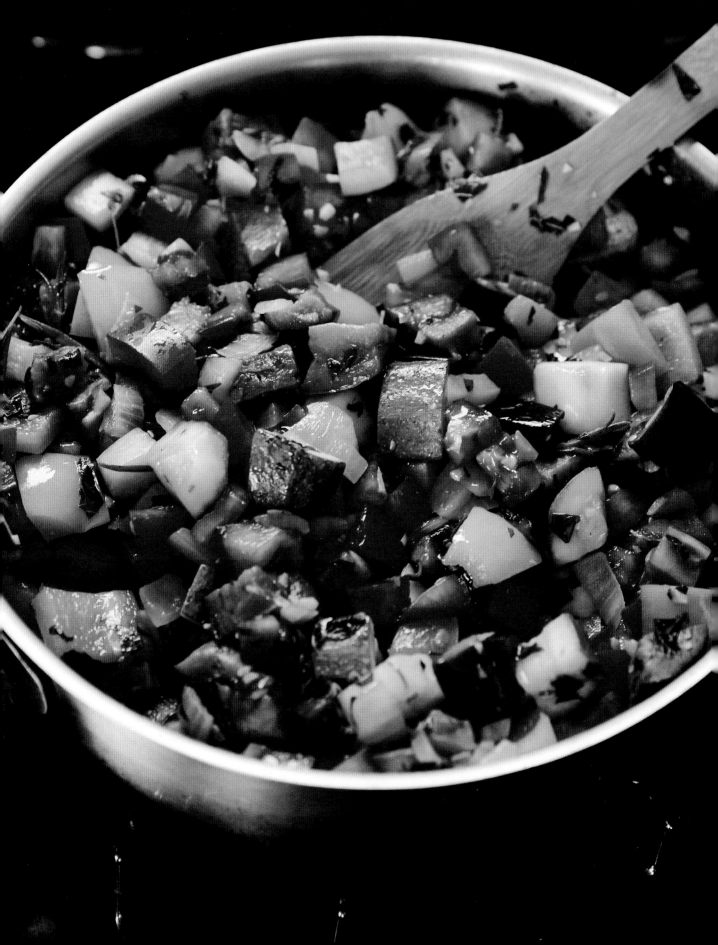

RATATOUILLE

Originating in France, ratatouille is a preparation of late-summer vegetables stewed with herbs. Variations exist, but the staple ingredients — eggplant, onion, zucchini, peppers, tomatoes, and herbs, especially basil — are a constant. As they ripen in the hot sun, these vegetables and herbs store that warmth in their rich, flavorful bodies. According to Chinese medicine, eating the gifts of summer's harvest is one of the ways in which we can collect and store the warmth we need for the colder, darker seasons to come. This dish is an offering to the body of the nourishment of summer's sun. May you soak it up.

◆ YIELD: 4 SERVINGS ◆

3 tablespoons olive oil

1 large or 2 small eggplants, chopped into 1-inch cubes (about 2 cups total)

Salt and freshly ground black pepper

1 large or 2 small yellow onions, chopped into ½-inch pieces (about 1 cup total)

2 medium or 3 small zucchini, chopped into 1-inch cubes (about 2 cups total)

2 large or 4 small bell peppers of any color, chopped into 1-inch pieces (about 2 cups total)

1 cup finely chopped fresh basil, plus whole or chopped leaves for garnish

2 tablespoons fresh rosemary or 1 tablespoon dried

2 tablespoons fresh marjoram or 1 tablespoon dried

6 garlic cloves, chopped (about ¼ cup total)

3 cups diced tomatoes

Shaved Parmesan cheese or sliced fresh mozzarella, for serving (optional)

Grated lemon zest, for garnish (optional)

I. Heat 2 tablespoons of the oil in a large saucepan. Once the oil is hot, add the eggplant and sauté until just tender and browned on the edges, 5 to 7 minutes, adding more oil if necessary along the way. Remove the eggplant from the pan, sprinkle with salt and black pepper, and set aside.

2. Heat the remaining 1 tablespoon oil in the same pan, reduce the heat to low, and add the onions. Sauté, stirring often, until translucent, about 3 minutes. Add the zucchini and bell peppers and continue to sauté over low heat for 5 minutes longer. Return the eggplant to the pan, add the basil, rosemary, marjoram, and garlic, and cook until the basil and garlic become fragrant, 2 to 3 minutes.

3. Add the diced tomatoes, stir well, and bring to a simmer. Let simmer over low heat until the tomatoes release their juice, the mixture takes on the consistency of a stew, and the vegetables are cooked through, 10 to 15 minutes. Season with salt and black pepper to taste.

4. Serve hot, with some shaved Parmesan or a few slices of mozzarella, if using. Garnish with whole or chopped fresh basil leaves and lemon zest, if desired.

SHIITAKE MUSHROOMS IN TARRAGON CREAM SAUCE

Tarragon is classically combined with cream, milk, and cheese for good reason: its lovely anise-like flavor and aroma bring out the sweetness inherent to dairy while also complementing the savory arc of a meal. Shiitake mushrooms are highly medicinal, helping to regulate and support immune function — not to mention the fact that they are delicious. This rich, nourishing, satisfying sauce can be served with everything from steamed greens and other vegetables to cooked grains, pasta, and potatoes or other roots.

◆ YIELD: 4 SERVINGS ◆

2 tablespoons unsalted butter

1 cup finely chopped onion or shallot

2 teaspoons fresh tarragon or 1 tablespoon dried

Salt and freshly ground black pepper

2 large garlic cloves

½ pound shiitake mushrooms, sliced ¼ inch thick

1½ cups heavy cream

Chopped parsley and grated Parmesan cheese, for garnish

1. Heat the butter in a skillet over medium-low heat. Once the butter is sizzling, add the onion and reduce the heat to low. Add the tarragon, about ⅛ teaspoon of salt, and ¼ teaspoon of pepper, and let it all cook together until the onions are translucent and soft, 3 to 5 minutes. If the onions start to stick to the pan, reduce the heat. The tarragon will begin to smell sweet as it cooks.

2. Add the garlic and shiitakes and another ⅛ teaspoon of salt and cook over low heat, stirring often, until the shiitakes are tender, 7 to 10 minutes. It might seem that the pan is dry at this point, but just keep stirring; the shiitakes should release moisture as they cook. If things start to stick, reduce the heat.

3. Once the shiitakes are tender, add the cream, ½ cup at a time, stirring continuously until the ingredients are well combined. Cook for another minute or two, just to heat up the cream. Serve with a garnish of parsley and Parmesan.

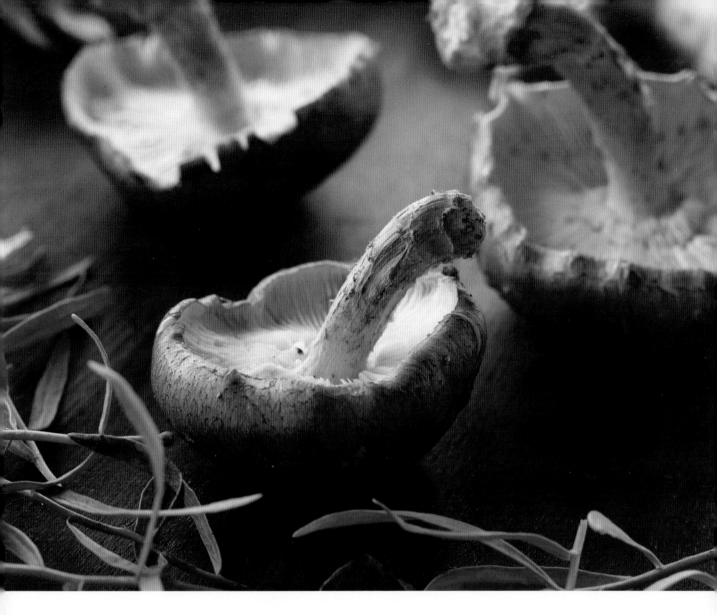

MUSHROOM MEDICINE

Mushrooms are the fruiting body of mycelia, the vegetative portions of fungi. Mycelia form a series of threadlike "roots" within whatever substance they inhabit, usually some type of organic material like soil or wood. They are great transformers, helping environments adapt by assisting the decomposition process, breaking down material and turning it into organic matter usable for other life forms, such as plants. The medicine of mushrooms is no different: mushrooms help the body to adapt by modulating the immune system and improving immune intelligence. They are excellent not only for building immunity against everyday colds and the flu, but also for assisting the body in responding to the effects of aging and exposure to toxins. Most mushrooms, including shiitake, have antitumor and anticancer properties, helping the body decipher between those organisms that do and do not benefit its inner ecosystem.

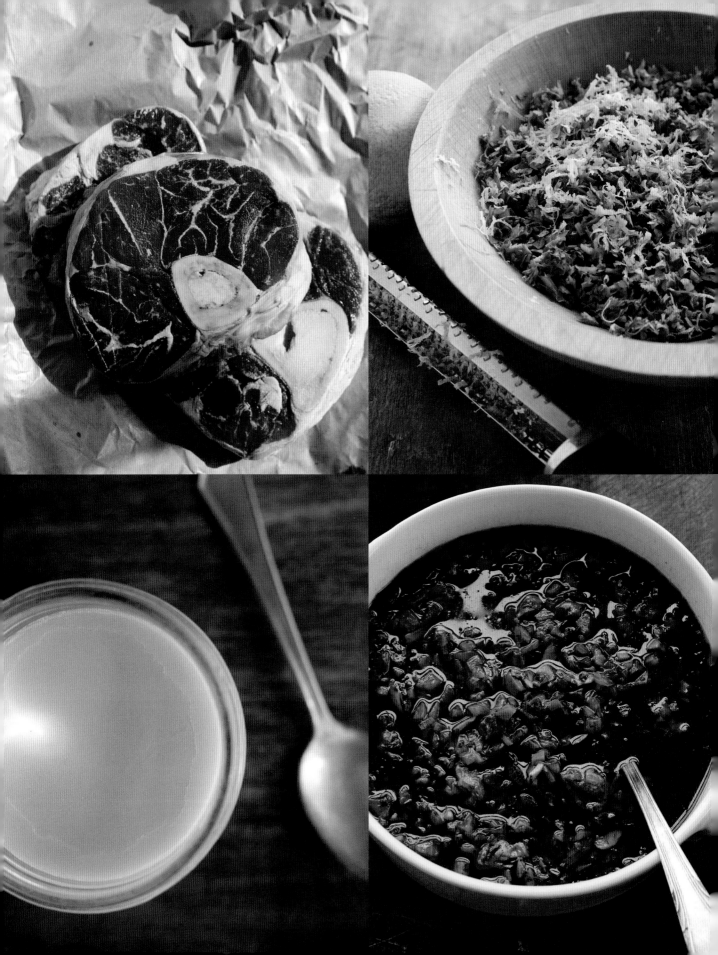

BRAISED BEEF SHANKS
WITH GREMOLATA

Braising is a long, slow cooking process that breaks down the gelatin in fat and connective tissue and renders otherwise tough cuts of meat more tender. Braises nourish us by keeping us close to home, by forcing us to be patient, and by nurturing our senses as the house fills with good smells. While this dish is braising, you might take a walk, read a good book in the sun, meander through other kitchen prep, or even get a little work done. The results will literally melt in your mouth.

The gremolata adds a fresh, light touch to the dish. Consider serving this dish alongside something that will soak up the delicious sauce, like rice, noodles, or polenta (see recipe, page 202).

◆ YIELD: 4 SERVINGS ◆

3 pounds beef, veal, or lamb shanks

Salt and freshly ground black pepper

4 tablespoons ghee (page 93) or a high-heat cooking oil

1 large onion, diced (about 1 cup)

2 tablespoons fresh oregano or 1 tablespoon dried

2 tablespoons fresh rosemary or 1 tablespoon dried

2 tablespoons fresh thyme or 1 tablespoon dried

3 bay leaves

2–3 carrots, diced (about 1 cup)

2–3 stalks celery, diced (about 1 cup)

4–6 ounces oyster, shiitake, or crimini mushrooms, diced

1 poblano pepper, diced

2 cups white wine

1 cup water

FOR THE GREMOLATA

1 bunch fresh curly parsley, finely chopped (1–1½ cups)

Zest of 1 lemon, finely grated

Zest of 1 orange, finely grated

2 garlic cloves, finely chopped

I. Generously coat both sides of the shanks with salt and pepper. Heat 2 tablespoons of the ghee in a saucepan over high heat. When the ghee is hot, reduce the heat to medium-high and add the shanks. Let sear for 2 to 3 minutes without moving, then flip and sear for 2 minutes on the other side. Remove the shanks from the pan and set aside. If all the shanks do not fit in your pan at once, sear them in batches, adding more ghee if needed.

2. Once you have seared the shanks, reduce the heat to medium and add the remaining 2 table-spoons ghee. Once it's hot, add the onion, oregano, rosemary, thyme, and bay leaves, and cook for 2 to 3 minutes. Then add the carrots, celery, mushrooms, poblano, and 1 teaspoon of salt. Cook, stirring frequently, until the veggies begin to soften, about 4 minutes.

3. Nestle the shanks into the veggie mixture and pour in the wine and water. Bring to a boil, then cover, reduce the heat to low, and let simmer gently for about 45 minutes. Flip the shanks and let simmer gently for another 1 to 2 hours, until the meat is tender and falling apart.

4. While the meat is braising, prepare the gremolata: Combine the parsley, lemon and orange zest, and garlic in a bowl and mix well.

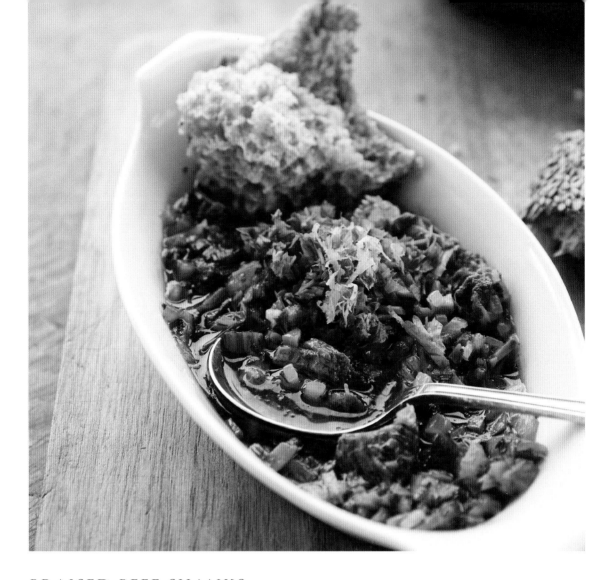

BRAISED BEEF SHANKS *continued*

5. When the meat on the shanks is thoroughly tender and falling off the bone, remove the shanks from the pan and allow to cool. Then remove the meat from the bones, shred it, and return it to the pan. Remove the marrow from the shank bones with a fork or knife and add to the pot as well.

6. Heat through and serve, with the gremolata as a garnish.

SLOW BRAISES

By breaking down connective tissue, gelatin, and other components, braising allows our body to access a host of nutrients we can't normally digest on our own. The resulting dish is rich in amino acids, calcium, iron, and other minerals. Slow-cooked, gelatin-rich meat dishes are very healing to mucous membrane tissues, particularly those along the digestive tract, and nourishing to our own bones, muscles, and connective tissues.

GHEE

Ghee is a form of clarified butter that's traditional to Ayurvedic medicine and Indian cuisine. The butter is cooked until the water evaporates and the milk proteins solidify and begin to caramelize. The proteins are then strained out, leaving behind the pure butterfat called ghee.

Ghee is highly nourishing, providing fat-soluble vitamins (A, D, E, and K) in an easy-to-absorb form. It is excellent for the nervous, endocrine, and digestive systems, healing the tissues of the GI tract and reducing inflammation. In Ayurveda, it is considered a carrier: when your meal includes ghee, the fat helps deliver the nutrients in the food you're eating to the cells of the body.

◆ YIELD: 2 CUPS ◆

1 pound unsalted butter

1. Melt the butter in a saucepan over medium heat. Once the butter is completely melted, reduce the heat to the lowest setting your stove will allow and cook, uncovered, to allow the water to evaporate.

2. As it cooks, the butter will bubble and its proteins will form a foamy white layer on top. This foamy white coat will eventually begin to solidify and fall to the bottom of the pan. The butter will sputter less and less as it cooks, indicating that the water has evaporated, and when the sputtering has mostly stopped and the ghee is clear with a rich golden color, it is ready. If necessary, use a spoon to push the foam to the side to see the color of the ghee beneath. (If it is brown, it has burned. Ghee usually only burns when it cooks too long — the proteins that settle to the bottom of the pan burn and discolor the rest of the ghee.) This entire cooking process usually takes 20 to 30 minutes.

3. Let the ghee cool for a few minutes, then strain it through fine cheesecloth or cotton muslin. Pour the strained ghee into a glass jar and let cool completely before putting the lid on. Store the ghee in an airtight container at room temperature. It will keep for 6 months. Always use a clean utensil when you scoop some out.

USING GHEE

Ghee has a high smoke point, up to 485°F (250°C), which makes it ideal for high-heat cooking. It can be used for searing, sautéing, roasting, or frying, or it can be used like butter in your cooking — fry an egg in ghee, or put a dab of ghee on steamed veggies or a bowl of oatmeal. It has a mild, nutty flavor that goes well with many foods.

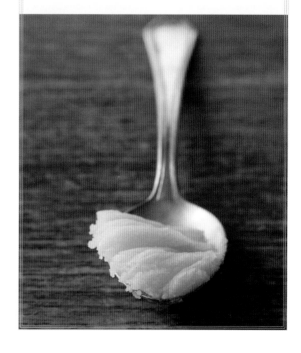

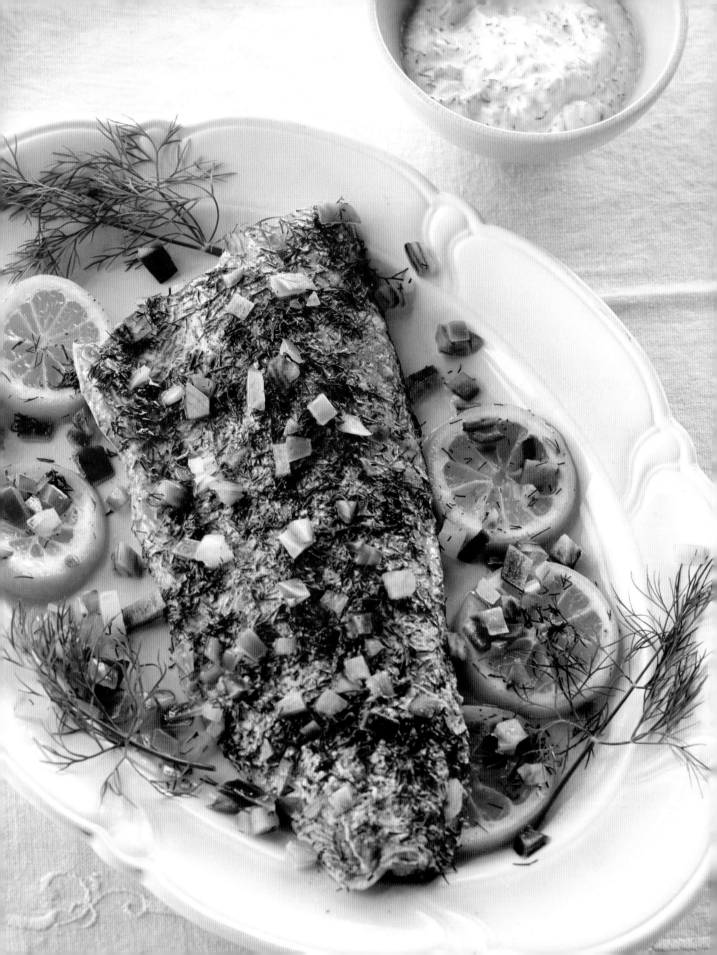

OVEN-POACHED SALMON WITH CRÈME FRAÎCHE AND CAPER DRESSING

This dish is a great example of how culinary traditions can so brilliantly support health and nutrition. The pungent dill and sour citrus (two flavorings commonly served with fish) support the digestion of fats and protein. Crème fraîche is a mild cultured cream, similar to but thinner and less sour than sour cream. It contains live probiotic bacteria that support the digestion of nutrients and feed our gut flora and overall health. Crème fraîche and other fermented foods not only make the food we eat easier to digest but also feed our digestive vitality, nourishing us deeply and holistically.

This dish makes an excellent main course served alongside seasonal vegetables. It can also be served cold, with bread or crackers, as an appetizer.

◆ YIELD: 2 SERVINGS AS A MAIN COURSE ◆

FOR THE SALMON

- ½   lemon, sliced into ¼-inch rounds
- ½   cup coarsely chopped red onion
- 4   sprigs fresh dill
- 1   pound wild salmon fillet
-     Salt and freshly ground black pepper
- 3   tablespoons finely chopped fresh dill
- 2   tablespoons olive oil
- ½   cup dry white wine, such as sauvignon blanc

FOR THE DRESSING

- 2   cups (16 ounces) crème fraîche or sour cream
- ¼   cup capers, chopped
- 1   tablespoon caper juice
- 1   tablespoon grated lemon zest
- 2   tablespoons finely chopped red onion
- 4   tablespoons finely chopped fresh dill
-     Salt and freshly ground black pepper
-     Sprig of fresh dill and wedge of lemon, for garnish (optional)

1. Preheat the oven to 375°F (190°C).

2. Prepare the salmon: Arrange the lemon slices, half of the chopped onion, and the dill sprigs in the bottom of a glass baking dish. Sprinkle both sides of the salmon with salt and pepper and place, skin side down, in the pan. Distribute the rest of the onion and the chopped dill on top and pour the oil and wine over all. Cover the dish with a lid or aluminum foil and bake for 20 minutes, or until the fish is cooked through. In my experience, a 1½- to 2-inch-thick piece of fish will be done in about 20 minutes. To see if the fish is done, cut into the fillet to see if the center has changed from translucent to opaque — the entire cross section should be the same color throughout.

3. While the fish is cooking, prepare the dressing: Combine the crème fraîche, capers, caper juice, lemon zest, onion, and dill in a bowl and mix well. Season with salt and pepper. Garnish with a sprig of fresh dill and a wedge of lemon, if desired.

4. Let the fish cool, uncovered, for at least a few minutes. Serve warm or cold, with the dressing on the side.

BURGERS WITH SWEET PEPPER AND MINT SALSA

Ground meat is a convenient and affordable foundation for a nice meal. Even excellent-quality organic or grass-fed ground meat is more affordable than so-called better cuts of conventionally raised meat. Herbs, spices, and fresh salsa not only build up the flavor but also make the burgers more nourishing, giving the body the tools to digest the meat and assimilate its nutrients. Not to mention, ground meat is already relatively easy to digest, because it is already partially broken down. Frying these patties in the skillet will fill your house with a rich, spicy aroma that nourishes your whole being even before the food hits the plate.

◆ YIELD: 4 SMALL BURGERS ◆

FOR THE SALSA

- 1   red or yellow bell pepper, finely chopped
- ½   cup loosely packed fresh mint, finely chopped
- 2   small garlic cloves, finely chopped
- ⅛   teaspoon salt
-     Pinch of freshly ground black pepper
- ½   teaspoon red wine vinegar
- 1–2   teaspoons olive oil

FOR THE BURGERS

- 1   pound ground lamb, turkey, or beef
- 1   small onion, finely chopped (about ½ cup)
- 2   tablespoons fresh oregano or 2 teaspoons dried
- ½   teaspoon salt
- ¼   teaspoon freshly ground black pepper

1. Prepare the salsa: Combine the bell pepper, mint, garlic, salt, black pepper, vinegar, and oil in a bowl and mix well. For best flavor, let the salsa sit and the flavors meld for 15 to 30 minutes before serving.

2. While the salsa is sitting, prepare the burgers: Combine the ground meat, onion, oregano, salt, and pepper in a bowl and mix well. Divide the seasoned meat into four equal parts and form each part into a patty.

3. Preheat a grill or set a heavy skillet over medium-high heat. Cook the patties to the point of about medium-rare, when the center is still pink but not bloody and the meat thermometer in the center registers 165°F (330°C); you'll need about 4 minutes per side depending on how thick you made them. The burgers will continue to cook after they have been removed from the heat, so remove them just before you think they are quite done. Let sit 5 minutes, then serve with the salsa.

MIX AND MATCH

This sweet pepper and mint salsa is excellent on burgers, but it is also good on other cuts of meat. The fresh flavor and crunchy texture offer a nice complement to rich flavors. I particularly like it on lamb, since mint and lamb are such a classic and complementary team.

CHICKEN LIVER PÂTÉ

Waste not, want not, as the saying goes. Foods such as pâté likely came from efforts to use all parts of an animal without letting anything go to waste — both for the sake of frugality and as a sign of respect and appreciation for the animal that gave its life so we could be nourished. Organs such as liver were highly valued in traditional diets for their nutrient content. Rich in iron, vitamins A, D, E, K, and B_{12} and other B vitamins, liver is one of the most nutrient-dense foods on the planet. Sauté it lightly with shallots and herbs and it becomes a delicacy you wouldn't want to waste. This recipe calls for chicken livers, but lamb, beef, and pork livers are also excellent and can be substituted.

I like to serve pâté with crackers or bread and coarsely ground mustard. Fermented vegetables and dried, pickled, or preserved fruit make a nice addition as well.

♦ YIELD: 6 SERVINGS ♦

2   tablespoons bacon fat or butter

2   large or 3 small shallots, finely chopped

2   garlic cloves, finely chopped

1   teaspoon dried rosemary, finely chopped

1   teaspoon dried thyme, finely chopped

½   teaspoon freshly ground black pepper

1   bay leaf

    Pinch of ground cinnamon

1   pound chicken livers, cut into 2- to
    3-inch pieces

½   teaspoon salt

1. Warm the bacon fat in a skillet over medium heat. Add the shallots and sauté until translucent, about 5 minutes. Add the garlic, rosemary, thyme, pepper, bay leaf, and cinnamon, and cook until just aromatic, 30 to 60 seconds. Then add the chicken livers and salt and cook, stirring often, until the centers are just pink and not bloody, 4 to 7 minutes. Remove the skillet from the heat and let sit for 10 to 20 minutes.

2. Once the livers have cooled, remove the bay leaf and scrape the contents of the skillet into a food processor. Blend until well combined and mostly creamy, with just a few chunks remaining. The mixture should hold together like a dip or spread but still have some texture.

3. Serve at room temperature. Store any leftovers in the refrigerator, where they will keep for 5 days. Or freeze, wrapped in plastic, for up to 3 months.

LAVENDER FIZZ

This flowery, slightly sweet drink is a cross between soda and champagne and can contain a very small amount of alcohol. The carbonation is a natural by-product of the fermentation process, a sign that the fizz is active and alive. Naturally fermented beverages are energizing and excellent for digestion. Lavender, a calming aromatic herb from the mint family, helps soothe anxiety, restlessness, anger, tension, and depression. Let the bubbles in this drink lift you up!

◆ YIELD: 8 CUPS ◆

7½ cups water

½ cup raw honey

1 tablespoon white wine vinegar

4 tablespoons fresh or dried lavender flowers

1 lemon, sliced into ¼-inch rounds

I. Combine the water, honey, vinegar, lavender, and lemon in a clean half-gallon mason jar, cover with a lid, and shake well until all the honey has dissolved. Set the mixture aside to ferment, covered, at room temperature for 2 days.

2. After 2 days, strain out the lavender and lemon. Transfer the liquid into glass or plastic bottles with tight-fitting lids, leaving about ½ inch of headroom in each bottle. (The lids need to be tight fitting to contain the carbonation that is going to develop. If the lids do not fit tightly, the carbonation will escape from the bottles, leaving you with a still delicious yet noncarbonated beverage.)

3. Set the bottles aside in a cool, dark place to ferment for 3 days. Then open one of the bottles to taste it. If the soda is still not carbonated, put the lid back on and let the bottles continue fermenting. Taste regularly. The length of time needed to produce carbonation will vary depending on the temperature and the activity of the yeasts in your fizz.

4. Once the soda reaches the desired carbonation, transfer the bottles to the refrigerator. The cold temperature will slow the fermentation process and keep the carbonation level as it is.

NOTE: Sometimes a bit of mold can form on the surface of the soda during the fermentation process. This is just surface mold, and the soda is still good; simply remove the mold and proceed.

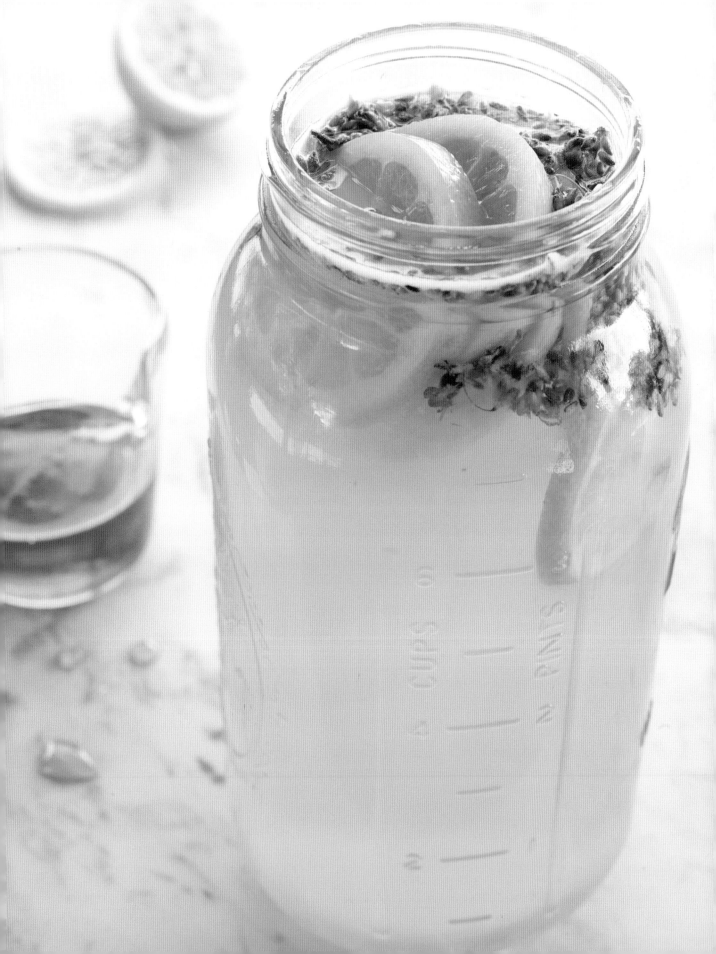

LAVENDER AFTER-DINNER TEA

I like to think of soothing, calming lavender as an ally in helping to make space in the mind — space to reflect, think, listen, feel, and simply be. What could be more relaxing at the end of a long day than permission and support to just *be*? Lavender, along with chamomile and peppermint, helps support digestion and assimilation of nutrients, making space for you to better absorb and utilize the nourishment of your dinner, too.

◆ YIELD: 3 CUPS ◆

2   tablespoons fresh or dried chamomile flowers

2   teaspoons fresh or dried lavender flowers

2   teaspoons fresh or dried peppermint

3   cups boiling water

Combine the chamomile, lavender, and peppermint in a teapot or jar and pour the boiling water over them. Cover with a lid and let steep for 5 to 15 minutes. Strain and enjoy.

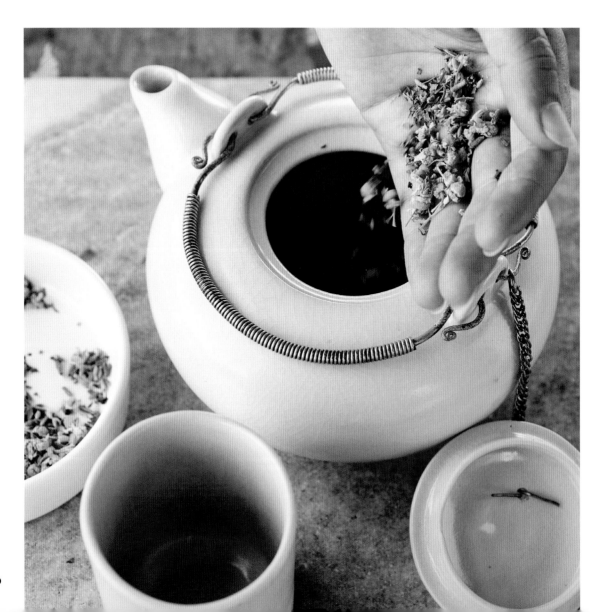

NOURISHING ROSEMARY HAIR RINSE

Rosemary stimulates circulation to blood vessels and capillaries. When applied topically to the scalp, it stimulates hair follicles, supporting the growth of strong, healthy hair. I love to use rosemary tea or rosemary-infused vinegar as a rinse on my scalp during the summer months, when the herb is abundant in the garden. I apply it liberally, letting my hair soak it in and then rinsing it out.

Rosemary tea: Rosemary tea can be made using the fresh or dried leaves, steeped for 15 minutes or longer. Use 2 cups boiling water with ¼ cup fresh rosemary or 2 tablespoons dried rosemary.

Rosemary-infused vinegar: Vinegar is a good choice for a hair rinse because it, too, is good for the scalp and hair. Simply combine ¼ cup dried or ½ cup fresh rosemary leaves with 1 cup raw apple cider vinegar. Let the mixture steep for 4 weeks, then strain. (If you're using a jar with a metal lid, put a piece of waxed paper between the lid and the vinegar. Otherwise the vinegar will erode the metal of the lid.) Infused vinegars will keep at room temperature for at least 3 months; if you refrigerate them, they'll keep for at least a year.

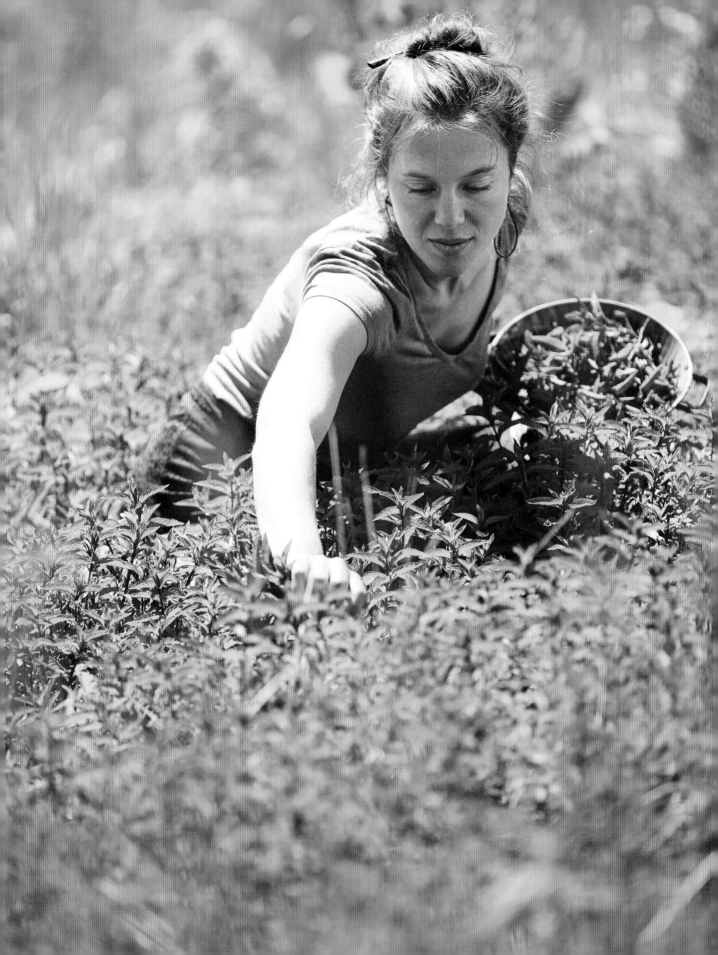

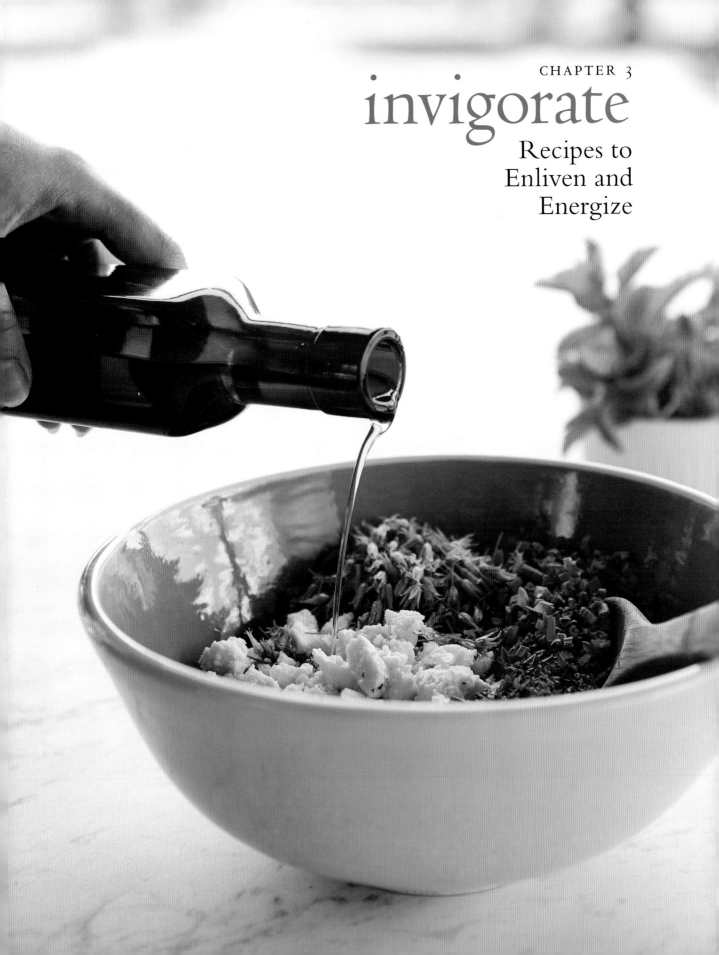

invigorate

Recipes to Enliven and Energize

Try doing a few jumping jacks. That's what I often do before I start writing. Movement is one of the ways in which we invigorate our bodies — it stimulates circulation and increases our intake of oxygen, which gives us energy and supports cellular metabolism. To *invigorate* is to enliven, energize, and excite, and certain foods, just like jumping jacks and other forms of movement, can stimulate these kinds of reactions in the body.

One of the many gifts of culinary herbs is that they invigorate the body. Their diverse and complex flavors have a stimulating, metabolically active effect. The strongly flavored herbs of the pungent/spicy, sour, and bitter families are particularly enlivening. They often stimulate physiological processes, such as the release of acids and enzymes in the stomach, the release of bile from the liver and gallbladder, or a boost to the circulation of blood and other body fluids. And, not insignificantly, they make eating more exciting by diversifying the plate and stimulating the senses.

Invigorating our senses and our body does not create energy but calls it up from the deep reserves of energy that live within us. These reserves comprise our vital energy, or vitality. While having energy may be a marker of vitality, energy does not imply vitality. We can also derive energy from unsustainable sources. Stress, for example, can give us energy, as can intense exercise, but if we rely on our stress response or overexertion to give us energy, we end up exhausted and depleted. Sugar and caffeine can also create an energy rush, but it does not last forever, and it is usually followed by an energy crash.

We build our vital energy by nourishing ourselves on all levels. It begins with high-quality, nourishing food, but it also calls for a host of more intangible factors: getting adequate rest, not working too much, spending time outside, exercising regularly, enjoying time with friends or family — the exact recipe will be different for each of us. We all want to feel energized, and so it is important to cultivate the link between energy and vitality. Invigoration is a union of the two, energizing the body in a way that helps to build lasting, sustained vitality.

On a basic physiological level, the most important way to make food invigorating is to cook with herbs, particularly the pungent, bitter, and sour ones. They bring an astounding diversity of bioactive constituents to the plate and encourage the smooth functioning of a wide range of systems. Culinary herbs, for example, support digestive processes and improve our absorption of nutrients, building deep vitality in the body.

Another important factor is to focus on the quality of the food we eat and how it is prepared. High-nutrient foods, for example, prepared in ways that make them easy to digest — such as soaked or sprouted nuts and seeds, long-simmered soups and stews, and fermented foods — provide the building blocks we need to support both energy and vitality. The same can be said for fresh, living foods, like just-picked fruits and vegetables, raw honey, and raw apple cider vinegar, which are alive with nutrients and biologically active enzymes that invigorate the body. Whether spicy, rich, sour, or fresh, these foods give us energy by wildly stimulating the senses,

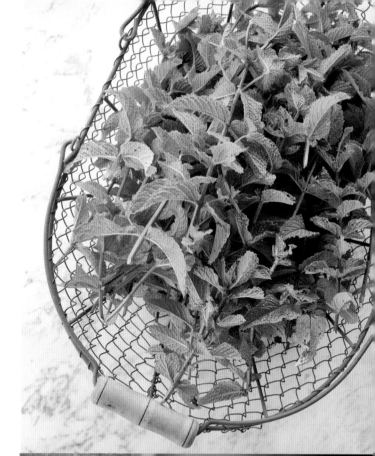

I like to think of invigoration as an awakening . . .

dynamically activating the body's biomechanisms, and helping to both stimulate and nourish our vital energy.

I like to think of invigoration as an awakening. An awakening of the senses of the body — taste, touch, sight, smell, and sound — that fosters self-awareness, inner inspiration, and creativity. What stimulates our senses has a powerful effect on the body through the nervous system. Long before we sit down to eat, the sights, sounds, and smells of the kitchen make our mouths water. Any time we stimulate and inspire the senses, we invigorate our body. And when that sensory stimulation comes from cooking food with love and intention, full of diverse and invigorating flavors, we are invigorating our sense of self-worth and our understanding of how we build vitality in our body and our life.

Food — growing it, gathering it, cooking it, and eating it — is a sensory experience. It holds the potential to enliven and inspire the senses and to awaken our vital life force. Invigoration of the body with flavorful food is important to our mental, emotional, and physical well-being . . . and it is enjoyable to eat, so make your food exciting!

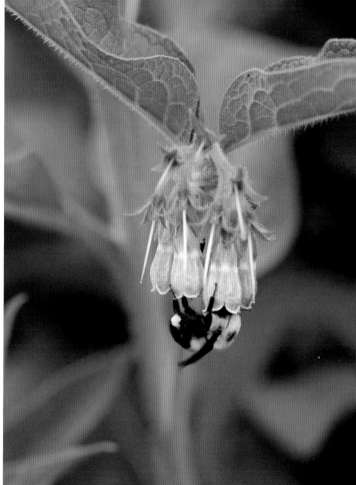

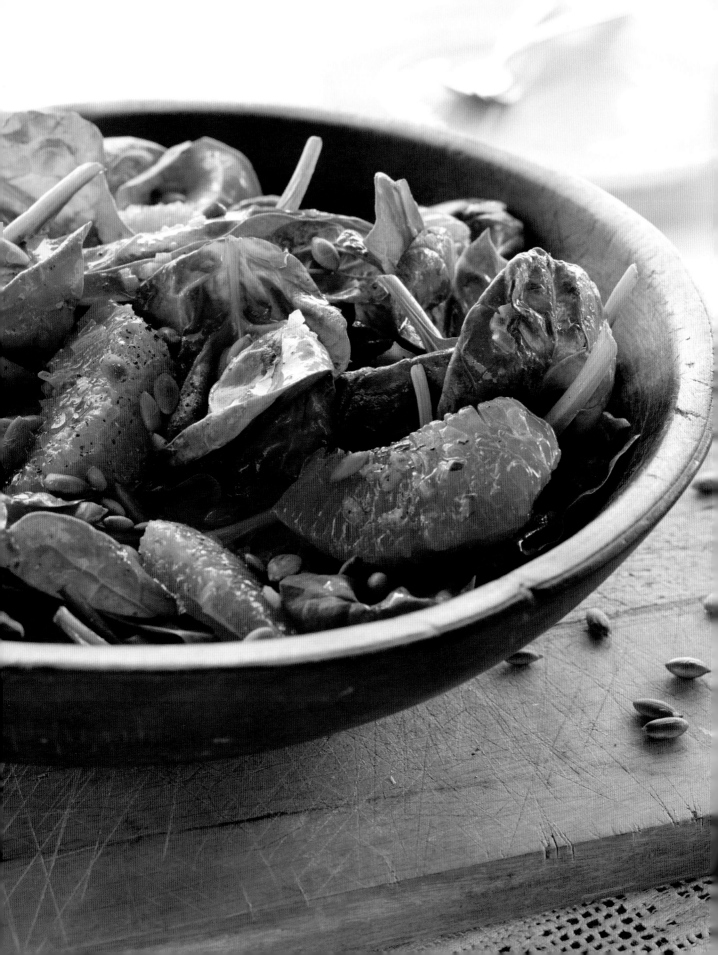

SPINACH AND GRAPEFRUIT SALAD WITH TOASTED PUMPKIN SEEDS

A welcome treat in winter months when color and flavor are in short supply, citrus fruits can invigorate any number of winter meals. The floral notes of tarragon in the dressing and the juicy, sour grapefruit invigorate the senses and wake up the digestive processes — an important example of the ways in which disparate flavors can come together to form a dish that feels exotic and bright during a quiet and dark time of the year.

◆ YIELD: 4-6 SERVINGS ◆

8   ounces spinach (about 4 packed cups)

1   large or 2 medium grapefruit

½   cup pumpkin seeds

FOR THE DRESSING

½   cup olive oil

1   tablespoon lemon juice

1   tablespoon white wine vinegar

1   teaspoon Dijon mustard

1   tablespoon finely minced shallot

1   teaspoon finely chopped tarragon

     Pinch of salt

I.   Tear the spinach into bite-size pieces, if necessary, and place in a large bowl.

2.   Section the grapefruit: Cut the top and bottom off the grapefruit so that the flesh of the fruit is exposed and it will sit flat on a cutting board. Cut the peel and pith from the fruit using a sharp knife or vegetable peeler. Set the grapefruit on one of its flat ends on a cutting board. The sections of the fruit will face up. Cut out the sections, slicing from the outside toward the center of the fruit, just inside the membranes. You can leave the sections whole or cut them into bite-size pieces.

3.   Toast the pumpkin seeds in a skillet over medium heat, stirring often, until they are lightly browned, have puffed up, and begin to pop, 4 to 7 minutes.

4.   Prepare the dressing: Combine the oil, lemon juice, vinegar, mustard, shallot, tarragon, and salt in a bowl and whisk together. Stir in any grapefruit juice that may have puddled on the cutting board while you were sectioning the fruit.

5.   Pour the dressing over the spinach. Depending on how much dressing you like, you may have some left over, and it will keep in the fridge for up to 1 week. Toss the spinach well, then add the grapefruit and pumpkin seeds and toss gently again to combine.

SERVING SUGGESTION: Grapefruit's sour flavor stimulates liver metabolism and helps the body digest fats and oils. Consider this salad alongside a heavier dish, such as Steak with a Lavender–Black Pepper Crust (page 120).

COMPOSED SALAD WITH MARJORAM VINAIGRETTE

A composed platter of vegetables and herbs, with an herb-laden vinaigrette for dipping, is a fun, easy, and unique appetizer. Simple enough in action, yet loaded in practice, dipping can represent indulgence and enjoyment in the same bite. The cultural stigma that demonizes double-dipping teaches us that we should not share, that food — and health — is a sterile object we must exert control over. With this dish, you get to dip (and double-dip, if you are at my house!) and use your hands, composing a different, flavorful arrangement of herbs and vegetables with every bite. The herbs you'll use here enliven the flavors of the raw vegetables and also make them more digestible, as they do for so many dishes. As the seasons change, use whatever vegetables are available, allowing your creative palate to guide you.

◆ YIELD: 6 SERVINGS AS AN APPETIZER ◆

FOR THE SALAD

- ½ pound red radishes or small hakurei turnips, sliced
- 2 carrots, sliced on the diagonal
- 3 scallions, trimmed, cut in half lengthwise, then cut into 2-inch lengths
- ½ cup fresh whole mint leaves
- ½ cup fresh parsley sprigs
- ½ cup radicchio leaves
- ½ cup walnut halves
- ⅓ pound feta cheese, thinly sliced
- ¼ cup pitted kalamata olives, halved

FOR THE DRESSING

- ½ cup olive oil
- 2 tablespoons red wine vinegar
- 2 tablespoons finely chopped shallots
- 2 garlic cloves, thinly sliced
- 2 tablespoons minced fresh marjoram or oregano

  Salt and freshly ground black pepper

I. Arrange the radishes, carrots, scallions, mint, parsley, radicchio, walnuts, feta, and olives on a platter.

2. Prepare the dressing: Whisk together the oil, vinegar, shallots, garlic, marjoram, and salt and pepper to taste. Place the dressing in a bowl or jar on the platter with the vegetables and serve.

3. To eat, you can dip the vegetables in the dressing on their own, but also try wrapping the veggies and other goodies in mint, parsley, or raddichio leaves and dipping them that way — delicious!

THYME AND JALAPEÑO PICKLED CARROTS

Preserving summer vegetables is a process of beauty. I love transforming the landscape of the kitchen with creative production, then watching as things bubble and ferment, only to open these treats later on and enjoy their colors, textures, and flavors all over again as I garnish a plate or pack a lunch. It's late fall, and I've reached the end of a long day of writing. The sun is slanting in through the window, and I just want to finish up so I can go outside for a walk. I need a little something to wake me up and keep me engaged. It's the perfect time for a pickled carrot.

The thyme gives these pickles a unique smoky flavor and the jalapeño lends a spicy kick. For less spice, cut the jalapeño in half and remove the seeds. This will give you a milder pickle without losing the jalapeño flavor. If you really do not like spicy, you could omit the jalapeño entirely.

◆ YIELD: 1 QUART ◆

1	jalapeño pepper
8–10	fresh thyme sprigs
4	garlic cloves, peeled and halved lengthwise
1	teaspoon whole black peppercorns
4–5	medium carrots, cut into 3-inch-long, ¼-inch-thick sticks

FOR THE BRINE

2	cups nonchlorinated water
1	tablespoon noniodized salt

1. Place the whole jalapeño, thyme, garlic, and peppercorns into a clean 1-quart mason jar. Put the carrot sticks in on top of the herbs and spices, packing them in tightly. Leave ½ to ¾ inch of headroom at the top of the jar.

2. Prepare the brine: Warm ¼ cup of the water, add the salt, and stir until dissolved. Stir that salty water into the rest of the water.

3. Pour enough brine over the carrots to cover them by ¼ inch. (You should have enough brine, but make more if you need to.) Put the lid on the jar and set aside to ferment at room temperature. I leave my fermenting carrots on the kitchen counter by the sink to make the next step easier.

4. As the fermentation progresses, gas will form inside the jar. Without actually taking the lid off, loosen the lid of the jar to release the pressure. I do this over the sink, as sometimes the jar contents will bubble up and some of the brine can leak out. Leave the lid loosened until the bubbles stop, then tighten the lid back down and let the jar ferment for another day. Do this daily for the first week.

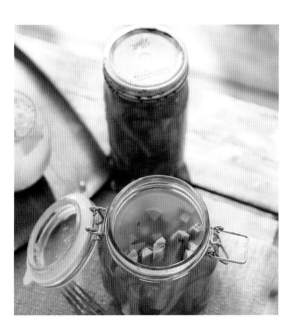

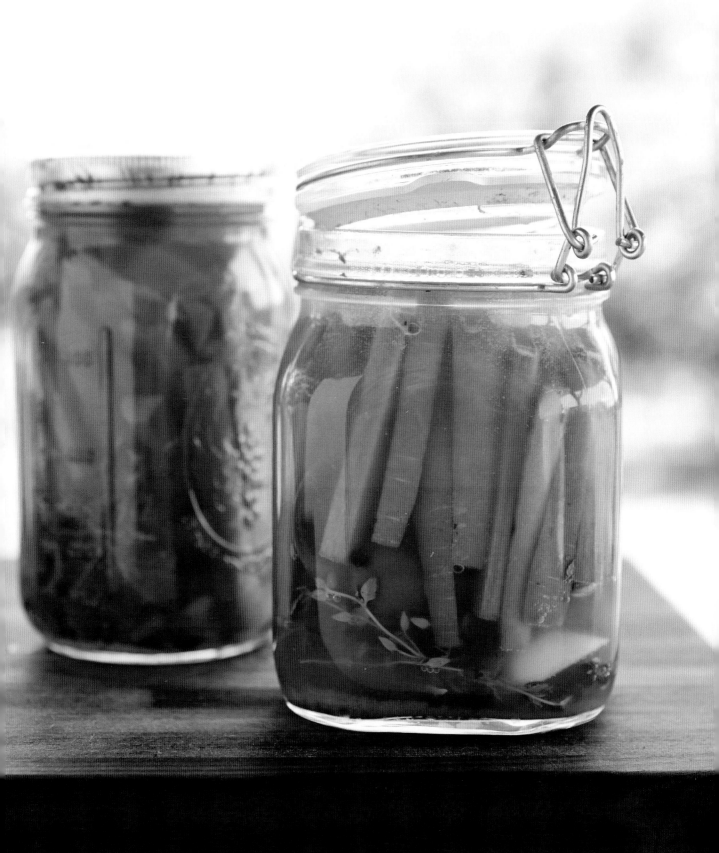

5. At the end of the week, remove the lid completely to make sure the brine still covers the carrots by ¼ inch; any carrots exposed to air may mold. Add more brine as needed and tighten the lid back on the jar.

6. Now set the carrots aside in a cool, dark spot to ferment for 4 weeks. Check them every week to make sure there is still sufficient brine covering the carrots and to release any pressure. It is common for a powdery-looking film, called kahm yeast, to form on the surface of the brine. You may also see spots of mold, which will usually form in a thicker layer and may look hairy or textured. The brine itself may also grow cloudy, which is normal. As long as the mold growth is on the surface of the ferment and hasn't penetrated the vegetables themselves, you can simply use a clean spoon to scrape off the mold and as much of the yeast as you can, and it's perfectly safe to continue to ferment or to eat the vegetables.

7. Begin to taste the carrots after 4 weeks. They should be sour, spicy, and a little smoky tasting (that comes from the thyme!). They should still be crunchy, but not as much as a raw carrot. If they still seem raw, or you want them softer, they have not fermented long enough; replace the lid and give them another 1 to 3 weeks. The speed of fermentation will vary depending on the ambient temperature. They will ferment faster in warmer temperatures and slower in cooler temperatures.

8. When you like the taste, store the carrots in the refrigerator, where they will keep for 6 months. Once they are refrigerated, the carrots do not have to be submerged beneath the brine; the cold will keep them from spoiling.

LACTOFERMENTATION

This lactofermentation pickling technique differs from vinegar pickling. Lactofermentation is a microbial process where lactic acid bacteria break down starches and sugars in plant material in an anaerobic environment. By-products of this microbial process include alcohol, acetic acid, and more lactic acid, biopreservatives that help preserve food. These acids are also responsible for the sour taste that gives fermented foods such a unique flavor and place in cuisine, cleansing the palate and invigorating digestion and liver function. Lactic acid bacteria are probiotic, supporting digestive health, energy, vitality, immune health, and emotional well-being.

MINT AND FETA BRUSCHETTA WITH CHIVE BLOSSOMS

As the sun sets, it casts a warm light on the garden. The bees buzz excitedly around the chive blossoms, harvesting the pollen and, I imagine, enjoying this smell — somehow oniony and floral, pungent, and sweet at the same time. I join them, collecting the tops and tender stems. Another fragrance joins my nose and I stop to pick some mint before I head into the kitchen. I won't wash these fresh, aromatic greens — like the bees, I want to enjoy the vitality of the garden: soft leaves, fragrant oils, and fresh pollen.

◆ YIELD: 4 SERVINGS AS AN APPETIZER ◆

½ cup fresh chive blossoms

1 French baguette

½ pound feta cheese, crumbled

1 cup chopped fresh mint

½ cup minced chives

2–4 tablespoons olive oil

Salt and freshly ground black pepper

1. Preheat the oven to 325°F (170°C).

2. While the oven is heating, pull apart the chive blossoms, removing the central stem and plucking the tiny purple florets.

3. Set the baguette in the hot oven and bake for 7 to 10 minutes, until the edges are crispy but not browned.

4. Meanwhile, combine the feta in a bowl with the mint, minced chives, and chive florets. Add enough of the oil to moisten, and season with salt and pepper to taste. Mix well.

5. Remove the baguette from the oven and slice along the diagonal. Arrange on a platter with 1 to 2 tablespoons of the bruschetta mixture on each slice. Drizzle with a little more oil and serve.

SOFT OR CRISPY?

I like to make bruschetta with the bread soft on the inside and crispy on the outside.
If you prefer the bread to be crisp throughout, slice it on the diagonal to start with, brush each piece with olive oil, and bake on a baking sheet at 325°F (170°C) for 5 to 7 minutes, until crispy.

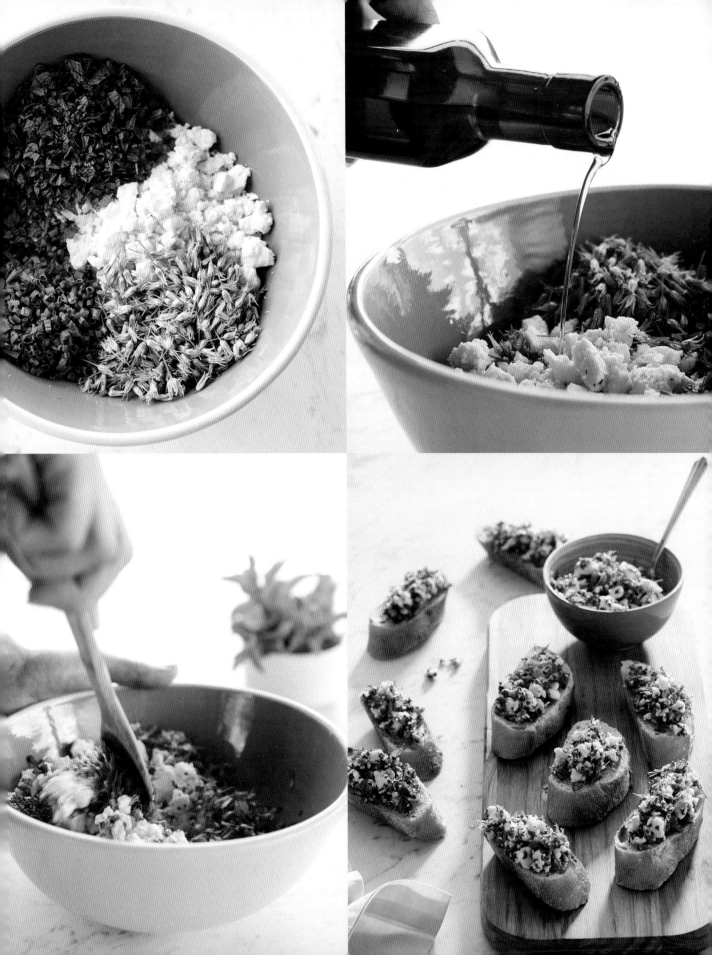

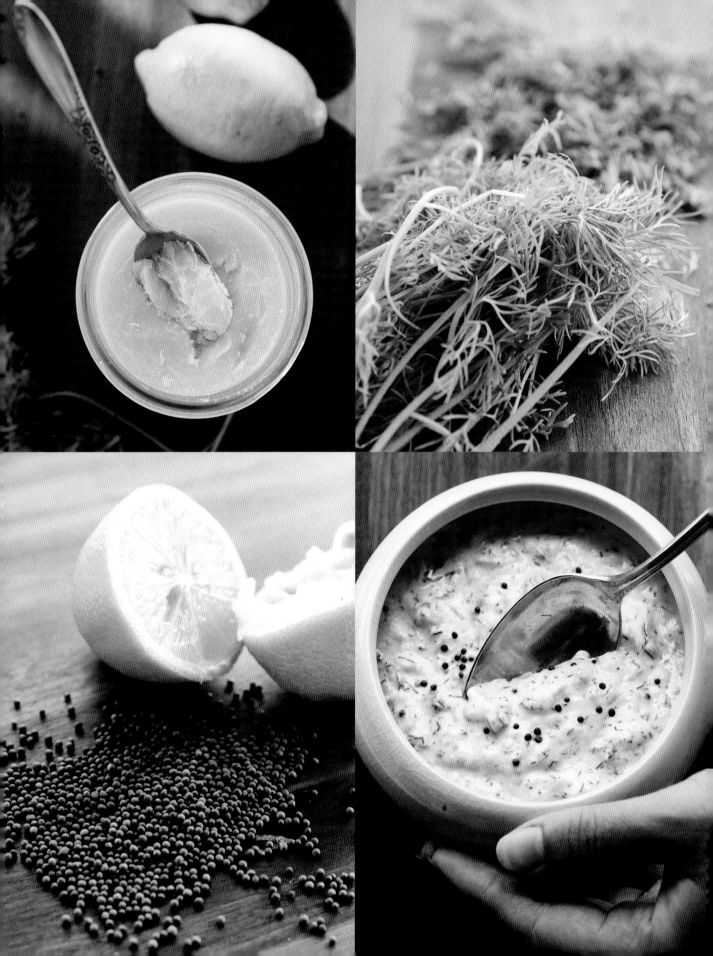

CUCUMBER RAITA
WITH DILL AND
BLACK MUSTARD SEEDS

Refreshing and cooling, raita is often served as a palate cleanser with spicy, rich-flavored foods — it can be a sauce, dip, or salad. Raita comes from the hot climates of India, Pakistan, and Bangladesh, where it is known to refresh the senses on a hot day and stimulate the appetite when heat has withered it. The sour flavor of the yogurt, alongside the herbs and citrus, invigorates digestive and liver function. Yogurt, as a fermented dairy product, is not only easier to digest than unfermented dairy but is a rich source of probiotic bacteria.

◆ YIELD: 4 SERVINGS AS A SIDE DISH ◆

2   tablespoons ghee (page 93)

½   teaspoon whole black mustard seeds

2   small cucumbers

½   cup minced fresh dill

¼   cup chopped scallions

1   cup plain whole-milk yogurt

1   tablespoon lemon juice

I. Heat the ghee in a small skillet. Once it's hot, add the mustard seeds. Cook, stirring often, until they begin to pop. Remove from the heat and set aside to cool.

2. Roughly peel the cucumbers, if you wish. (I leave the tender skins on when I use pickling cucumbers; otherwise I peel them.) Coarsely grate the cucumbers, place the gratings in a colander, and set aside to drain for 5 to 10 minutes.

3. Meanwhile, combine the dill and scallions in a bowl with the yogurt, lemon juice, and ghee.

4. Squeeze the grated cucumber, wringing out as much liquid as possible. Add the cucumber to the yogurt mixture, mix well, and serve.

SERVING SUGGESTION: This makes a tasty, cooling side dish or condiment alongside spicy food or rich fare. Try it with Roasted Red Lentil Dhal (page 80), or Vegetable Curry with Thai Basil (page 118), or serve it alongside a salad on a hot summer day. Sometimes, when serving the raita as a side dish, I like to stir in a grated raw beet; it adds nice texture, sweetness, and beautiful color.

VITAL ROOTS KIMCHI

Roots can grow deep into the earth — determined, focused, and driven. They can also meander between and around rocks and other roots — flexible, adaptable, and open to change. Roots are foundational and elemental. When we think about our own roots as people, we look to our origins, our identity, and the ideas and values that we hold central. Just as roots provide nutrition and structure for a plant, having solid roots as a person nourishes, supports, and provides the structure we need for growth. As food, roots provide foundational, blood-building nutrition — the kind of nutrition that builds vitality. This fermented root-based kimchi, full of probiotic goodness and warming herbs like garlic and ginger, offers excellent support for the digestive system, that central place where we take in food and experience, sort through its inevitable waste, and break it down to absorb its infinite wisdom.

♦ YIELD: ABOUT 8 CUPS ♦

1 medium green cabbage (about 3 pounds)

3 medium carrots, grated (about 1 cup)

¾ pound daikon, red, or watermelon radishes, quartered and thinly sliced (¾–1 cup)

¾ pound sunchoke, halved and thinly sliced (¾–1 cup)

¾ pound burdock root, thinly sliced (about ½–¾ cup)

8–12 scallions, cut in half lengthwise and then sliced into 2-inch-long pieces

1 head garlic, cloves separated and grated or chopped (⅛–¼ cup)

2-inch piece fresh ginger, grated (about ⅛ cup)

1–3 red chiles, chopped (optional)

3–4½ teaspoons noniodized salt

FOR THE BRINE

2 cups nonchlorinated water

1 tablespoon noniodized salt

I. Remove and compost the outer leaves of the cabbage. Cut the head into quarters and slice ⅛ inch thick. (You can remove the core before slicing, but I don't usually bother.) Combine the sliced cabbage in a large bowl with the carrots, radishes, sunchoke, burdock, scallions, garlic, ginger, and chiles (if using). Sprinkle 3 teaspoons of the salt over the cabbage mixture and massage with your hands by squeezing and flipping for 10 to 20 minutes. Taste the mixture at this point. It should taste salty, but not be unpleasantly salty. Add more salt as desired. Let the vegetables rest for 10 minutes or so, then massage for another 5 to 10 minutes. By this point the vegetables should have begun to sweat, with juice collecting at the bottom of the bowl.

2. Pack the vegetable mixture into a clean half-gallon mason jar or crock. Pour any juice remaining in the bowl into the jar. If that juice is enough to cover the vegetables by 1 inch, you do not need to prepare the brine.

3. Prepare the brine: Warm ¼ cup of the water, add the salt, and stir until dissolved. Stir that salty water into the rest of the water.

4. Pour enough brine over the vegetables to cover them by about 1 inch. (You should have enough brine, but make more if you need to.) To keep the vegetables submerged beneath the brine, set a ziplock bag on top of the vegetables and fill it with water, so it spreads out and seals off the jar or crock. Or set a smaller glass jar filled with water as a weight on top of the vegetables.

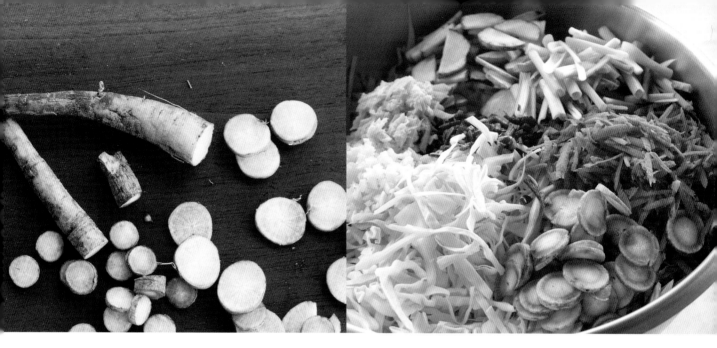

If you are using a crock rather than a jar, you can put a plate on top of the vegetables inside the crock and put a jar full of water on top of the plate to weigh it down. With either method, be sure the vegetables are submerged below the salty brine; any vegetables exposed to air may mold.

5. Let the kimchi ferment at room temperature until the flavor reaches your liking, 2 to 3 weeks. Check it every other day during the first week to make sure the vegetables stay submerged beneath the brine; any vegetable exposed to air may mold. Push the weight down and add more brine if necessary.

6. Begin to taste the kimchi after a week or so. The longer it ferments, the more sour the flavor and the softer the vegetables. The speed of the fermentation will vary depending on the ambient temperature. A ferment made during a heat wave in August might take only 10 days to be as sour as you like it, whereas a ferment made in October could require 3 weeks.

7. When you like the taste and texture, transfer the kimchi to smaller containers and store in the refrigerator, where it will keep for 3 to 6 months. Once it is refrigerated, the kimchi does not have to be submerged beneath the brine; the cold will keep it from spoiling.

PREBIOTICS AND PROBIOTICS

Fermented vegetables and other types of fermented foods contain probiotic bacteria that support the health of our microbiome. The roots of burdock and sunchoke (also called Jerusalem artichoke) both contain inulin. Inulin is a prebiotic — a starch that feeds probiotic bacteria already in the gut and thus supports digestive health. Burdock is also excellent for liver health, and consistently eating the root or taking it medicinally can improve immune health, energy levels, and skin issues. If you do not have access to sunchokes or burdock root, you can substitute other root vegetables or use more radish and carrot in their place.

VEGETABLE CURRY WITH THAI BASIL

Our senses come alive in the kitchen. Aromatic herbs are our helpers, keeping us engaged as we process, chop, grind, sauté, simmer, or bake. As the smells permeate the air, they tickle us with anticipation of the meal to come: our tummy rumbles, our mouth waters. Through herbs, we experience our cooking viscerally and emotionally — the tears from chopping onions, the joy of smelling fresh lemongrass and aromatic basil, and the flash of a renewed outlook just from zesting a lime.

This curry, redolent with pungent herbs and chock-full of vegetables, is an inspiration for the senses. To make it vegetarian, leave out the fish sauce and use extra lime juice and a bit more salt in its place.

◆ YIELD: 4-6 SERVINGS ◆

FOR THE CURRY PASTE

2 pieces lemongrass

½ bell pepper

3 medium shallots or 1 large onion

2 red chiles, ideally Thai chiles

1 cup packed cilantro leaves

¼ cup grated cilantro root (optional)

3 garlic cloves

2-inch piece fresh ginger, grated

1 teaspoon ground coriander

Zest of 1 lime

FOR THE VEGETABLE CURRY

2 medium zucchini, sliced into thin spears

1 medium onion, cut into ¼-inch-thick half moons

½ head cauliflower, cut into bite-size florets

½ bell pepper, chopped

2 (12-ounce) cans coconut milk

2 cups packed fresh Thai or sweet basil

1 tablespoon fish sauce

Juice of ½ lime

Salt

Hot cooked rice, for serving

Lime wedges, for garnish

I. Lemongrass can be fibrous and tough. To use it in the curry paste, you'll need a food processor with a sharp blade. If you don't have that, leave the lemongrass out of the paste and cook it in the actual curry instead. To prepare the paste, remove the outer leaves of the lemongrass and slice the tender parts (usually half of the stalk) into ¼-inch rounds. (Set the tougher parts aside to cook in the actual vegetable curry.) Combine the lemongrass slices in the food processor with the bell pepper, shallots, chiles, cilantro leaves, cilantro root (if using), garlic, ginger, coriander, and lime zest, and blend until smooth. Set aside.

2. Prepare the curry: Cut whatever lemongrass you have left into 2-inch pieces. Combine the lemongrass with the zucchini, onion, cauliflower, bell pepper, and coconut milk in a saucepan, bring to a simmer over medium heat, then reduce the heat to low and simmer until the vegetables are tender, about 20 minutes.

3. When the vegetables are tender, remove and compost the lemongrass pieces and add the curry paste, basil, fish sauce, and lime juice. Cook for 1 to 2 minutes, then season with salt to taste. You don't want to overdo it with the salt, but you also don't want to skimp, because the salt really brings the diverse flavors of the curry together and enlivens the dish.

4. Serve over rice and garnish with a wedge of lime.

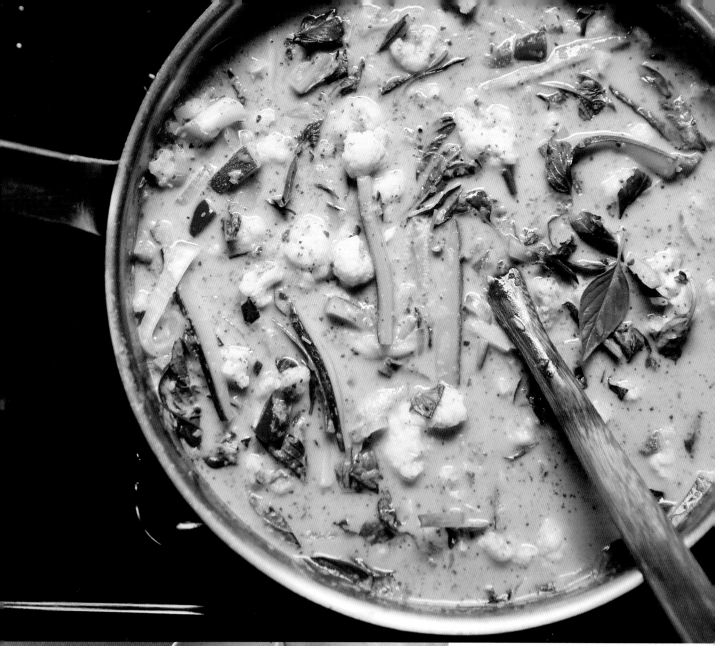

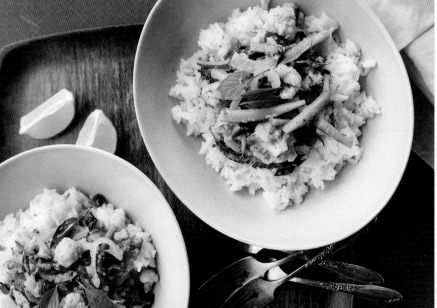

COOKING WITH THE SEASONS

Which vegetables you use in the curry can depend on what's available. Some of my favorite seasonal variations include

- FALL: sweet potato with chickpeas and spinach

- WINTER: white potato and parsnip with kale or collard greens

- SPRING: asparagus and green onion

- SUMMER: eggplant and sweet peppers

STEAK WITH A LAVENDER–BLACK PEPPER CRUST

Cooking with lavender brings me outside, to images of rolling purple fields, bees buzzing, children laughing, and clouds moving quickly along the horizon. Lavender's rich, floral aromatics are so strong that sometimes you can catch them in the breeze — gentle and evocative, yet hard to capture, with a fleeting arrival and departure. The fragrance of lavender relaxes the senses, eases tension, and makes space in the mind. When you have space in your mind, challenges shrink, obstacles bow down, and life is more laughable. Beneath its light, flowery first impression, lavender carries a bitter taste, a grounding quality that helps anchor the body and grant perspective within experience. Lavender's lessons are life's lessons: to enjoy, accept, love, and let go.

◆ YIELD: 2 SERVINGS ◆

2   teaspoons dried lavender flowers

2   teaspoons freshly ground black pepper

2   teaspoons olive oil

1   pound skirt steak or New York strip steak

    Salt

    Fresh parsley sprigs, for garnish

I. Finely powder the lavender flowers in a spice grinder or with a mortar and pestle. Combine the powdered lavender with the pepper in a small bowl. Drizzle 1 teaspoon of the oil on one side of the steak, sprinkle generously with salt and half of the lavender mixture, and rub the seasonings into the meat. Flip the steak and repeat on the other side. Let this rub infuse the meat with its flavor for at least 1 hour and up to 24 hours.

2. When you're ready to cook, pat the meat dry of any moisture. Heat a cast-iron skillet over medium-high heat. When it's hot enough that a drop of water flicked in the skillet jumps right up, place the meat in the pan. Reduce the heat slightly to prevent smoking. Let the steak cook, undisturbed, to your desired doneness. (To cook a 1½-inch steak to medium doneness, 4 to 5 minutes per side is about right.) Flip the steak and cook on the other side.

3. Remove the steak from the pan and let rest for 3 to 5 minutes before slicing and serving. For a hint of green, garnish with fresh parsley.

LAVENDER SALT SCRUB

A potent antimicrobial, lavender has long been valued as a bath herb. In fact, the Latin name for lavender, *lavandula*, comes from the Greek word *lavar*, meaning "to wash." In a salt scrub, lavender puts its aromatherapeutic magic to work, relieving tension and anxiety and helping us to relax at the end of a long day. At the same time, the salt helps to exfoliate the skin and stimulate the lymphatic and immune systems, thoroughly invigorating and refreshing the body.

This lavender salt scrub is excellent for detoxification and can help prevent and support recovery from cold, flu, sinus infection, ear infection, and other common illnesses. All you need is

- ¼ cup lavender flowers, powdered (see page 39)
- 1 cup finely ground sea salt
- 3 drops lavender essential oil (optional)

Combine the powdered lavender with the salt in a bowl and mix well. Then add the essential oil (if using) and mix again. Store in a jar with a tight-fitting lid away from heat and light.

To use the scrub, put a few table-spoons of the salt mixture in a bowl and add enough olive oil, or a body oil of your choosing, to form a paste. Gently massage the paste, a pinch at a time, into moist skin for 30 to 60 seconds, then rinse. You can apply the salt scrub in the shower or tub. Because the scrub will leave a light oily, slippery residue, be careful when you next use the shower or tub, or wipe it out immediately after using.

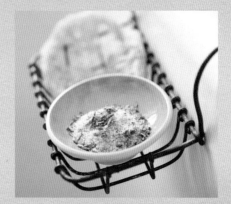

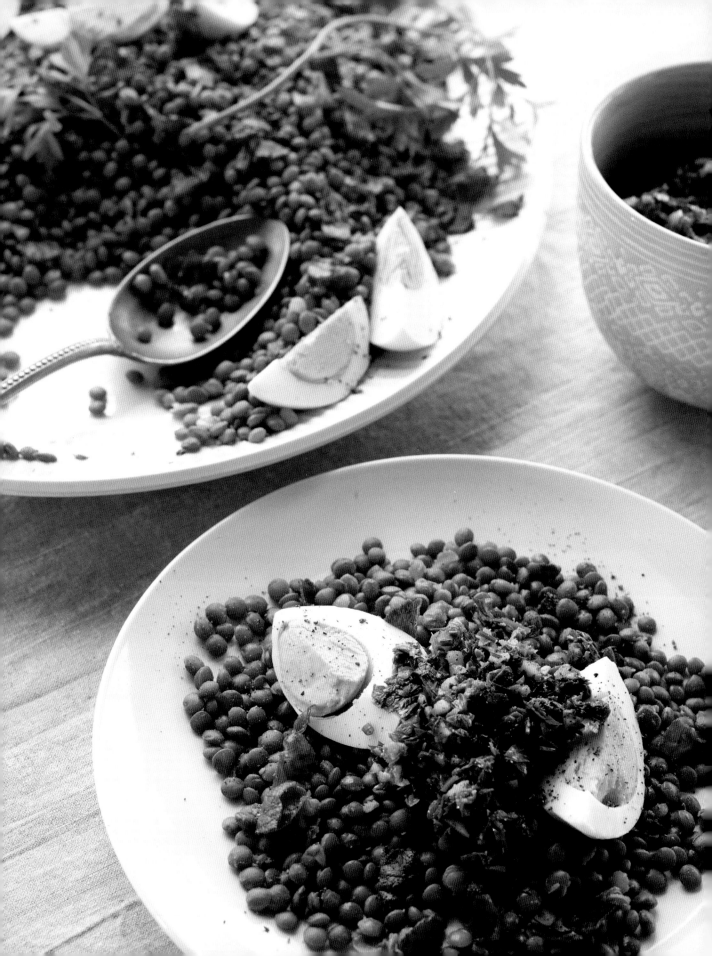

LENTILS, PROSCIUTTO, AND BOILED EGGS WITH SALSA VERDE

Salsa verde is reminiscent of sitting in the sun with your eyes closed — you can bask in its rich, complex, and vibrant flavors. It has long been one of my favorite palate cleansers — I crave the parsley, the capers, and the brightness of the lemon zest. It is great as part of an appetizer spread, on boiled eggs, as a garnish for soups, or with meat, beans, and grains. This particular application is inspired by a potluck dish I once made for my students on a summer day. I can't think of a better way to learn about the medicinal benefits of parsley than to thoroughly enjoy it.

◆ YIELD: 4 SERVINGS ◆

2 cups French lentils

5 cloves

2 bay leaves

½ cinnamon stick

⅛ pound prosciutto, chopped

Olive oil

Salt

2 hard-boiled eggs, peeled and quartered

Fresh parsley sprigs, for garnish

FOR THE SALSA VERDE

2 cups packed flat-leaf parsley leaves and tender stems, finely chopped

½ cup capers, coarsely chopped

2 garlic cloves, finely minced

Zest of 1 lemon, finely grated

½ cup olive oil

Salt and freshly ground black pepper

1. Soak the lentils overnight in enough water to cover by 6 inches.

2. Drain the lentils and combine them in a saucepan with the cloves, bay leaves, cinnamon, and enough water to cover by 1 inch. Bring to a simmer, then reduce the heat, cover, and let simmer, stirring occasionally, until the lentils are just tender, 5 to 15 minutes. Turn off the heat, remove the lid, and let the lentils cool in their cooking liquid.

3. While the lentils are cooking, prepare the salsa verde: Combine the parsley, capers, garlic, lemon zest, and oil in a bowl and mix well. Season to taste with salt and pepper.

4. Heat a skillet over medium heat. Add the prosciutto and cook, stirring constantly, until browned, 3 to 5 minutes. Set aside to cool.

5. Strain the lentils from their cooking water and remove the cloves, bay leaves, and cinnamon stick. Place the lentils in a large serving bowl or on a platter. Drizzle with oil and sprinkle with salt. Arrange the egg wedges around the edges and scatter the prosciutto over the lentils, along with any oil left in the skillet. Garnish with a few sprigs of fresh parsley and serve with the salsa verde. The ratio of salsa verde to lentils should be generous, about ¼ cup of salsa verde for every 1 to 1½ cups of lentils.

APRICOT-CASHEW BARS WITH COCONUT AND ROSEMARY

Snack food has largely become an empty-calorie affair, full of starches and simple sugars that increase blood sugar short term without providing the building blocks to support lasting vitality. Blood sugar issues can contribute to sugar cravings, fatigue, mental fog, anxiety, and mood swings. A much better option is a balanced snack containing fat and protein and low in processed sugars; this nutritional profile gives the body the fuel it needs for sustained energy. These apricot-cashew bars are a good example, and they can be made for a fraction of the price you would pay to buy energy bars in the store. Sesame seeds are high in calcium, an essential nutrient for muscular, skeletal, and nervous system health. The rosemary helps invigorate the sweet fruit and nutrient-dense nuts and seeds.

◆ YIELD: 16 (2-INCH) SQUARES ◆

1¼	cups raw cashews
½	cup raw sesame seeds
1	cup dried Turkish apricots
1	tablespoon coconut oil
1	tablespoon raw honey
¼	cup fresh rosemary leaves, finely chopped
¼	cup shredded coconut, plus some for garnish
	Zest of 1 orange, finely grated
	Coarsely ground salt or salt flakes

1. The night before, soak the cashews and sesame seeds in enough water to cover them by a few inches.

2. The next day, chop the apricots in a food processor until they are in small pieces; scrape out into a bowl and set aside.

3. Warm the oil and honey in a saucepan over low heat until melted, stirring frequently. Then stir in the rosemary and remove from the heat.

4. Strain the cashews and sesame seeds from their soaking water. Combine the cashews and sesame seeds in the food processor with the shredded coconut and the honey mixture. Blend until smooth, then add the apricots and blend until combined.

5. Pour the mixture into an 8- by 8-inch baking dish and press evenly and firmly into the dish. Top with the orange zest, a few pinches of shredded coconut, and salt; press these toppings into the bars to help them stick, if needed. Refrigerate for 20 minutes.

6. Cut into bars. Eat immediately or store in the refrigerator in an airtight container. The bars will keep for up to 5 days. They can also be frozen for 1 to 3 months and defrosted as needed.

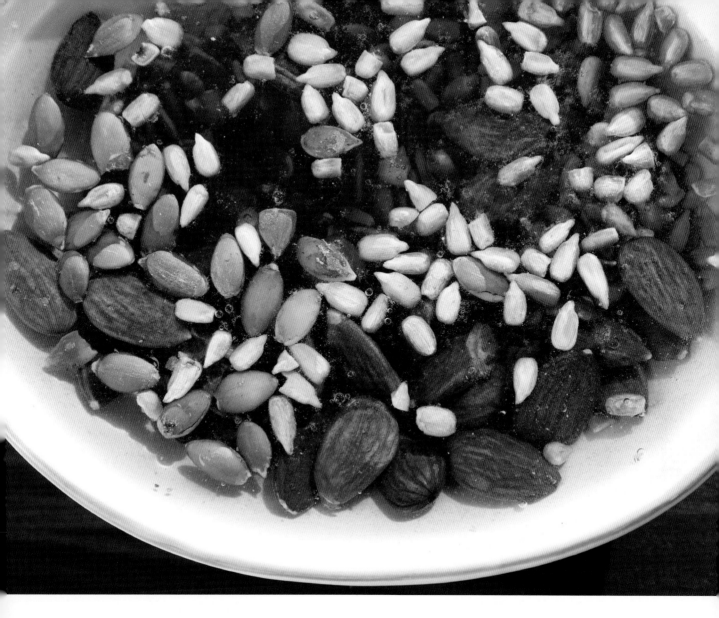

SOAKING NUTS AND SEEDS

All seeds — including what we call nuts, grains, and legumes — contain phytic acid. Phytic acid locks nutrients into the seed and protects them until the seed needs the nutrients to germinate. This allows a seed to sit in the dirt through winter or in a seed packet without rotting or losing the nutrition necessary for sprouting. When a seed is given germination conditions (warmth and moisture), the phytic acid breaks down and the nutrients become available to the germinating seed. For those of us who eat nuts, seeds, grains, and legumes, soaking them before cooking mimics germination conditions and neutralizes the phytic acid, making the nutrients in the seed more bioavailable to our body. How long to soak them? It depends on the seed, but generally speaking, at least 6 hours and as long as 12 (what I call overnight). I soak seeds of all types the morning before for use that evening and the night before for use the next morning. Toasting nuts and seeds is also thought to help neutralize phytic acid.

SAGE HONEY

Whether made with fresh sage right from the garden on a hot, sunny day or with the dried plant from the pantry on a winter evening, this infused honey melds soothing sweetness with the stimulating, bitter, and pungent actions of sage. While summer and winter can feel like opposites, there is always some spark of each season within the experience of the other, like yin and yang. In its diversity — sweet and bitter, moistening and drying — sage honey challenges our notions of duality. It can both calm the nervous system and invigorate the senses and the mind; it can soothe a sore throat and stimulate immunity. Excellent as medicine by the spoonful, in a cup of tea, or used in cooking, sage honey is an important remedy for the kitchen pharmacy. It may also help you find use for what seem to be opposing forces.

◆ YIELD: 1 CUP ◆

1 cup raw honey

½ cup chopped fresh sage or ⅓ cup dried

There are two ways to prepare this honey: the first is to prepare it well in advance and allow it to steep, while the second allows you to make it in just an hour or two and is a great option for last-minute situations.

METHOD 1: PLAN AHEAD

I. Combine the honey and sage in a jar and mix together well. Push down on the herbs in the jar to remove any large air bubbles. Make sure all the sage leaves are completely submerged beneath the honey; any plant material exposed to air may mold. (The risk of mold is lessened by using dried herbs.) The more air that is in the jar, the more likely mold will form on top; for this reason, use a jar that is just big enough to hold all the ingredients (a half-pint jar works best for this recipe).

2. Put the lid on the jar and set aside to infuse in a cool, dark place for 2 to 4 weeks. The longer the honey steeps, the stronger the herbal flavor. Check the honey every week or so to make sure all the plant material is still submerged. If mold does form on top of the honey, remove it with a spoon, make sure all the sage is submerged beneath the honey (adding more honey, if necessary), and secure with a lid again.

3. When the honey is to your liking, strain out the sage leaves by pouring the honey through a fine-mesh strainer into a glass jar with a tight-fitting lid. If the honey is too thick to pour through a strainer, heat it slightly in a double boiler, then strain it. If you do heat the honey before straining, allow it to cool in the storage jar before putting on the lid; otherwise condensation will form inside the jar, which may cause mold to grow.

4. Store the jar, labeled with the date and contents, in a cool, dark place. The honey will keep for up to a year.

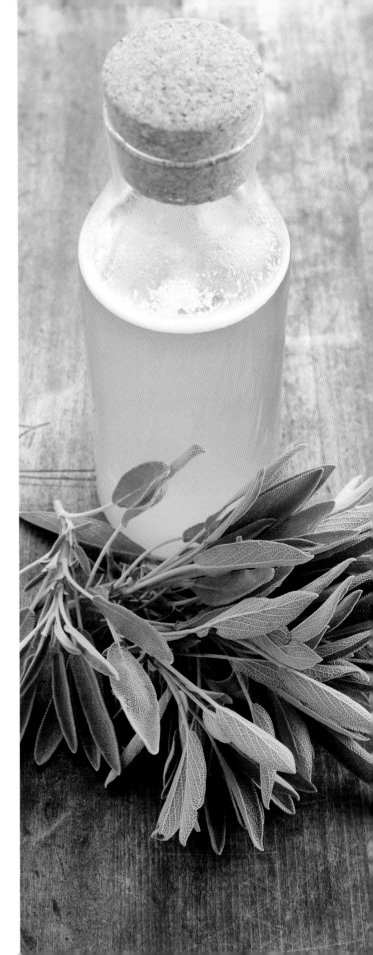

METHOD 2: I NEED IT NOW

I. Combine the honey and sage in the top of a
    double boiler. Bring an inch or two of water
    in the lower pan to a boil, then reduce the heat
    to low and let the honey and sage infuse for
    45 to 60 minutes. Do not let the honey get too
    hot or the herbs will burn. Stir the mixture every
    5 to 10 minutes. You will smell the sage's deli-
    cious aroma as it infuses into the honey. Add
    more water to the bottom pan along the way,
    if necessary.

2. When the honey is to your liking, strain it
    through a fine-mesh strainer into a glass jar.
    Let cool, then cover with a tight-fitting lid.
    Label with the date and contents and store in
    a cool, dark place. It will keep for up to a year.

AVOID WASHING

If you make this preparation using fresh sage
leaves, it is best not to wash the leaves before
using them. Sage contains potent volatile
oils that are part of the flavor and medicine,
and washing can remove these oils. Washing
will also introduce extra moisture into the
honey and increase the chances of mold.

The same holds true for most other herbs
you might use in either of these methods.
And there's a wide variety that infuse beautifully in honey, including rosemary, thyme,
tarragon, lavender, basil, and mint!

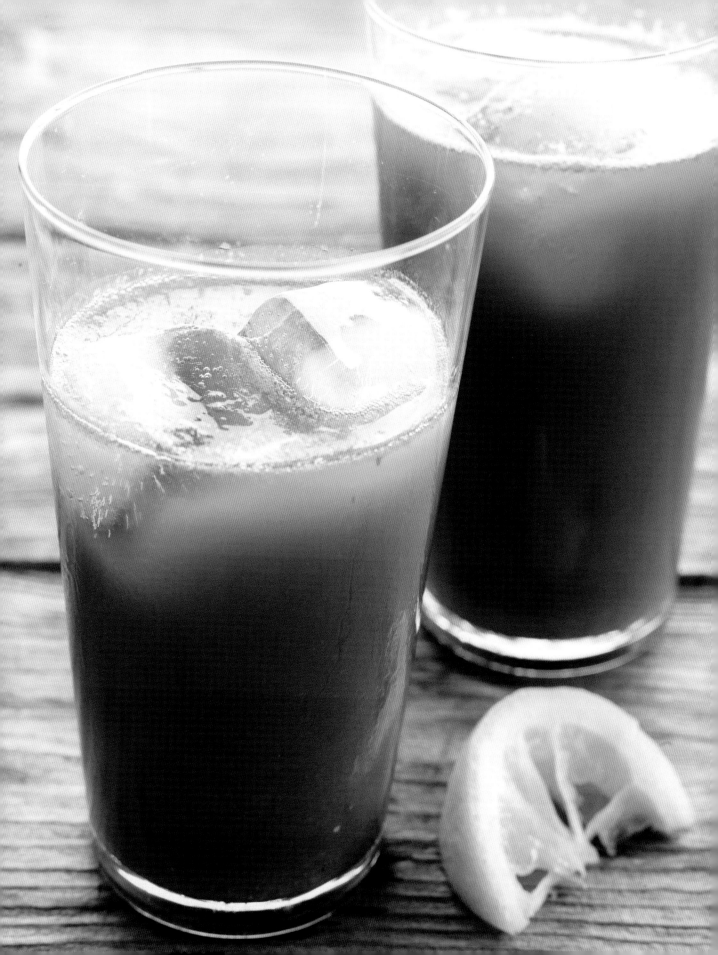

CILANTRO LEMONADE

Cilantro lemonade is hydrating, detoxifying, and invigorating. The combination of cilantro's cooling and detoxifying properties with the high amounts of vitamin C found in the lemon juice, the enzymes and sugars from the honey, and a little pinch of mineral-rich salt help replenish the body on a hot day. Cilantro lemonade is excellent plain or over ice. You can even use it as a base for fun summer cocktails.

◆ YIELD: ABOUT 3 CUPS ◆

1   bunch cilantro (about 2 cups packed)

¼   cup freshly squeezed lemon juice (from 1–2 lemons)

2   tablespoons raw honey

¼   teaspoon salt

2   cups water

Combine the cilantro with the lemon juice, honey, salt, and water in a blender and purée for 3 minutes. The drink will be a rich green color with a beautiful white foam on top. I enjoy drinking the lemonade as it is, with the cilantro pulp, but you can strain it through a sieve or tea strainer before serving, if you like. It will keep in the refrigerator for up to 3 days.

CILANTRO FOR GENTLE CLEANSING

You can drink cilantro lemonade on a daily or weekly basis to stay cool in hot weather or to support liver and digestive function and gentle detoxification. It also makes a nice seasonal tonic to help the body transition from colder to warmer weather.

MINT HYDROSOL

Rich in volatile oils and wonderfully aromatic, hydrosols are steam distillations made from fresh plants. They are easy to make at home if you have access to an abundance of fresh aromatic plants. Mint hydrosol has a mild flavor and aroma, reminiscent of, but not as strong as, the flavor and aroma of mint tea. Like the herb itself, mint hydrosol is cooling and invigorating, enlivening the senses and stimulating circulation. It is an excellent addition to summer beverages, imbuing them with refreshing mint undertones. As a spray, it energizes and promotes mental clarity. It can also help relieve tension and symptoms of headache and nausea. Try bringing some in the car with you on your next road trip!

◆ YIELD: 1–2 CUPS ◆

2   cups water

2   pounds fresh peppermint (or other mint), on the stems

1   tray ice cubes (about 12 cubes)

1. Center a clean, flat rock or a brick (2 to 3 inches high) in the bottom of a large soup pot. Set a soup bowl on top of the rock; the top of the bowl should be 2 to 3 inches below the top of the pot. Pour the water into the pot and place the mint in the bottom of the pot around the rock and bowl, fitting in as much of the mint as you can without it rising above the edges of the bowl. Put the lid of the pot on upside down, so that the low point or handle of the lid is above the bowl.

2. Turn the heat on medium-high. As soon as the water comes to a simmer and condensation begins to form on the underside of the lid (a pot with a glass lid works well because you can see what is going on inside the pot; otherwise just listen for the sound of boiling water), put half of the ice cubes into the lid of the pot. The ice will make the lid cold and cause the steam to condense and run down the lid and into the bowl. The water that collects in the bowl is the hydrosol.

3. As the ice cubes melt, add more, keeping the lid as cold as possible. The hydrosol is usually done 10 to 15 minutes after the water has begun simmering. To check, gently lift the lid ½ inch or so and smell. If the steam smells very minty and aromatic, let it go for a few minutes longer; if it smells more mild, as if the volatile oils in the steam are no longer as rich, it is likely done or almost done. You must turn off the heat before all the water evaporates from the bottom of the pot.

4. If you intend to use the hydrosol for internal consumption, store it in a glass jar with a tight-fitting lid in the refrigerator and use within 1 week. For use as a room spray or for the skin, hydrosols can be stored in a spritzer bottle (also called an atomizer) at room temperature for up to 1 month or in the refrigerator for up to 3 months.

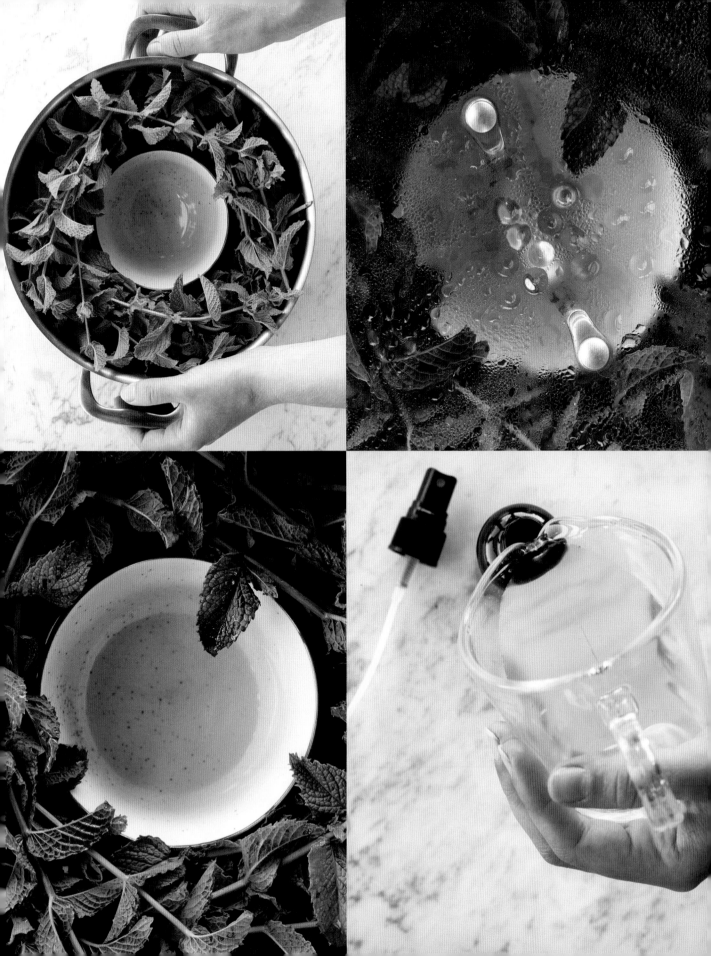

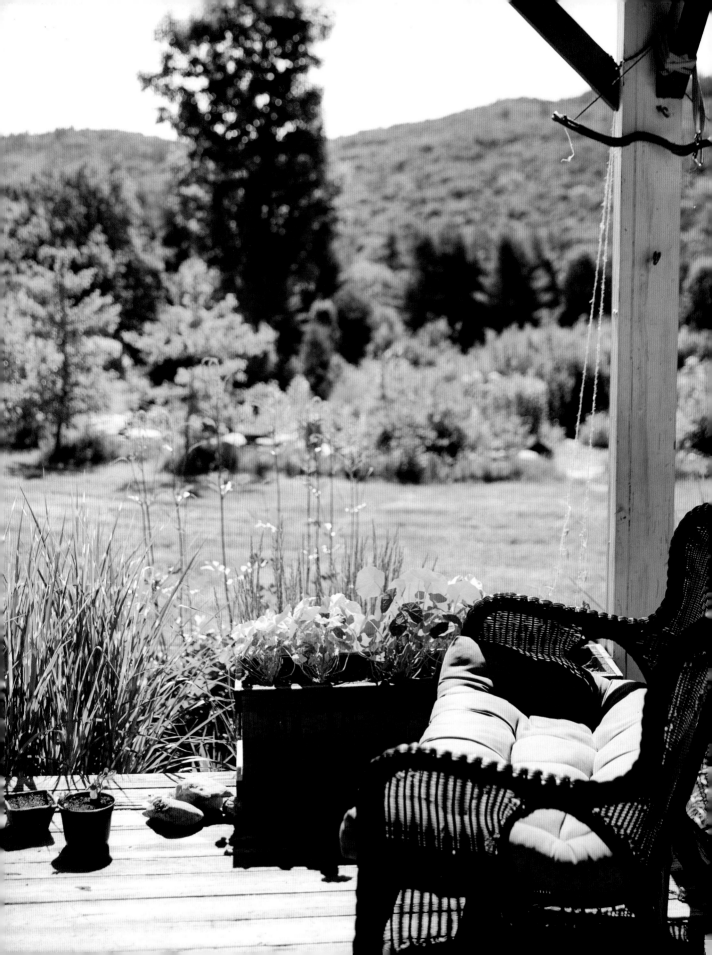

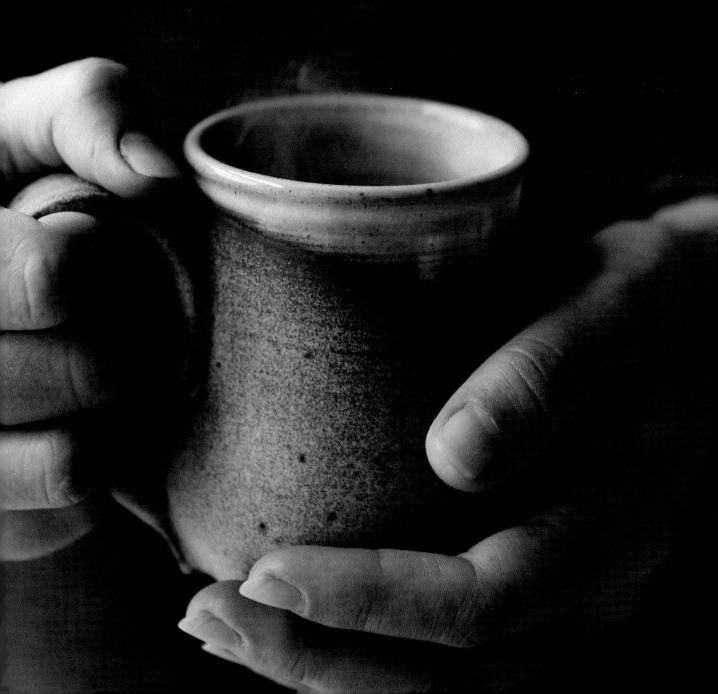

CHAPTER 4
comfort
Demystifying the Body's Cravings

Comfort foods are those foods that help us feel secure, relaxed, content, and cozy. Depending on our tastes, we may crave sweet or salty, crunchy or creamy, or something different entirely. Oftentimes our comfort associations with foods are rooted in feelings of nostalgia: they remind us of something we had during our childhood, perhaps, or of some particular time and place in which we felt happy or loved. We might seek comfort in a food that actually has a comforting story behind it; Sunday dinner was always roast chicken, for example. Or maybe just because it is familiar — habit alone is comforting, so just the familiarity of a food is enough to make it comforting.

We usually crave comfort foods in times of difficulty, whether minor or major — at the end of a long day, or when we're cold or wet, or during a hard emotional time. What is it about comfort foods that make them so satisfying and so . . . comforting? Why do we crave them? Why do we crave anything? I think it is important to unpack the concept of cravings so that we can learn to understand what our body is asking for and perhaps fulfill a deeper craving at its core.

Idiosyncrasies aside, for most people comfort foods fall into the sweet or salty flavor families. As we discussed in chapter 2, sweet foods make up most of humankind's traditional staple foods, including grains, nuts, root vegetables, meats, milk, butter, and cheese. These foods are rich in nutrients and calories. They are heavy, making us feel full, satisfied, and grounded. The salty flavor is also heavy and grounding, and salty foods — unrefined salt itself or salty-tasting vegetables — contain minerals that provide valuable nutrition.

Feelings of anxiety, restlessness, anger, frustration, and confusion are all light emotions. In hard times or moments of insecurity, when we are confronted with these feelings, it is natural to gravitate toward heavier foods to help ground the body and the emotions. Heavy, grounding foods that make us feel full and satisfied are absolutely comforting. Being well fed fulfills a basic survival need, which puts the body at ease and allows it to relax, relieving the uncomfortable feelings that may have caused the craving in the first place.

Cravings for comfort foods are completely natural. After all, these foods help us to nourish ourselves, self-soothe, and put the body at ease. However, issues can arise if cravings for comfort lead us to foods that actually deplete us rather than nourish us. Highly processed "snack foods" that are full of sugar or salt, sugary drinks like soda and juice, sweets like cookies and candy, and refined carbohydrates like crackers and chips fill the body up without providing any real nutrition. Your taste buds might feel like the comfort craving has been fulfilled, but the body has not. In fact, since these foods provide quick energy with nothing for the body to store for later, the body is left feeling even more insecure since it didn't get any real nutritional building blocks, leading to further cravings for quick-energy foods.

One way to look at cravings is to see them as a sign that the body is seeking good-quality nutrition that will provide enough fuel for the moment and sufficient nutrients for the body to store some energy for later. When addressing cravings, rather than focus on eating less of the foods you crave, focus instead on eating the kinds of foods that will give the body what it needs to feel satisfied, so that your cravings are truly satisfied. Look to foods that provide excellent-quality nutrition. Make sure your meals and snacks alike contain all the nutrient groups — fat, protein, and carbohydrates, with vitamins and minerals. Aiming to have all the flavors at each meal will also help create balance. Serving comforting dishes like Shepherd's Pie (page 259) or Crispy Sage and Roasted Garlic Risotto (page 144) with a salad of bitter greens or a side of a sour lacto-fermented vegetable, for example, will leave us feeling more satisfied and help reduce cravings overall.

In the same way that good-quality, nutrient-dense food is comforting because it provides good nutrition, eating regular meals on a schedule is comforting. It puts the body at ease because the body can feel secure knowing that it will be well fed. If you eat irregularly and the body does not know when it can expect food, it will experience a constant level of stress and insecurity. Eating regular and balanced meals is one of the best things you can do to comfort the body, support overall balanced health, and help manage stress and anxiety. It's also important to eat mindfully. Many of us overeat when we eat for comfort, because being full contributes to that heavy, grounded feeling we seek. Try to eat slowly, reminding yourself that you can be safe, secure, and satisfied without being uncomfortably full and that you can eat these delicious comfort foods again tomorrow.

Many cravings are rooted in a desire to more deeply connect with our human

Cravings for comfort foods are completely natural. After all, these foods help us to nourish ourselves, self-soothe, and put the body at ease.

instincts. Human beings have evolved to gather, grow, store, cook, and eat food together. We have evolved alongside that process; the process comforts us, grounds us, provides feelings of safety, accomplishment, fulfillment . . . it feeds us in the ways we cannot measure. In today's world, however, physical nourishment has been separated from emotional nourishment. Many of us eat on the go or at our desk. As a society we consume vast quantities of packaged or preprepared dishes; we seldom cook together. Many of us rarely sit down together to share a meal.

In the modern trap, not only does our diet lack nutrients on a chemical level, but we have become separated from the sense of love and care that can come from food. When we desire to be comforted by food, we are also craving the comfort of a kitchen full of good smells, a meal prepared with care and attention, and a shared table giving rise to laughter and love. We all crave that feeling of nourishment that comes when we prepare a meal for others or when someone prepares a meal for us — it's true comfort for the soul.

ROASTED ONIONS WITH SAGE BUTTER

The smell of onions cooking is enticing. Promising a warm, home-cooked meal, it calls us to the kitchen. Onions make up the sauté base of many popular dishes — those of us who cook know how many times we begin the process by peeling and chopping an onion! Beyond their comforting aroma, onions are a superfood, rich in flavonoids, including quercetin, sulfur compounds, and other phytonutrients. Onions have clearly made their way into so much of our cooking for reasons of nutrition as well as flavor. Perhaps the comfort of the smell is part familiarity and part magnetic attraction to their magical healing properties. Given all they have to offer, sometimes they deserve to be featured all on their own.

This recipe calls for retaining most of the onion skins. The skins keep the onions moist and juicy while they're cooking and help them hold their shape. The outer layers have also been show to contain the most nutritional value. I like to use some red and some yellow onions if I have both — the colors of this dish are beautiful that way.

◆ YIELD: 4 SERVINGS AS A SIDE DISH ◆

6 small to medium onions

8 tablespoons (1 stick) unsalted butter, softened

2–3 tablespoons finely chopped fresh sage

1 teaspoon finely grated lemon zest

¼ teaspoon freshly ground black pepper

¼ teaspoon salt

1. Preheat the oven to 375°F (190°C).

2. Peel off the loose outer layer of each onion's skin, leaving the majority. Slice the onions in half lengthwise and place them faceup on a baking sheet or in a roasting pan. Roast uncovered for 30 minutes, then cover and roast for another 30 minutes.

3. While the onions are cooking, combine the butter with the sage, lemon zest, pepper, and salt, and mix until well combined.

4. When done, the onions will be soft and cooked through, but still juicy. I like them to be just slightly browned on top. If they are not browned, you can finish them off under the broiler for 2 to 3 minutes. Remove from the oven and put 1 to 2 teaspoons of the compound butter on each onion. It will melt into the layers and disappear. Serve the remaining butter at the table. (Any leftover butter will keep in the refrigerator for 5 to 7 days.) Serve the onions in their skins. While it is easy to separate the skins and set them aside, they also tend to soften as they cook, so I eat them skin and all.

ONION MEDICINE

Onions are excellent for cellular health on many levels. They support healthy cell growth, prevent the growth of abnormal cells, and reduce inflammation. Like garlic, onions are members of the allium family and share many of the same benefits to the cardiovascular system: they help reduce cholesterol, increase the elasticity of the blood vessels, and may have anticlotting benefits.

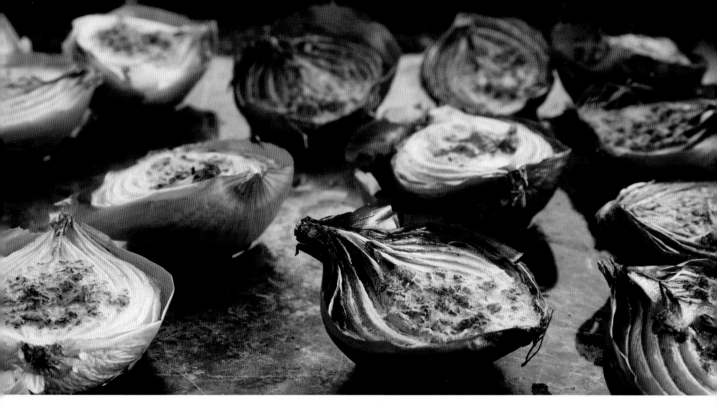

KITCHEN AROMATHERAPY

Aromatherapy is the ancient practice of using fragrance to affect the physical, emotional, and spiritual body. Smells can relax and ease tension, invigorate and inspire, encourage circulation, ease pain, and remind us of another time and place. Smelling fresh aromatic herbs is the most basic form of aromatherapy; simply walking by an aromatic plant or plucking a leaf and sniffing it affects the nervous system. So does inhaling the aromatic steam as you sip a cup of hot tea, or burning aromatic herbs to release their oils, two traditions long used in ritual and ceremony to shift consciousness and promote connection with the divine.

Cooking may just be the most common and humble form of aromatherapy practiced the world over. In fact, scent is the very basis of much of cooking: we sauté aromatic plants (onions, garlic, celery, herbs, and spices) in fat until the aroma is released, then add other ingredients and cook. When we cook at home and our house fills with the fragrance of sautéing onions and garlic, stewing vegetables, roasting meat, and aromatic herbs, it physically prepares the body for food by stimulating the secretion of digestive enzymes and acids. This *cephalic phase* of digestion, where the smell, sight, thought, and taste of food stimulate digestive function, can be responsible for up to 20 percent of the digestive secretions associated with eating. In our minds and in our hearts, a space full of good aromas helps us feel comfortable and at home, soothed and nourished.

Each time we cook, we are practicing the art of kitchen aromatherapy. This simple practice has the ability to shift our consciousness, transforming a bad mood, a misunderstanding, or a sore subject, and to connect us to our physical body, to our emotional selves, and to one another. Cooking is simple, but the results are far from it.

CHEDDAR AND DILL CRACKERS

One of the things I learned through talking with friends while writing this chapter is that people's favorite comfort foods are often reminiscent of their childhood. Answers to questions like "What are your favorite comfort foods?" will often sound something like "Oooh, I love pot roast — the way we used to have it growing up." As with so many things, the comfort is in the familiarity. And that concept extends to commercial "snack foods" that come from a bag or a box. When we crave comfort, we may feel the same longing for a particular brand of chips, cookies, or candy that we feel for the homemade pot roast from our childhood. One of the things that inspires me is the possibility of creating homemade versions of these processed, low-nutrition foods, fulfilling our cravings, and getting the same comfort out of cooking for ourselves that we got from enjoying food with our family as children. These crackers are an attempt to quench the craving for a crunchy, cheesy morsel — the kind that could come from a box, but is so much better when homemade.

◆ YIELD: 24 CRACKERS ◆

½ cup white wheat or spelt flour

½ cup rye flour

2 cups grated extra sharp or sharp cheddar cheese

3 tablespoons cold butter

2 tablespoons finely chopped dill, fresh or dried, or 1 teaspoon ground dill seeds

Freshly ground black pepper

2½–3 tablespoons milk or water

Sea salt or flaked salt

1. Preheat the oven to 375°F (190°C). Grease a baking sheet.

2. Combine the flours, cheese, butter, dill, and pepper in a food processor and pulse until combined. Then add the milk and pulse until all the flour is incorporated. The mixture may not be a uniform dough, but it should be moist enough to stick together.

3. Roll out the dough on a floured work surface to ⅛ to ¼ inch thickness. Prick the dough all over with a fork and garnish with salt or salt flakes.

4. Cut the dough into 2-inch squares with a knife, pastry cutter, or pizza cutter. (For a bite-size snack cracker, you might want them smaller than 2 by 2 inches; to serve with dips or snacks, you might like them a little bigger. You can also use cookie cutters to make fun-shaped crackers.)

5. Transfer to the prepared baking sheet. Bake for 10 to 15 minutes, or until golden and cooked through. The bottoms are usually a little crunchy, which I like. If you don't want a crunchy bottom, take them out earlier. The cooking time will depend on how thin or thick you rolled the dough.

6. Let cool on the baking sheet. Once cool, store in an airtight container; they will keep fresh for 2 to 3 days.

COOKING WITH PURPOSE

The lengthy list of ingredients on most boxed foods includes lots of artificial flavors and/or preservatives. Artificial flavors stand in for the flavor that you don't find in poor-quality, overly processed foods. They're unnecessary when you cook for yourself with good-quality ingredients because good-quality food naturally tastes good. Preservatives support a larger American lifestyle choice — they allow us to be on the go, to have food preprepared and on the shelf without spending time in the kitchen or the garden. They justify a lifestyle with less intention, where we pay less attention to ourselves, each other, land and agriculture, and our health. The choice to cook for yourself at all, and especially to make your own snacks, saves you from these unhealthy ingredients, but it also provides a nice sense of purpose. It is rewarding to the taste buds and gives you satisfaction to know that you are caring for yourself.

NAAN with GHEE, GARLIC, and CILANTRO

Making your own bread is a process of hands, heart, and patience: mixing up the dough, kneading it, setting it to rise, shaping it, baking it. In the traditional manner, naan would be baked in a *tandoor*, a hot clay oven. I use a cast-iron skillet and my broiler, and though my setup is not as authentic, the naan come out beautifully.

The yogurt for this recipe should be thick yet pourable. If your yogurt is too thick, thin it with the whey (the liquid on top) or a bit of water. For the flour, you can substitute up to 1 cup whole-grain flour, but more than that will make the dough too heavy.

◆ YIELD: 8 FLATBREADS ◆

3¾ cups flour

1 teaspoon baking soda

½ teaspoon salt

1¾ cups plain yogurt, at room temperature

FOR THE TOPPING

½ cup finely chopped cilantro

4 garlic cloves, finely chopped

2 tablespoons ghee (page 93), at room temperature

1. Combine the flour, baking soda, and salt in a mixing bowl and whisk until well combined. Add the yogurt and mix until a dough begins to form. Turn the dough out onto a floured work surface and knead gently for 2 to 3 minutes. Return to the bowl, cover with a towel, and leave to rise at room temperature for 1 to 2 hours.

2. Divide the dough into eight pieces. Roll each piece into a circle about ⅛ inch thick.

3. Prepare the topping: Combine the cilantro, garlic, and ghee in a bowl and mix into a paste.

4. Preheat the broiler. Warm a cast-iron skillet over medium heat. When it's hot enough that a drop of water bounces when flicked on the pan, lay one of the dough disks in the skillet. Don't move it for the next 30 to 60 seconds. When the naan has puffed up in parts and the bottom has begun to brown (1 to 3 minutes), transfer the skillet to the oven and broil until the top is golden brown.

5. Remove the skillet from the oven. Flip the naan onto a plate and rub the top with a portion of the herbed ghee. Set the skillet back on the stovetop and cook the next flatbread. If you have two skillets, that will speed up the process.

SERVING SUGGESTION: You can serve the naan hot right from the oven, but this can be challenging if you want to eat at the same time as everyone else. I usually allow it to cool and then warm all the naan in the oven, wrapped in aluminum foil or in a covered dish. If you heat the flatbreads uncovered, they will dry out. Naan is delicious on its own and makes an excellent accompaniment to stews, thick curries, and Roasted Red Lentil Dhal (page 80). It can also be served with Baked Ricotta (page 143), White Bean Spread with Rosemary and Mellowed Garlic (page 272), or other dips and appetizers.

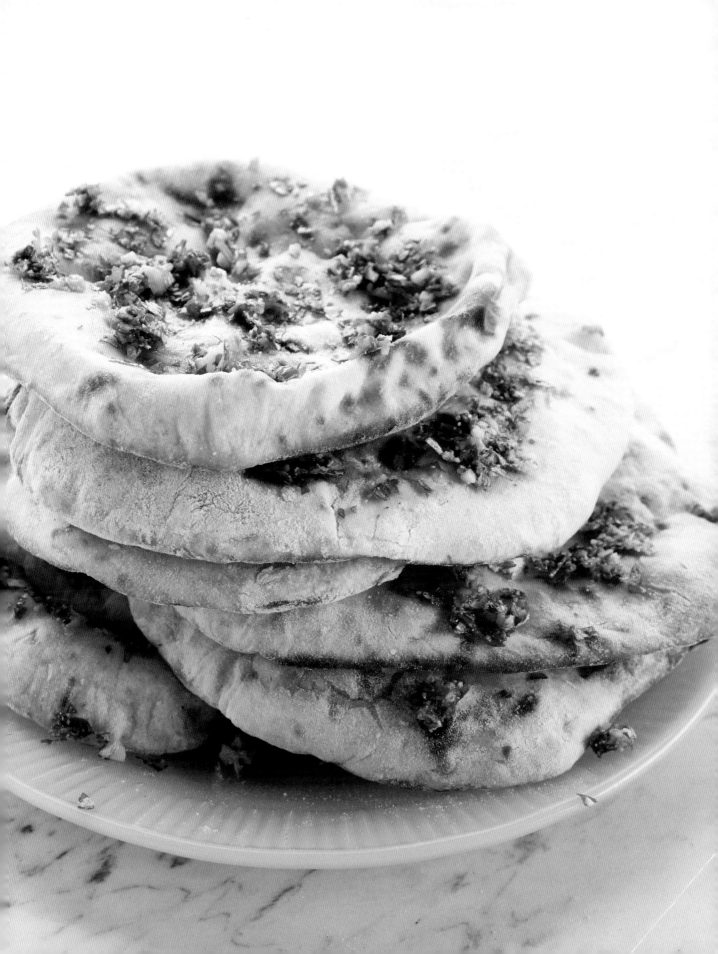

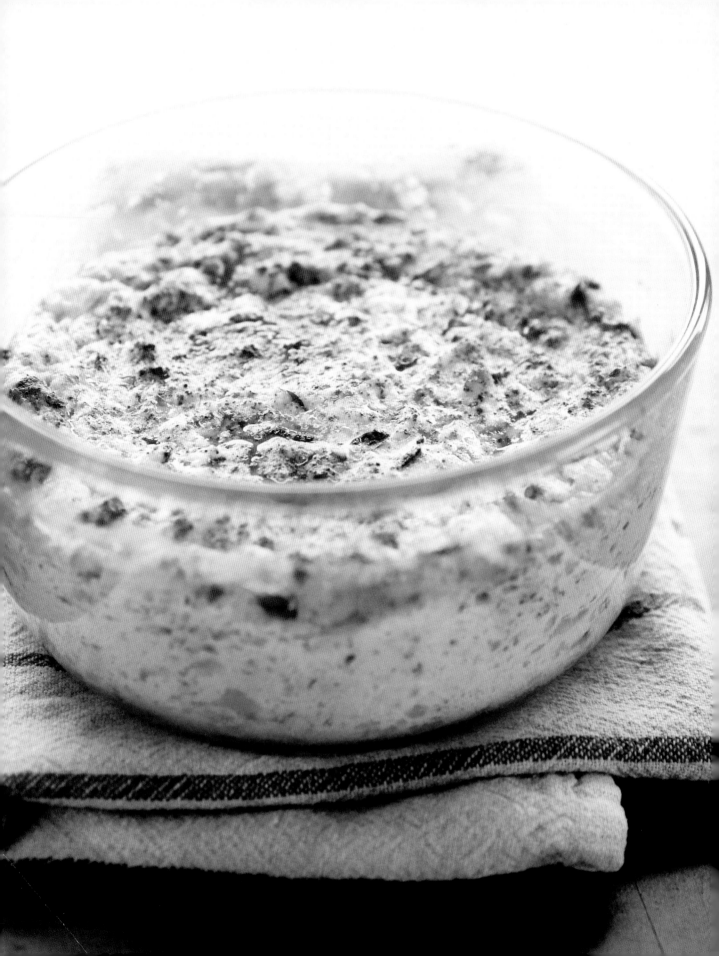

BAKED RICOTTA

I tend to be an improvisional cook, viewing recipes as a source of inspiration and using whatever I have on hand in the refrigerator or garden. Creamy, comforting, and full of flavor, this is one of those basic recipes that lends itself well to many combinations of herbs and flavors. Fresh herbs really shine here, so prioritize using them if you have them. Serve with toasted bread or crackers.

◆ YIELD: 4-6 SERVINGS AS AN APPETIZER ◆

Olive oil

1 pound (about 2 cups) whole-milk ricotta cheese

1 tablespoon chopped fresh oregano or 1 teaspoon dried

1 tablespoon fresh thyme or 1½ teaspoons dried

2 teaspoons chopped fresh rosemary or 1 teaspoon dried

1–2 tablespoons chopped garlic (2–4 cloves)

Zest of 1 lemon, finely grated

¼ cup thinly sliced sun-dried tomatoes (optional)

Salt and freshly ground black pepper

1 egg, lightly beaten

Ground paprika, for garnish

1. Preheat the oven to 375°F (190°C). Use a drizzle of oil to grease a 2-cup baking dish.

2. Combine the ricotta with the oregano, thyme, rosemary, garlic, lemon zest, sun-dried tomatoes (if using), and a few grinds of pepper. Mix well and season generously with salt (I usually start with ¼ teaspoon). Add the egg and mix thoroughly.

3. Transfer the mixture to the prepared baking dish. Sprinkle the top with paprika and a drizzle of oil. Bake for 20 to 30 minutes, or until the top puffs up slightly and the mixture is hot and bubbling. Let cool for 10 minutes before serving.

NOTE: The ricotta has to be well drained; if it is too liquidy, the finished product will be soupy. Most ricotta comes strained, but if the ricotta you have has any liquid on top, pour it off rather than mixing it in.

COOKING FROM SCRATCH

Ricotta is one of the easiest cheeses to make. Unlike hard cheeses that have to age, ricotta is a fresh cheese that can be eaten almost immediately after preparing. Making your own cheese — or bread, crackers, jam, pickles, sauerkraut, or any other pantry staple — puts new meaning into the popular term "cooking from scratch." In fact, I think one of the many reasons we are seeing a resurgence of people wanting to learn to grow and cook their own food is because there is comfort in it, a sense of calm and personal satisfaction that derives from learning to do things for ourselves. It leaves us feeling empowered and self-aware: aware of what goes into making and eating and of what it takes to support our life.

CRISPY SAGE AND ROASTED GARLIC RISOTTO

I remember the time during college when my friend Beth came home from a trip to the ocean to make risotto. It had been a windy, chilly day, wild feeling and alive. Risotto, she said, was just what she was craving to warm herself up and "get cozy." I can still picture her in the kitchen, telling me how she liked to make it. It was an introduction to her world of comfort food, a glimpse into what made her feel comfy and at home at the end of an adventurous day.

Risotto can be simple, mostly rice with stock and herbs, or it can be loaded with greens and vegetables, meats, and more. You can use this recipe as a base, adding other ingredients as you are inspired.

+ YIELD: 4 SERVINGS +

2	heads garlic, cloves separated, peeled, and sliced ⅛ inch thick
¼	cup plus 1 tablespoon olive oil
1	cup whole sage leaves
5–6	cups Bone Broth (page 203) or some other type of broth or stock
	Salt
1	cup finely chopped shallots or onions
2	cups Arborio rice
	Freshly ground black pepper
1	cup dry white wine (I usually use sauvignon blanc)
¼	cup heavy cream
½	cup freshly grated Parmesan cheese

I. Combine the sliced garlic and ¼ cup of the oil in a small skillet over low heat. Cook, stirring often, being careful not to let the garlic burn or even brown much, until the garlic is softened and aromatic, 10 to 15 minutes. Set both the softened garlic and the oil aside.

2. Crisp the sage leaves: Heat the remaining 1 tablespoon oil in a small pan over medium heat (you may need more oil if you use a larger pan). Once the oil is hot, add the sage, keeping the leaves separated as best you can to increase their contact with the pan. Keep them moving to prevent them from burning, flipping them as needed. They are done when they are crispy but still bright green, 1 to 2 minutes. Watch carefully, because the transition from bright green to brown happens very fast. If some leaves turn brown, however, they can still be used. When the sage leaves are crisped, remove them from the pan immediately and set aside. Set aside any remaining oil in the pan as well.

3. Bring the broth to a gentle simmer in a covered saucepan on a side burner. Season to taste with salt.

4. Transfer the garlic, and its oil, along with any remaining oil from cooking the sage leaves, to a large saucepan and heat over medium heat. Once the oil is hot, add the shallots and sauté until translucent, 3 to 5 minutes. Add the rice, season with a pinch of salt and a grinding of pepper, and cook, stirring almost continuously, until the rice is translucent, 2 to 3 minutes. Add the wine to deglaze the pan, scraping up any bits that may have stuck to the bottom of the pan. Continue to stir until the rice has absorbed the wine, 2 to 3 minutes. Reduce the

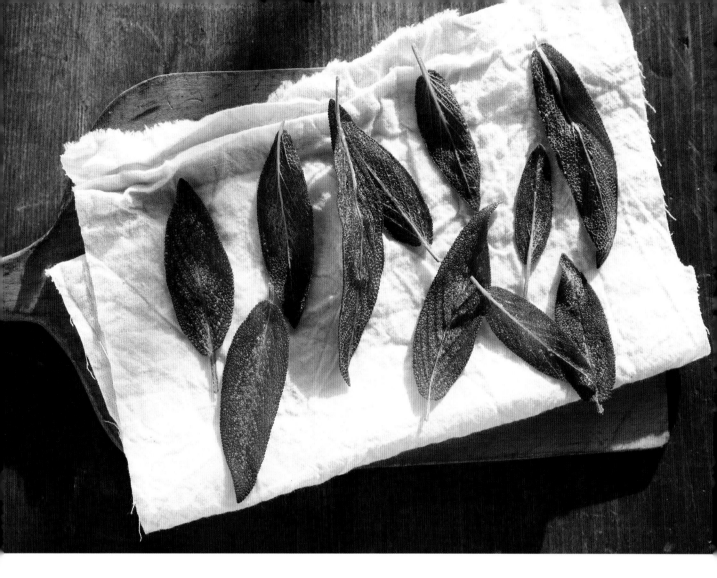

heat and begin to add the hot broth 1 cup at a time, stirring almost continuously until the rice has absorbed the broth before adding more. If the rice is sticking to the pan, stir it more, reduce the heat, or both. When done, the risotto should be al dente and creamy, but not runny. In total, this can take 20 to 25 minutes.

5. When the risotto is done, stir in the cream, Parmesan, and crispy sage leaves. Season to taste with salt. If you want, use some of the crispy sage leaves as garnish.

LEFTOVERS

Leftover risotto can be reheated with a little stock, milk, or water. Or you can add an egg to the leftovers, form into patties, and sauté in olive oil or butter to make risotto cakes.

BRAISED CHICKEN with SHALLOTS and FIGS

In some styles of cooking, you chop things as tiny as possible so that their flavors blend together harmoniously but are not detectable individually in the finished dish. On the other end of the spectrum are stews, braises, and roasts, where vegetables are left whole or just roughly chopped. Food prepared in this rustic style draws more attention to the hands that prepared it and to the food itself as we break it apart to eat. I find these processes of chopping, cooking, and eating comforting through and through. Preparing this dish warms my heart as deeply as it nourishes. I savor the beauty and deliciousness of each ingredient as I chop, sauté, and arrange, and the steamy, sweet aromas that fill the house as the dish cooks.

◆ YIELD: 6 SERVINGS ◆

2½ pounds bone-in chicken pieces (breasts, thighs, or legs), with the skin

Salt and freshly ground black pepper

2–3 tablespoons olive oil

4 large red or white shallots, peeled and quartered

1 head garlic, cloves separated, peeled, and crushed (halve them if they are large)

½ cup fresh or dried figs, quartered

6 sprigs fresh thyme or 2 teaspoons dried

2 sprigs fresh sage or 1 teaspoon dried

1 sprig fresh rosemary or ½ teaspoon dried

1 bay leaf

1½ cups dry white wine

2 tablespoons Dijon mustard

I. Generously season the chicken with salt and pepper on all sides. Heat 2 tablespoons of the oil in a large skillet over medium heat. When hot, reduce the heat to medium-low, place the chicken in the pan skin side down, and sear until brown, 5 to 7 minutes. Do not move the chicken pieces once you have dropped them in the pan; this disrupts the sear. Flip and repeat on the opposite side, then remove the chicken from the pan and set aside.

2. If the pan is dry, add another tablespoon of oil. Add the shallots, garlic, figs, thyme, sage, rosemary, and bay. Sauté until aromatic and golden brown, about 5 minutes. Season with salt. Reduce the heat as needed to maintain a gentle sauté; the pan should not be so hot that ingredients are burning or sticking to the pan.

3. Pour the wine into a small bowl and whisk the Dijon mustard into it. Return the chicken to the pan, arranging the pieces among the garlic, shallots, and figs. Add the wine mixture. Bring to a gentle simmer, then cover and let simmer until the chicken is cooked through, 15 to 25 minutes, depending on the size of the chicken pieces. The chicken is cooked through when the meat closest to the bone is opaque and the juices run clear, or the internal temperature of the meat nearest the bone reads 165°F (75°C) on a meat thermometer.

4. Remove any herb sprigs and the bay leaf. Season the broth with salt, if necessary. Serve immediately.

SERVING SUGGESTION: This dish is lovely served over rice, polenta, greens, or anything else that will soak up the flavors of the broth. If you have more fresh herbs, consider using them to garnish the dish.

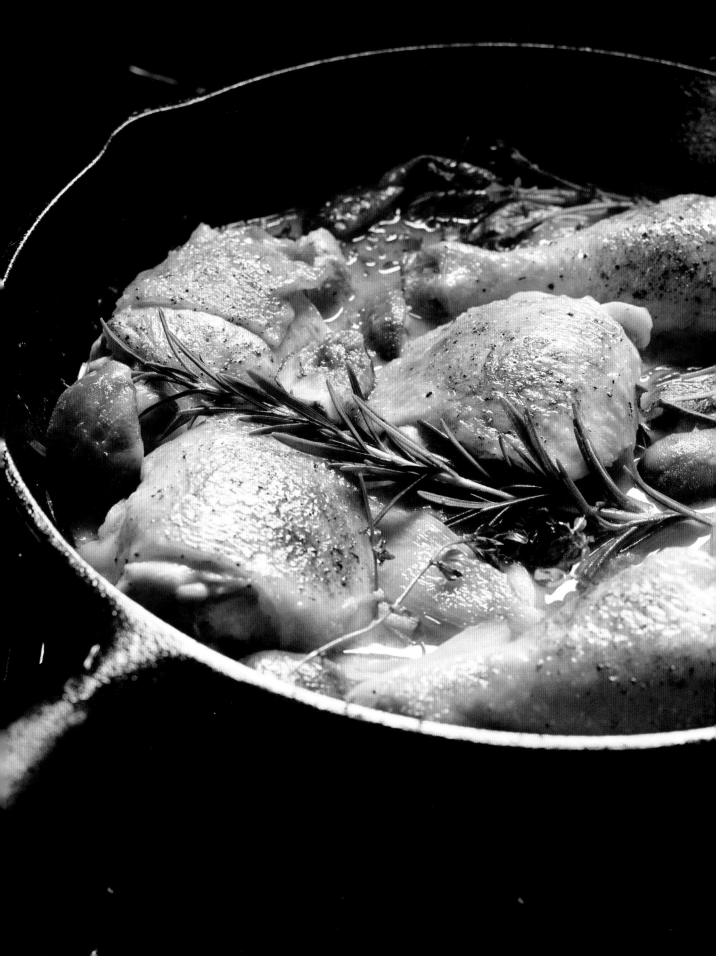

GARLIC-STUFFED ROAST PORK

This is how pork roasts were always cooked when I was growing up: the garlic cloves were stuffed into the meat and found on your plate later, full of flavor, sometimes even still a little crunchy. The garlic flavor infuses into the meat and the meat flavor into the garlic — both flavors comforting and satisfying.

Roasts are easy to prepare and a great way to feed a lot of people. Their very presence on the table exudes a feeling of bounty — a situation itself worth celebrating, even if there is no occasion other than gathering together for a meal.

This recipe assumes that you have a spice grinder. If you don't have one, use preground coriander, and grind any other dried herbs in a mortar and pestle or blender, or chop them.

◆ YIELD: 6-8 SERVINGS ◆

6   large or 8 small garlic cloves

1   (4- to 5-pound) bone-in pork butt or shoulder roast

1   teaspoon fresh or dried sage

2   teaspoons fresh or 1 teaspoons dried thyme

½   teaspoon fresh or dried lavender flowers

1   teaspoon coriander seeds

    Salt and freshly ground black pepper

    Olive oil

I. Preheat the oven to 325°F (170°C).

2. Peel the garlic cloves and slice bigger ones in half or even thirds lengthwise. Using the sharp tip of a paring knife, cut a slit into the meat about ¾ inch deep. Wedge a piece of the garlic into the slit. Repeat until you've stuffed all the garlic pieces into the meat, spreading them out somewhat evenly over the top and sides of the roast.

3. If you're using dried sage, thyme, or lavender, combine them with the coriander in a spice grinder and process until finely ground. If you're using fresh herbs, finely chop them. Combine all the herbs to make a dry rub.

4. Generously coat all sides of the pork with salt and pepper, then rub the herb mixture into all sides of the meat. If needed, add a bit of oil to help the herbs stick to the roast.

5. Place the roast on a wire rack set in a roasting pan. Bake until the internal temperature reaches 150 to 155°F (65 to 70°C). This is usually 20 to 25 minutes per pound for bone-in meat.

6. Remove the roast from the oven and let rest for 20 minutes. (The roast will gain a few degrees of temperature while it rests.) Then slice as desired. Pour the drippings over the meat before serving.

NOTE: You could also use a boneless roast, but keep in mind that it will likely take less time to cook.

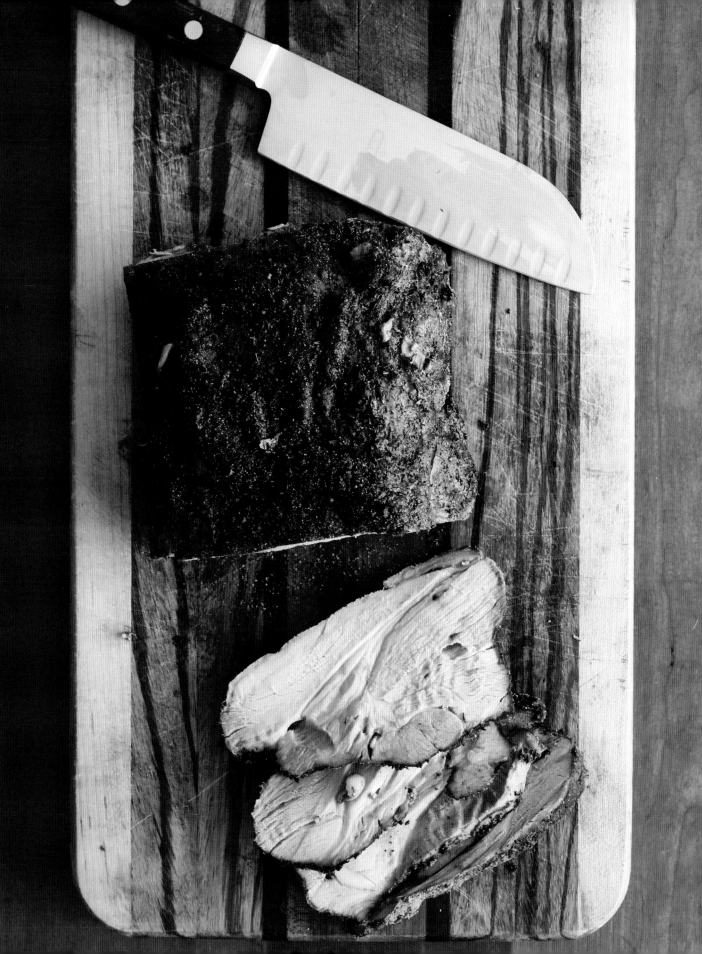

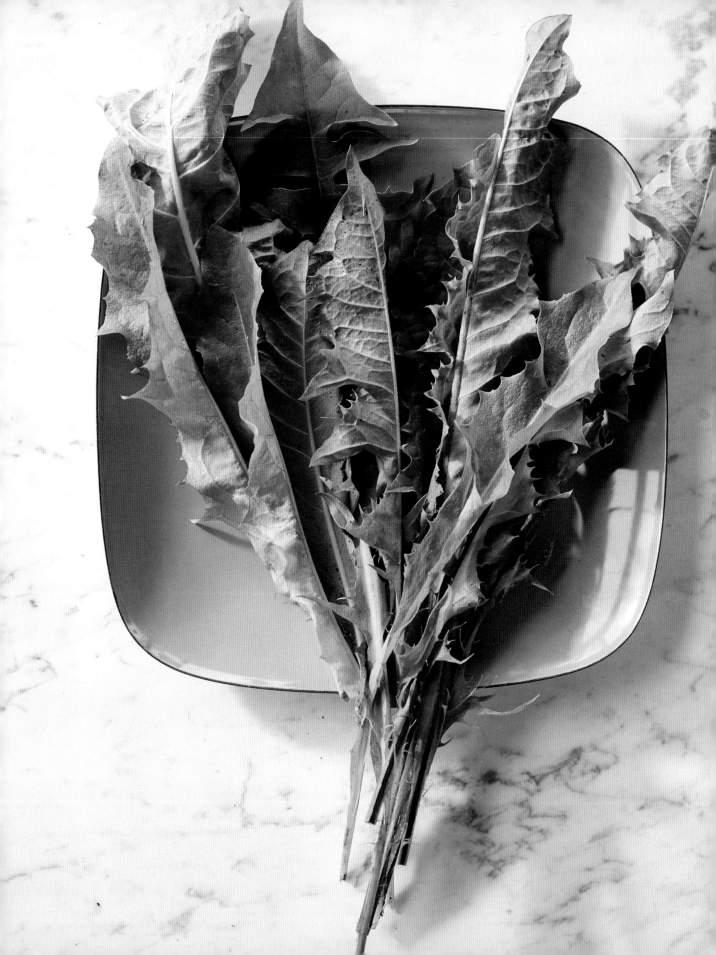

CANNELLINI BEANS AND POTATOES WITH DANDELION GREENS AND PARSLEY

Both bitter and salty, dandelion greens and parsley are high in a variety of minerals that nourish the blood, bones, and kidneys, including iron, calcium, and magnesium. Their bitter flavor cleanses and detoxifies the body while also enhancing the digestibility of the sweet, dense potatoes and white beans, making this a nourishing, comforting dish for almost any season of the year.

Other greens can be substituted for the dandelion. I was originally inspired to make a dish similar to this by a student whose husband specializes in Mediterranean nutrition. In the Mediterranean region, people call all greens *horta* (meaning weeds or wild mountain greens), and they freely substitute different wild greens in dishes depending on what is available.

✦ YIELD: 4 SERVINGS ✦

½ cup dried cannellini beans (to make about 1½ cups cooked)

1 pound young potatoes, red or white, cut into 1-inch cubes with the skins

2 cups chopped dandelion greens, in 1- to 2-inch pieces

2 cups chopped fresh flat-leaf parsley

3 garlic cloves, sliced

½ cup olive oil

½ cup water

½ teaspoon paprika, plus more for garnish

½ teaspoon salt

½ teaspoon fresh ground black pepper

Juice of ½ lemon (about 1 tablespoon)

Edible flowers (such as calendula, comfrey, rose, violet, chive blossom, and/or lilac), for garnish (optional)

1. Soak the beans overnight in enough water to cover by 8 inches.

2. Strain the beans and combine them in a saucepan with enough water to cover by 2 to 3 inches. Bring to a boil, skim off any foam, reduce the heat, and cover; simmer over low heat, stirring often, until the beans are tender, 45 to 75 minutes. Set aside to cool in the cooking water.

3. Combine the potatoes, dandelion greens, parsley, garlic, oil, water, paprika, salt, and pepper in a large saucepan. Bring to a boil, then reduce the heat and let simmer, covered, stirring often, for 30 minutes.

4. Strain the beans from their cooking water and add to the pan, along with the lemon juice. Simmer, uncovered, stirring almost continually, for 5 minutes. Serve hot, garnished with paprika and edible wildflowers, if desired.

FOOD SYNERGY

In the Mediterranean and other parts of the world, greens are often prepared with lemon juice. Not coincidentally, the high vitamin C content of the citrus improves the body's absorption of the iron found in the greens.

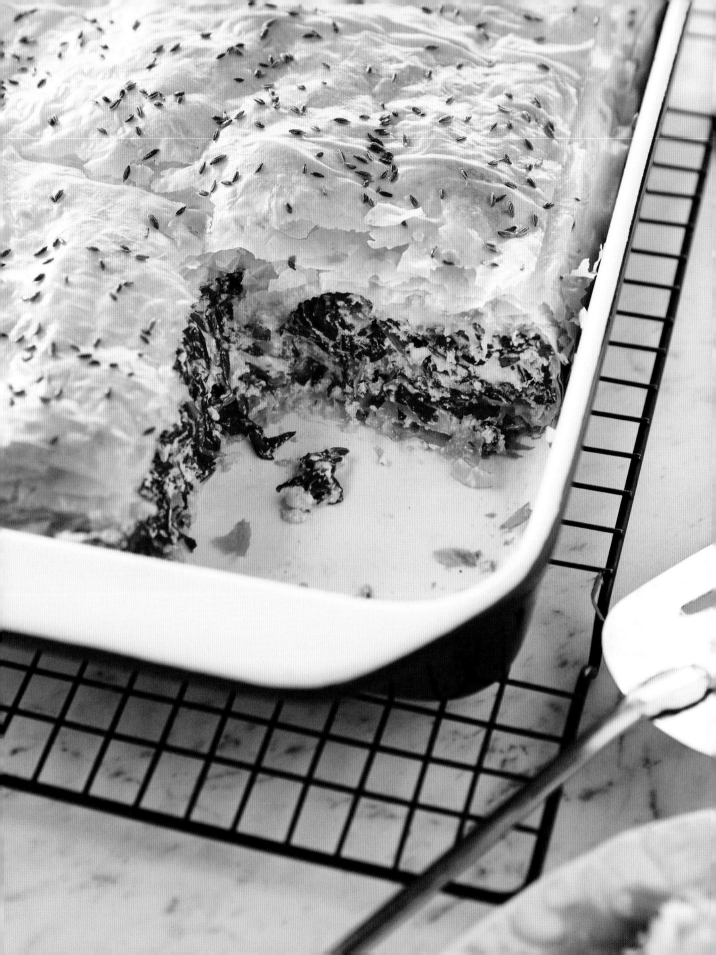

SPANAKOPITA WITH FRESH HERBS AND WILD GREENS

When I was growing up, whenever someone had a baby or was sick, a community of family and friends would organize a schedule and bring meals to those who needed to be nourished. I remember when both my brothers were born, and later when my mom had cancer, being fed by this village. The food was a big help, but so was the joy, warmth, and support brought by these visitors. It was comforting to see familiar faces, to dote over new life, to watch people care for one another, and to be reminded of all the love we shared with our family and friends. On one such occasion, a friend brought spanakopita, delicious, mouthwatering bites of cooked greens and cheese wedged between crunchy sheets of dough. Later, when I got into herbs and wild foraging, spanakopita became one of the many traditional dishes that tempted me to eat my weeds.

◆ YIELD: 8 SERVINGS ◆

2   tablespoons olive oil

2   cups chopped onion, leeks, scallions, or a combination

2   pounds greens, chopped into bite-size pieces

Salt

4   eggs, beaten

2   cups cottage cheese or ricotta cheese

1½ cups crumbled feta cheese (about ½ pound)

1   head garlic, cloves peeled and chopped

½   cup chopped fresh basil

½   cup chopped fresh parsley

2   tablespoons chopped fresh oregano

Freshly ground black pepper

¾   cup (1½ sticks) butter, melted

1   (1-pound) package frozen phyllo dough, defrosted

Ground paprika, dried chives, dill seeds, fennel seeds, or sesame seeds (optional)

I. Preheat the oven to 375°F (190°C).

2. Warm the oil in a large soup pot over medium heat. Add the onion and sauté until translucent, 3 to 5 minutes. Add the greens in several layers, salting lightly as you go. I use a large soup pot because 2 pounds of greens is a lot, and it usually fills the whole pot. Put the lid on and cook over medium-low heat, stirring every 2 to 3 minutes, until the greens have cooked down to about one-quarter of their original volume. Put the greens in a colander to drain and set aside to cool. I like to set the colander over a pan and collect the drippings; they are flavorful and nutritious and can be used like broth in your cooking.

3. Combine the eggs with the cottage cheese, feta, garlic, basil, parsley, and oregano, and season generously with pepper. Once the greens have drained and cooled, stir them into the mixture.

4. With a pastry brush, grease the inside of a 9- by 13-inch baking dish with some of the melted butter. Lay a sheet of phyllo dough in the dish so that only half of it covers the bottom of the pan, with the extra hanging over one of the long ends of the pan. Brush the half of the sheet that's in the pan with melted butter. Lay another sheet on top, again with only half the sheet covering the bottom of the pan, setting it exactly on top of the first sheet, and brush with

SPANAKOPITA *continued*

butter. Continue this process until you have laid out and buttered 8 sheets, then repeat with another 8 sheets, only with the extra spilling out over the opposite side of the pan.

5. Add the filling, spreading it out evenly to the edges of the pan. Fold the pieces of phyllo dough over the top, alternating between sides, brushing each layer with butter. Layer any remaining phyllo dough on top, folding each piece to fit the pan and brushing with butter between each layer. Continue layering the phyllo dough until you run out of space in the pan, phyllo dough, or butter! Dust the top with paprika, dried chives, and dill, fennel, or sesame seeds, if desired.

6. Bake for 45 minutes, or until the filling is bubbling and the top is golden brown. Cut into pieces and serve hot (although it is also yummy cold).

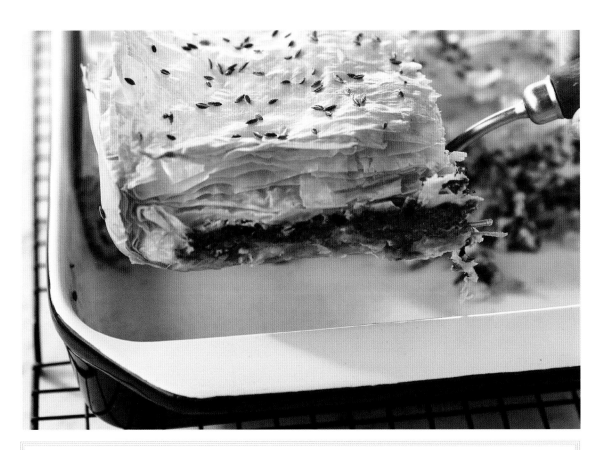

GREEN SUBSTITUTIONS

For this dish I like to combine wild greens like dandelion, nettle, galinsoga, lamb's quarters, and sorrel with cultivated greens like spinach, Swiss chard, kale, and tatsoi, but you can use whatever you have available. If you do not have fresh herbs, you can substitute 1 tablespoon dried basil, 1 tablespoon dried parsley, and 1 teaspoon dried oregano.

SWEET POTATO RICE

I made this for the first time during college when I was living in San Francisco. Since then I have prepared it many times, and it has been much loved by my family and friends. Some have even begun to claim it as their own. I can hear my brother's voice: "Brit, we made sweet potato rice last night — so good!" And then he tells me about his latest rendition. One of his favorites is to sauté jalapeño and garlic with the sweet potato and garnish the dish with cilantro. Sometimes the most comforting foods are those that we lovingly return to time and again, adapting them as we go to fit the season, the meal, and the mood.

◆ YIELD: 4 SERVINGS ◆

4   tablespoons butter or ghee (page 93)

2–2½   cups grated sweet potato, with the skin (1 medium sweet potato)

¼   cup finely chopped fresh rosemary or 1 tablespoon plus 1 teaspoon dried

2   cups white basmati rice

3½   cups water

   Salt and freshly ground black pepper

1. Melt the butter in a saucepan over low heat. Add the sweet potato and rosemary and mix well. Season generously with salt and pepper. Cook, stirring continuously, until the sweet potatoes are completely coated with the butter and begin to deepen in color, 1 to 2 minutes.

2. Add the rice and cook, stirring continuously, for 30 to 60 seconds. Then add the water. Season to taste with salt.

3. Bring to a simmer over medium heat, cover, reduce the heat to low, and simmer until the rice has absorbed all the water and is soft, 20 to 25 minutes.

4. The rosemary and sweet potato have a tendency to end up on top of the rice; just fluff the rice with a fork to mix it all together before serving.

SERVING SUGGESTION: This technique is a great way to jazz up plain rice and make it a little more special. It goes well with beans and legumes, vegetable dishes, meats, and eggs. I particularly enjoy the leftovers reheated for breakfast with over-easy eggs.

CREAMY FETA AND HERB DRESSING

So often when we have a craving for something comforting, we reach for heavy, dense, sweet, and salty foods. Unintentionally, our limited comfort-food palate can mean that we don't consider greens and vegetables at just the point when we may most need their flavor, fiber, and energy-boosting, nutritive power. In fact, there is no reason why vegetables can't be transformed into comfort foods. This rich and creamy dressing has all the satisfaction of a comfort food, and it helps make the vegetables you put it over more digestible. The oils and acids in dressings help break down fibrous plant material, and the fat makes the nutrition in the vegetables more bioavailable. Yes, dressings taste good, but they also make the food more usable — everything has a reason.

◆ YIELD: ABOUT 2 CUPS ◆

1   cup olive oil

3   tablespoons raw apple cider vinegar

2   tablespoons feta brine (or 1 tablespoon water plus a pinch of salt)

1   cup coarsely chopped scallions or ½ cup coarsely chopped yellow onion

½   cup fresh parsley

½   red bell pepper, seeded and roughly chopped

1   ounce feta cheese, crumbled (about ¼ cup)

2   garlic cloves, roughly chopped

Freshly ground black pepper

Combine the oil, vinegar, feta brine, scallions, parsley, bell pepper, feta, and garlic in a food processor and blend until creamy. Season to taste with black pepper. Use on salad or steamed greens or as a dipping sauce for veggies. Store any leftover dressing in the refrigerator, where it will keep for up to 1 week.

CENTERED AND FOCUSED TEA

One of the most important ways that we can comfort ourselves is by soothing the nervous system. Our nervous system becomes agitated and aggravated when we are in pain, when we are cold, hungry, or dehydrated, or when we are emotionally distraught. And, of course, when the nervous system becomes aggravated, all of those symptoms worsen. Many culinary herbs, with their aromatic oils, soothe and open up the nervous system while supporting circulation and mental clarity. This tea is perfect for helping us to stay focused and relaxed during times of relative calm or high stress.

◆ YIELD: 4 SERVINGS ◆

1 tablespoon dried linden leaf and flower (oatstraw or milky oat tops also work well)

2 teaspoons fresh or dried basil

2 teaspoons fresh or dried mint

1 teaspoon fresh or dried rosemary

1 teaspoon fennel seeds

4 cups boiling water

Combine the linden, basil, mint, rosemary, and fennel seeds in a teapot and pour the boiling water over them. Cover and let steep for 5 to 15 minutes, depending on how strong you like your tea. Strain and enjoy. As you sip the tea, let the aroma of it stimulate the senses and relax your body and mind.

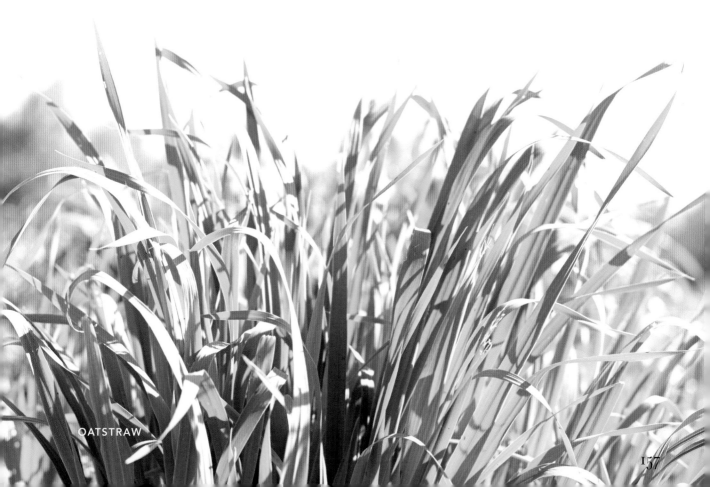

OATSTRAW

LAVENDER AND ROSE TAPIOCA

Many desserts are low in nutrition and high in sugar, which fills us up with empty calories and gives us a sugar rush before leaving us to crash. Good-quality desserts, on the other hand, contain real food, with an emphasis on the sweet flavor. Tapioca, for example, comes from the cassava tuber, a staple food in South America. Cassava is a nutritious, complex food that actually gives the body something to work with. Tapioca is traditionally prepared as a custard with egg and milk; the protein and fat complete our food groups here, providing the body with lasting, sustainable energy — a treat that will leave all parts of you feeling satisfied.

◆ YIELD: 4-6 SERVINGS ◆

1   tablespoon dried rose petals

1   teaspoon dried lavender flowers

⅓ cup quick-cooking tapioca

1   (14-ounce) can coconut milk

1   cup water

1–3 tablespoons maple syrup or honey, to taste (optional)

⅛ teaspoon salt

2   egg yolks

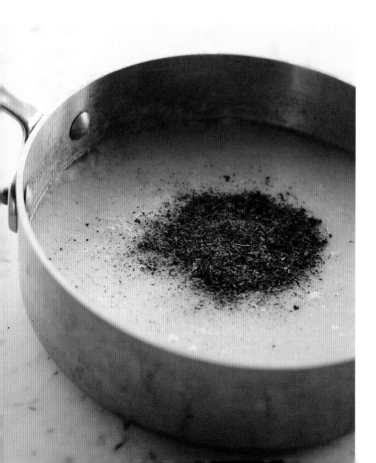

1. Finely grind the rose petals and lavender flowers in a spice grinder or mortar and pestle.

2. In a saucepan, whisk together the tapioca, coconut milk, water, maple syrup, salt, and ground rose petals and lavender flowers. Let sit for 10 minutes; it should begin to thicken.

3. Slowly bring the mixture to a simmer over medium-low heat, whisking often. Then reduce the heat and simmer gently, whisking often, until the tapioca is soft and translucent, about 5 minutes.

4. Whisk the egg yolks together in a separate bowl. Then temper the eggs: Measure out 1 cup of the hot tapioca mixture and add it to the egg yolks, 1 tablespoon at a time, stirring continuously. Then pour the egg yolk mixture into the saucepan, return to a simmer, and cook over low heat, whisking often, for 3 to 5 minutes. At this point, the mixture should be thick enough to coat a metal spoon.

5. Let sit for 15 to 20 minutes before serving. It will continue to thicken considerably during this time. Serve warm or cold.

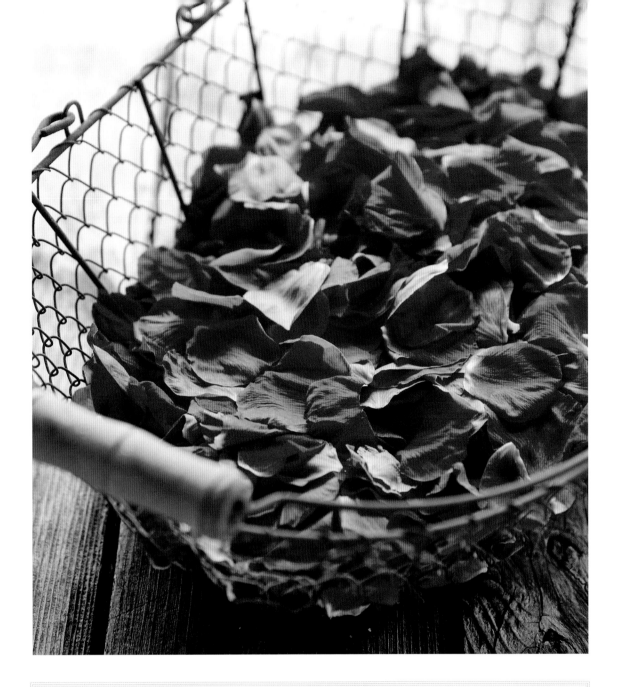

ROSE MEDICINE

Roses are iconic, their gently fragrant flowers and soft petals a symbol of love and long associated with the heart. The petals are a tonic for the cardiovascular system, toning arteries and blood vessels. Their fragrance, color, and gentle energy also soothe and soften the spiritual heart. The soft and open-hearted nature of their flowers stands in contrast to their thorns, which provide sharp, firm boundaries. Don't overstep your limits or walk out of line with the rose; it knows how to stand up for itself. There is comfort in the wisdom of limits and boundaries. *No* is not always a negative; often *no* opens new possibilities and makes space for more of something else.

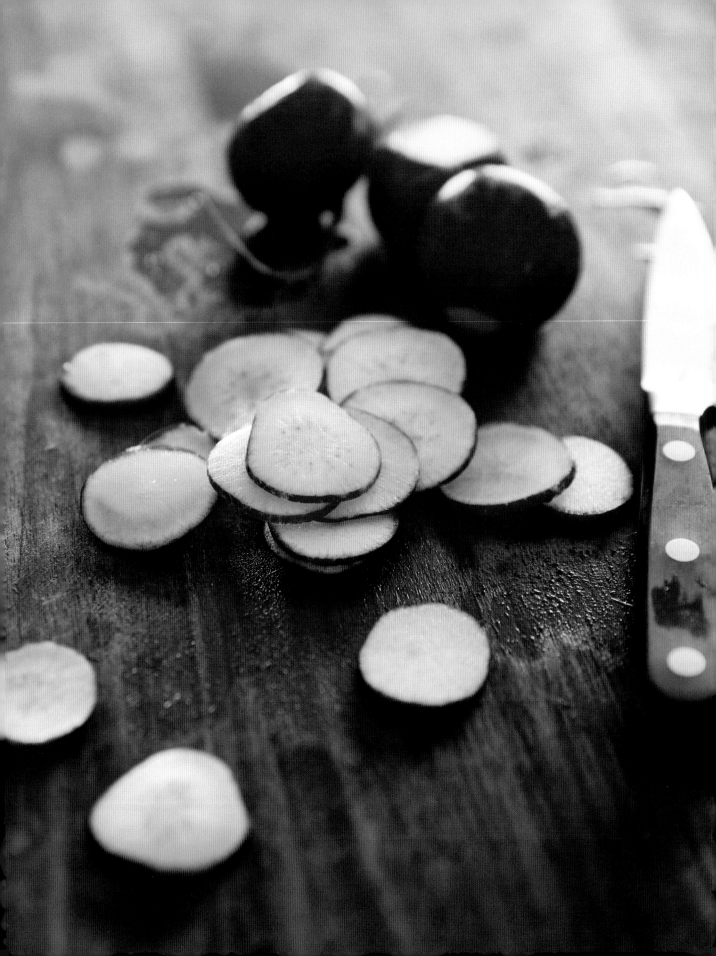

challenge

Satisfying Our
Survival Instincts

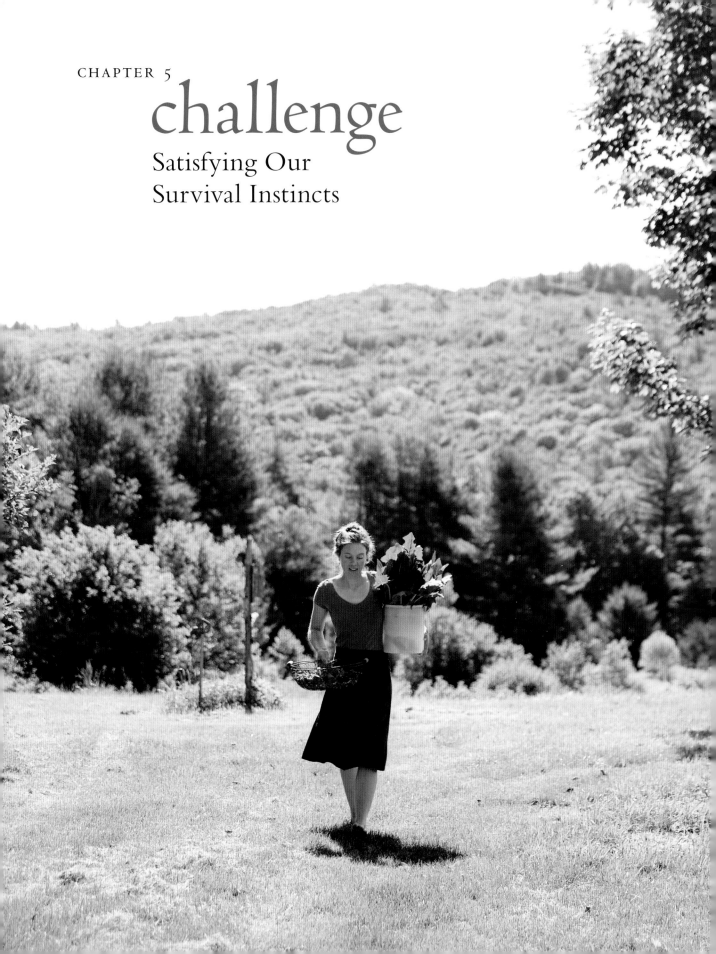

As EATERS IN TODAY'S WORLD, we face many challenges that are a far cry from those of our ancestors. Early humans had to identify their food correctly, find or grow enough of it, and store it properly; their survival was dependent on that. In our culture today, relationships with food are largely consumer relationships. Food is produced and marketed on a global scale, and we buy it as we need it. For many of us, food has become simply a commodity like any other. We don't know where it was made, who made it, or how it was made. We have no personal connection to it beyond the fact that we intend to consume it.

As consumers we are constantly asked to make choices — choices of brand, quality, origin, and price. When it comes to food and eating, our choices seem particularly charged with anxiety. Perhaps we carry an echo of our ancestors' insecurities in our psyches, telling us that a plant identification error or a crop storage failure might mean life or death. So when we're standing in the grocery store staring at rows upon rows of shiny produce and packaged goods, we're often struck with angst. How do we choose?

Under such pressure, many of us agonize over how to do it right — buy the right food, cook the right way, eat the right things. We try harder and harder to be better, more responsible, more health-conscious consumers. But how do we know what is right? Especially when there are countless experts and marketers out there telling us what they think!

The truth is that there are no right answers. There is no such thing as the healthiest or the most responsible or the most sustainable food,

because each option is infinitely influenced by processes difficult to unpack well enough to compare quality, value, and cost. Even if we could unravel it all, there would be a host of different interpretations of the results.

Consumerism is not inherently wrong. It is the disconnection, insecurity, and disempowerment that often accompany it that are problematic. The sheer range of choices in the grocery store and barrage of advice from news sources and social media leads to an underlying level of stress as we weigh the options of local, organic, sustainably harvested, raised without antibiotics, low fat, low calorie, sugar free, gluten free, GMO free . . . the list goes on and on, with our environmental, social, and personal morals waging war against our pocketbook. It is important to be a well-educated consumer — to know what labels mean and to read them. Yet amid such challenges, our best choices are those driven not by societal pressures but by our instincts. We have to learn to trust our instincts, to make choices that work for us and to let them be good enough. The biggest challenge we face today is not what choices to make, but finding the courage to let go of the static that surrounds consumer food culture and reconnect with our intuition.

Intuition is instinctive knowledge. It is the voice inside that tells you what the right choice is for *you*. It is awareness, insight, and perception. Intuition is like a muscle: the more you use it, the stronger it gets. With intuition there are no absolutes or "right" answers, because all decisions are individualized. When we look at health from an individualized perspective, it is not about whether

Our best choices are those driven not by societal pressures but by our instincts.

meat or grains, garlic or ginger, chia seeds or goji berries are healthy, it is a question of whether or not they are healthy for *you*. As you come to trust your intuition, you'll gain confidence in your ability to meet the challenges of your own unique situation.

Instinctive knowledge grants us permission to purchase the less expensive option, knowing that the financial pressure of the alternative would create more stress than not. Trusting we have made the right choice for ourselves at that given moment in time gives us permission to let go of potential guilt associated with our decision and instead focus on the empowered story of self-care that should be inherent in any decision that avoids stress and anxiety, including financial. But the point is that while one person may have more stress over the financial commitment to buy organic, the next person might have a comparable stress response to the thought of eating pesticides. Neither is wrong; the right choice depends on each individual and each individual situation at that moment in time.

Learning to trust and follow your intuition starts with reconnecting with your body and your instincts. One of the best places to begin is by engaging your senses: looking, watching, listening, smelling, tasting, and feeling. Much of this requires a shift from a

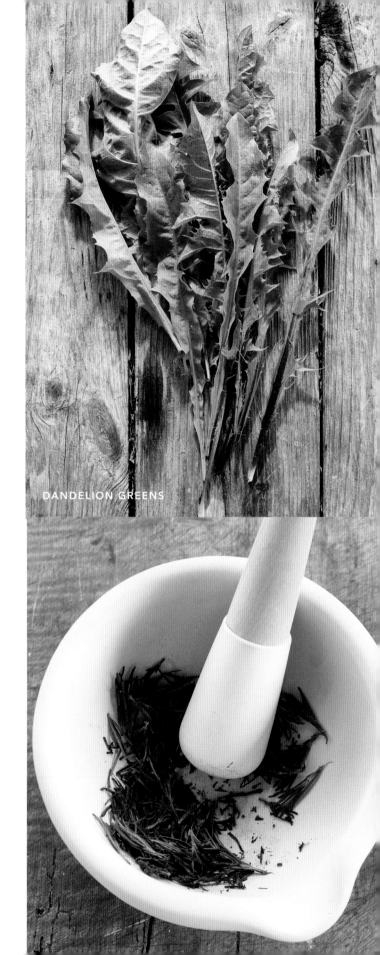

DANDELION GREENS

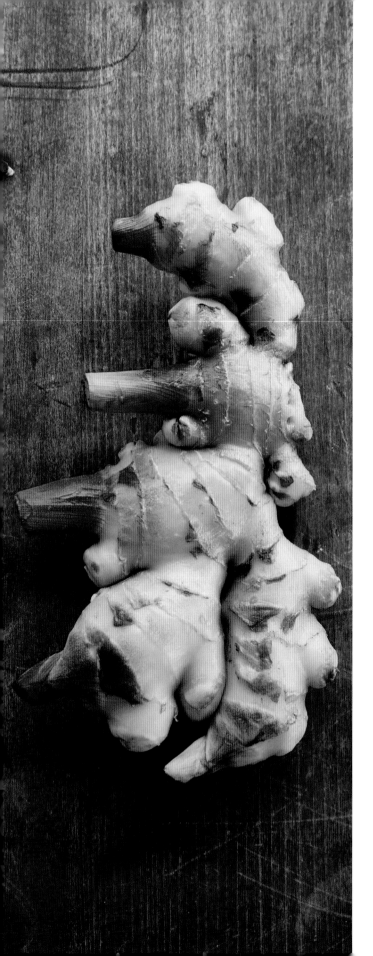

thinking-dominant perspective to a feeling-dominant perspective. When making food choices, for example, try to let go of *thinking* about which decision is better and tune in to which decision *feels* better. When you eat, instead of thinking about how the food *should* make you feel, according to the experts, focus instead on how it *actually* makes you feel, and how you feel throughout the day. Exercises such as these may seem difficult at first — it can be hard to ignore the critical voices in your head — but over time you will become more and more comfortable as you build trust in your intuition.

Eating foods with diverse and challenging flavors not only helps us develop our senses of taste and smell but also connects us to our intuition. Challenging flavors such as pungent herbs, spicy radishes, bitter greens, and carminative aromatics clear the palate, stimulate the enteric nervous system via the taste buds, and balance the stress response while simultaneously improving digestion, metabolism, and our overall biological function. Boosting our body's natural biological processes in turn helps cultivate a more accurate sense of inner knowledge or intuition that we can then allow to guide us. The recipes in this chapter focus on challenging flavors — wild foods, bitter greens and herbs, strongly flavored pestos, and so on — as impetus to help us reconnect with our intuition. And hopefully, as we reconnect, they will serve as a reminder that whether or not a food is "healthy" depends in large part on our own unique reaction to it and relationship with it. These recipes are an invitation to challenge yourself to engage your senses, to smell, taste, feel, and wonder, and to trust this inner knowledge wholeheartedly.

OREGANO PESTO

The joy of eating is in the known and unknown ways in which food inspires the taste buds and the spirit. So much of the food we eat today is bland, sweet, or salty, with little actual flavor. Herbs are used as accents rather than centerpieces. Yet herbs and spices often deliver the most distinct flavor profiles and can bring great diversity to a meal, whether they are used to enliven a dish or are featured on their own as a condiment or palate cleanser. This role is powerful, one that stimulates the senses, and it can transform our very relationship with food. The more different flavors we eat at a meal, the less likely we are to crave things later on. Break up your bland staple foods with something bitter and pungent like this oregano pesto, and you may find your afternoon cookie fix on the fritz. Let the flavors help you find the balance that your spirit craves.

◆ YIELD: ABOUT ¾ CUP ◆

2	tablespoons pumpkin seeds
2	tablespoons sunflower seeds
2	cups fresh oregano
2–3	cloves garlic
½	cup olive oil
1	teaspoon salt
	Freshly ground black pepper

I. Toast the pumpkin seeds and sunflower seeds separately in a heavy skillet over medium heat, stirring often so they do not burn, until golden brown, 3 to 5 minutes. The pumpkin seeds will pop and puff up when they are ready.

2. Combine the toasted seeds, oregano, garlic, oil, salt, and a healthy grinding of pepper in a food processor and blend until smooth. Taste and adjust the seasonings as necessary. The pesto will keep for 5 to 7 days in the fridge or for 6 months or more in the freezer.

SERVING SUGGESTION: Oregano pesto has a strong, pungent flavor that is a great complement to heavier foods. I like it with grilled meats and veggies, mixed into grain dishes, and alongside meat and cheese plates.

CURBING CRAVINGS

Cravings are fueled by real biological processes. One of the main chemicals the body uses for fuel is glucose, a monosaccharide, or simple sugar. You get glucose from your food, and primarily from carbohydrates. When you have excess glucose, the liver stores it by converting it to glycogen, a polysaccharide made up of complex strings of glucose molecules. (Glycogen is also found in complex carbohydrates.) Let's say you skip lunch and develop low blood sugar in the afternoon. The liver goes to the pantry and breaks some of that stored glycogen down into glucose, which gets dumped into the bloodstream to raise your blood sugar levels and prevent you from getting too "hangry" during your afternoon meeting.

If you consistently eat high-glucose foods, however, the body gets used to receiving glucose in abundance, and the liver becomes lazy and stops converting extra glucose to glycogen to store for later. Similarly, if you tax your liver and glucose supply by consistently skipping meals, then your glycogen pantry will run dry. If you have no glycogen to convert to glucose when you get low blood sugar, the body will naturally crave the simplest, easiest-to-access forms of blood sugar it can find: sugars and other simple carbohydrates (cookies, cakes, crackers, chips, popcorn, soda, juice). The more of these foods you eat, the more you crave them, because your body becomes dependent on a steady stream of simple sugars and carbs. Many people crave these same foods when they are tired to get an extra boost of energy.

I have a lot of clients who try to fight their cravings with willpower alone, which is just plain hard. Instead, we can use herbs and foods to support liver metabolism and help restore the glycogen pantry. Rather than focusing on what foods to avoid, I prefer to embrace the abundance model and have people focus on adding to their diet good-quality whole foods, with complex carbohydrates, fats, and protein. Meals and snacks should contain all of these important nutrient groups. A balanced diet supports the glycogen conversion mechanism and supplies the body with long-term stable energy. You can remain aware that you would like to reduce your consumption of the sugars and refined carbohydrates you crave, but focus simultaneously on adding these important complex food groups into your diet.

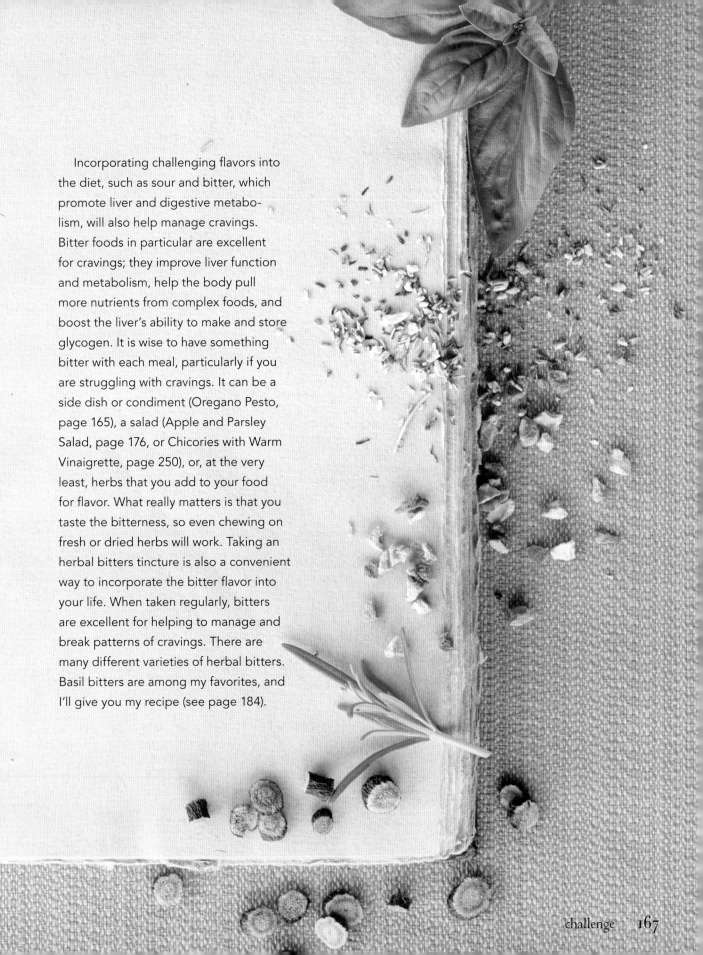

Incorporating challenging flavors into the diet, such as sour and bitter, which promote liver and digestive metabolism, will also help manage cravings. Bitter foods in particular are excellent for cravings; they improve liver function and metabolism, help the body pull more nutrients from complex foods, and boost the liver's ability to make and store glycogen. It is wise to have something bitter with each meal, particularly if you are struggling with cravings. It can be a side dish or condiment (Oregano Pesto, page 165), a salad (Apple and Parsley Salad, page 176, or Chicories with Warm Vinaigrette, page 250), or, at the very least, herbs that you add to your food for flavor. What really matters is that you taste the bitterness, so even chewing on fresh or dried herbs will work. Taking an herbal bitters tincture is also a convenient way to incorporate the bitter flavor into your life. When taken regularly, bitters are excellent for helping to manage and break patterns of cravings. There are many different varieties of herbal bitters. Basil bitters are among my favorites, and I'll give you my recipe (see page 184).

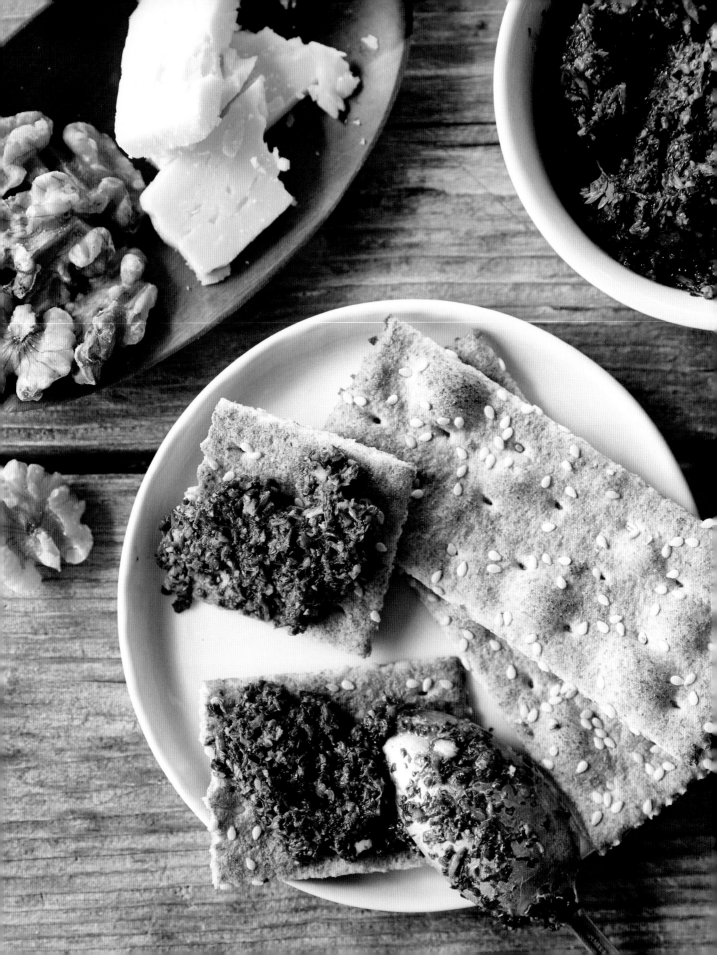

CILANTRO PESTO

What's the big deal with stems? Cilantro, parsley, kale, chard, spinach . . . so often we are told to remove the stems from our greens, but the stems have the same nutrition as the leaves. We want things to be so neat and tidy all the time — in our home, in our job, in our relationships, in our food — but life is a mess! Dirty, tough, painful, sad, and lonely *and* full of joy, wonder, beauty, amazement, and passion. These experiences do not have to be separate, but we often separate them like a leaf from a stem, thinking we can have one part without the other. But can you experience joy and beauty and wonder to the same capacity without pain and sorrow and loss? Can you enjoy the clean and the simple without an understanding of the dirty and the messy? I say, keep the flexible stems: let them hold the center, sway and adapt, nourish you, and challenge your sense of neat and tidy. May their presence make the texture richer, truer, and more nuanced.

⬧ YIELD: ABOUT ½ CUP ⬧

2 heaping tablespoons walnuts

2 cups packed cilantro leaves and stems (1 large bunch)

2 garlic cloves

2 tablespoons olive oil

Salt

Freshly ground black pepper

1. Soak the walnuts overnight in enough water to cover them. (Soaking the walnuts makes them easier to digest and helps remove some of the bitterness in the skin.)

2. Drain and rinse the walnuts. Combine them with the cilantro, garlic, oil, salt to taste, and a few grinds of pepper in a food processor. Blend until smooth. Taste and adjust the seasonings as necessary. The pesto will keep for 5 to 7 days in the fridge or for 6 months or more in the freezer.

USE AND STORAGE

Cilantro pesto has tremendous detoxifying properties and can be particularly helpful for those who may have been or are continually exposed to environmental pollutants or heavy metals, including the heavy metals found in seafood.

Some of my favorites things to top with cilantro pesto include scrambled eggs, sandwiches, tuna and other fish, toast, roasted beets and other root veggies, and grains . . . and it's delicious on its own by the spoonful!

PICKLED DAIKON WITH CILANTRO AND LIME ZEST

Condiments are an excellent way to introduce a variety of challenging flavor profiles into the diet, but we don't often go to the trouble of making them when we're in the midst of cooking. Having them in the fridge, ready to go, makes it a cinch to incorporate them into meals. Fermented foods bring the sour flavor into the diet, stimulating the digestive system and encouraging the breakdown and absorption of nutrients, including fats. Naturally fermented foods also contain probiotic bacteria that support the health of our gut flora and improve immunity, mental-emotional health, and the absorption of fat-soluble vitamins.

This recipe creates a deliciously sour, salty condiment that is excellent for challenging and invigorating the digestive system. You can use this simple technique to ferment any type of grated root vegetable, substituting or adding to the daikon. One of my other favorites is to do half daikon and half carrot.

◆ YIELD: 4 CUPS ◆

1 pound daikon radish, grated (with skin)

½ cup chopped cilantro

Zest of ½–1 lime, finely grated

FOR THE BRINE

1 cup nonchlorinated water

1½ teaspoons noniodized salt

1. Combine the daikon, cilantro, and lime zest, and toss to combine. Pack into a clean wide-mouthed 1-quart mason jar.

2. Prepare the brine: Warm ¼ cup of the water, add the salt, and stir until dissolved. Stir that salty water into the rest of the water.

3. Pour enough brine over the vegetables to cover them by at least ½ inch, pushing out any air bubbles as you go. (You should have enough brine, but make more if you need to.) To keep the vegetables submerged beneath the brine, set a ziplock bag on top of the vegetables and fill it with water, so it spreads out and seals off the jar. Or set a smaller glass jar filled with water as a weight on top of the vegetables.

4. Cover with a clean dishcloth and secure it around the edges of the jar with a rubber band or piece of string. Let the vegetables ferment at room temperature until the flavor reaches your liking, 7 to 14 days. Check the jar daily to make sure the grated roots stay submerged beneath the brine; any vegetables exposed to air may mold. Push the weight down as needed and add more brine if necessary.

5. Begin to taste the vegetables after 5 days. The longer they ferment, the more sour the flavor and the softer the vegetables. The speed of fermentation will vary depending on the ambient temperature. They will ferment faster in warmer temperatures and slower in cooler temperatures.

6. When you like the taste, remove the weight, put a lid on the jar, and store in the refrigerator, where it will keep for 3 to 6 months, if you don't eat it all first! Once they are refrigerated, the vegetables do not have to be submerged beneath the brine; the cold will keep them from spoiling.

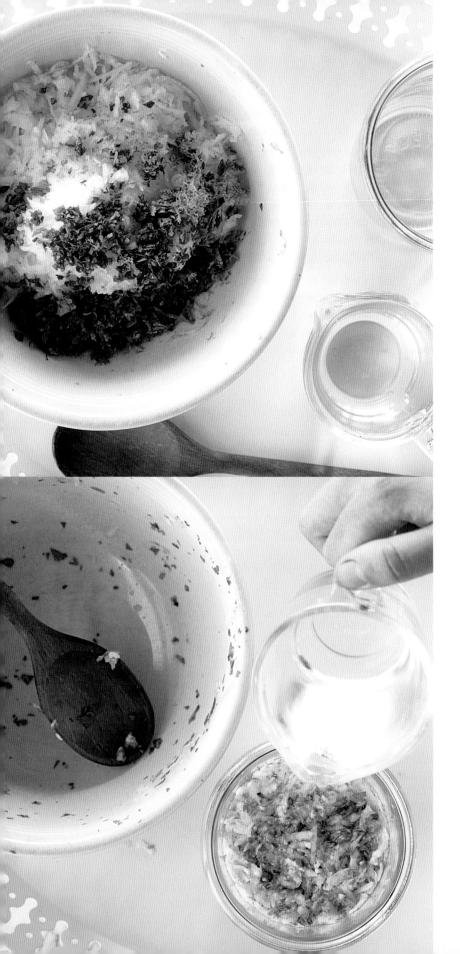

OTHER SOUR CONDIMENTS AND FERMENTS

Other recipes that utilize the processes of fermentation with a sour, salty result include Thyme and Jalapeño Pickled Carrots (page 109), Deep-Sea Purple Kraut (page 83), Lactofermented Dilly Beans (page 196), and Vital Roots Kimchi (page 116). You can also bring the sour and pungent flavors to salads and condiments without fermentation by the simple addition of lemon juice or vinegar, such as in Apple and Parsley Salad (page 176) or Dandelion Greens with Garlic-Mustard Vinaigrette (page 175).

WATERMELON RADISH SALAD
WITH FETA AND FRESH MINT

Color adds beauty to any plate. Color also serves as an indicator of nutrient content. Vibrantly colored foods almost always have high levels of antioxidants, vitamins, and minerals. One way to observe this is by watching greens and other vegetables as they age — they may turn from green to yellow, from dark purple to light purple, from vibrant to muted as their nutrient content declines. Of course, beautifully colored foods engage the senses for reasons beyond taste and nutrition. Beauty inspires. Adding color to the plate is one of the simplest ways to entice those who are eating. A colorful side dish, like this salad, or even just a simple garnish of edible flowers is a great way to get started. Take inspiration from the foods available to you seasonally; nature's palate always has something lovely to share.

⬥ YIELD: 4 SERVINGS AS A SIDE DISH ⬥

2 large watermelon radishes (or radishes of your choice)

2 tablespoons finely chopped fresh mint

½ cup crumbled feta cheese

1–2 tablespoons olive oil

Squeeze of fresh lime juice or a dash of red wine vinegar

I. Trim off the tails and tops of the radishes. The peel is spicier and stronger flavored than the insides, so if you prefer a milder flavor, peel the radishes, too. Cut each radish lengthwise into eighths and then thinly slice each section. (If you're using a different kind of radish, aim to have about 2 cups sliced.)

2. Combine the sliced radishes with the mint, feta, oil, and lime juice in a large bowl and toss together. Taste and add more lime if the dish needs more of a sour touch. Serve at room temperature.

ALTERNATIVES

The spicy, salty, and cool minty flavors of this salad can complement and enliven almost any meal. In winter, when watermelon radish season has outlasted mint season, you can make this with mint-infused vinegar or some other infused vinegar that you think will complement the flavors well. Consider using a little more vinegar to increase the pungency of the flavor. As always, you can substitute other fresh herbs for the mint.

WILTED DANDELION GREENS
WITH GARLIC CONFIT

Americans love their lawns and hate weeds. In fact, Americans use upwards of 90 million pounds of pesticides on lawns yearly. Yet despite all the efforts made against them, weeds still prevail, resorting to popping up through the cracks in sidewalks if they must, along roadsides, and in garden paths. Their resiliency is part of what makes them so special — they are up for a challenge and continue to thrive despite adverse conditions. Dandelion is one such hardy weed, tenacious and determined to overcome all obstacles. And while many hate it as a pestilent lawn invasive, dandelion is beloved by children, herbalists, and bees and has been revered as a food and medicine throughout history. In fact, European settlers purposefully introduced dandelions to the United States so that they could eat the leaves as a spring green.

◆ YIELD: 4 SERVINGS ◆

12   garlic cloves (about 3 heads)

Olive oil

½   pound dandelion greens

Salt and freshly ground black pepper

1   teaspoon fresh lemon juice

I. Peel the garlic cloves and trim off the ends. Place the cloves in a small saucepan or cast-iron pan; the pan should be just big enough that the garlic cloves can sit flat on the bottom without overcrowding. Add enough oil to cover them by half. Turn the heat on as low as possible. As the oil heats, the garlic will begin to smell delicious and turn a warm yellow color. After 5 minutes, flip the cloves. Continue cooking, flipping the cloves every 5 minutes, until they are soft and mushy. The total cooking time is usually 20 to 30 minutes, but it depends on how low you're able to set the heat on your stove, and the slower you cook them the better. If your stove will not go low enough and the oil gets so hot you think the garlic may burn, take it off the heat for a moment, let it cool, then return it.

2. While the garlic is cooking, chop the dandelion greens into 2-inch pieces.

3. When the garlic is done, transfer the cloves and the oil into a large skillet and mash them with a fork until they are broken down but still a little chunky.

4. Turn the heat to medium-low. Once the oil is warm, add the dandelion greens, sprinkle with salt and pepper, and cook, stirring continuously, until the greens have wilted, 5 to 8 minutes. Add the lemon juice and cook for another minute or two. Season to taste with salt and serve hot.

WEEDS AS PROTECTORS

While weeds may challenge some of our culture's more contemporary perspectives on lawn aesthetics, they also protect the earth. Bare earth wants to be covered, because uncovered soil loses nutrients, undergoes erosion, and offers less habitat for animals, insects, and microorganisms. Weeds will often grow when nothing else will, thriving in disturbed or compacted soil, and in this way they protect and nourish the land. Labeling a plant a "weed" implies that we do not have a use for it or that it is not wanted where it is — but in the natural world, everything has a purpose.

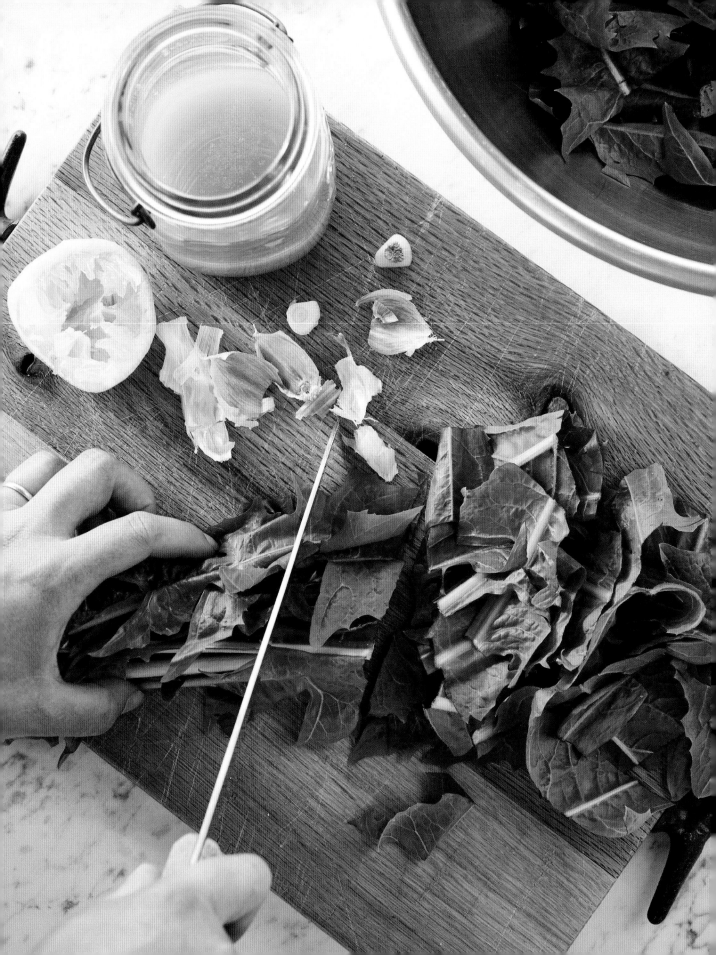

DANDELION GREENS WITH GARLIC-MUSTARD VINAIGRETTE

Dandelion greens are very bitter, challenging both the digestive system and the taste buds. They stimulate digestion and metabolism and increase liver function. The lemon and garlic in this dressing are strong enough to hold up against the dandelions' own strong flavor, making for an excellent side dish, palate cleanser, or first course. This dressing is best when made the day before and allowed to marinate overnight, which allows the flavors to meld and gives the garlic time to mellow. If you do not have time to prepare it ahead, though, make it anyway!

⋄ YIELD: 4-6 SERVINGS ⋄

½–¾ pound dandelion greens, chopped

FOR THE DRESSING

½ cup olive oil

2 tablespoons fresh lemon juice

2 tablespoons red wine vinegar

2 teaspoons prepared Dijon mustard

2 garlic cloves, thinly sliced

⅛ teaspoon salt

Freshly ground black pepper

1. Put the dandelion greens in a salad bowl.

2. To make the dressing, combine the oil, lemon juice, vinegar, mustard, garlic, salt, and pepper to taste in a jar or bowl and shake or whisk well.

3. Toss the salad with as much or as little dressing as you like just before serving. Store any extra dressing in the refrigerator, where it will keep for 5 to 10 days.

WILD FORAGING

There is always a challenge in the hunt. Hunting plants, or wild foraging, gets you outside in nature and also gets you into yourself. Once you find a good patch, the gathering process has a meditative, rhythmic quality that is relaxing, calming, and grounding. The entire process helps me connect to myself, to my food, and to my environment. When you sit down to eat, there is something more rewarding about meals made with wild foods. Just like with home cooking, it seems to taste better when you gather it yourself.

Dandelions grow just about everywhere, from fields to yards and gardens. Do not harvest the greens from areas that have been treated with fertilizers, pesticides, or herbicides. You can often find dandelion greens for sale at the store or farmers' market — but then you lose the fun of the hunt!

APPLE AND PARSLEY SALAD

Parsley is ubiquitous on restaurant plates across America. Most of us don't give it a second thought, but there's good reason it's become a common garnish: it is a rich source of metabolically active elements that stimulate digestion, promote kidney function, and aid in detoxification. It's also a nutritional powerhouse, rich in antioxidants and vitamin C and folate, alongside smaller but still significant amounts of copper, potassium, magnesium, and iron. It deserves to spend at least some time as the centerpiece of a meal. A fresh parsley salad provides a wealth of nutrition while simultaneously cleansing the palate, invigorating the taste buds, and stimulating digestion.

◆ YIELD: 4 SERVINGS ◆

1   large bunch fresh flat-leaf parsley, chopped (about 3 cups)

1   apple, chopped

4   scallions, chopped (about ¼ cup)

FOR THE DRESSING

3   tablespoons olive oil

1   teaspoon apple cider vinegar

1   tablespoon fresh lemon juice

    Salt and freshly ground black pepper

I. Combine the parsley, apple, and scallions in a large bowl and toss well.

2. Prepare the dressing: Combine the oil, vinegar, lemon juice, and salt and pepper to taste and whisk or shake well.

3. Toss the salad with the dressing up to 10 minutes before serving.

TIME VS. SPACE

People often feel that they do not have enough time to cook for themselves, to feed themselves well, to eat the "right" things. It is true that both time and energy are resources that may be tight in our lives. Yet in my experience, as often as we need *time* to prepare food and eat in a way that makes us feel good, we also need *space*.

Space can be physical — a kitchen, a table, a garden — but it can also be emotional and mental. When we have space in our mind, we can feel liberated from distractions and available to be in the moment: we are able to think about what we might want for dinner, make a thorough trip to the grocery store, or take something out of the freezer for dinner before we leave for work. I tend to make simple meals that are easy to prepare and don't take a lot of time, but they often require that I plan ahead. They also require that I have enough space in my mind to be creative with my cooking and with my use of time. Soaking a grain or getting something out of the freezer before I start my day doesn't take long, but I have to have the space to remember to do that and to not feel overwhelmed by it.

With this in mind, it's helpful to develop habits and practices that are time saving: Shop one day a week, and buy in bulk. Cook with the intention of having leftovers for another meal or snack. Make big batches of condiments like sauerkraut on the weekends or as an evening activity with family or friends. Make pesto, soups, and broth in large batches and freeze some for later.

Once you establish these practices and intentions, you will always have them to come back to. When you find yourself out of the habit of making time and space for your relationship with food, make a date with yourself to do some cooking and initiate that intentional, self-nourishing process.

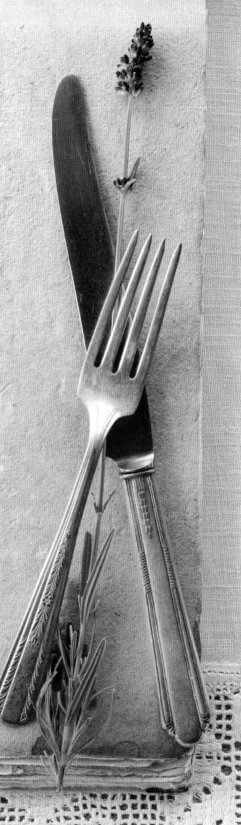

FRESH HERB DOLMAS

Dolmas are little leaf-wrapped bundles of spiced meat or rice. They can be wrapped in any number of wild greens or in cabbage leaves. Today most people associate dolmas with grape leaves, which lend themselves to being stuffed because their tough, fibrous texture holds up well to folding, rolling, and steaming.

There comes a time in mid- to late summer when the wind blows just right and my nose catches the sweet smell of wild grapes. Sometimes it is so brief I can't even tell where the fragrance is coming from. Other times the smell persists and I follow it, hoping I can find the fruit. It serves as a nice reminder to go out and forage some wild fruit and to bring home some leaves for supper. Stuffed grape leaves are a wonderful and simple way to enjoy wild food in the summer months and make a nice light meal; the fresh flavor of the herbs is refreshing and cooling on a hot summer's day.

◆ YIELD: 30 DOLMAS, OR 6-8 SERVINGS AS AN APPETIZER ◆

1 cup short-grain brown rice

30 grape leaves, wild harvested or canned

¼ cup toasted pine nuts

¼ cup chopped chives or scallions

¼ cup finely chopped fresh dill

¼ cup finely chopped fresh mint, plus extra for garnish

2 tablespoons dried currants

2–3 garlic cloves, finely chopped

2–4 tablespoons olive oil

2–4 tablespoons fresh lemon juice (about 1 lemon)

Salt and freshly ground black pepper

Red wine vinegar, for serving

1. Soak the rice in enough water to cover by 2 inches for 6 to 8 hours, or up to overnight.

2. Strain the rice from its soaking water and combine in a saucepan with 1½ cups of fresh water. Bring to a boil, then reduce the heat to low, cover, and simmer until all the water is absorbed and the rice is tender, about 45 minutes. Set the rice aside to cool slightly.

3. If you are using fresh grape leaves, you'll need to prepare them. (If you are using canned leaves, skip this step.) Cut off any stems at the leaf base. Stack the leaves in a large bowl, pour enough boiling water over them to cover, and place a dinner plate on top of the leaves to keep them fully submerged in the hot water. Let soak for 10 minutes, then drain and set aside.

4. Toast the pine nuts in a heavy skillet over medium heat, stirring often, until golden brown, 2 to 3 minutes. Remove from the heat and set aside to cool.

5. Once the rice has cooled slightly, combine it with the toasted pine nuts, chives, dill, mint, currants, garlic, 2 tablespoons of the oil, and 2 tablespoons of the lemon juice. Mix well and season generously with salt and pepper.

6. To stuff the grape leaves, lay one leaf shiny side down in front of you, with the stem end facing you. Place 1 to 2 teaspoons of stuffing at the bottom (stem end) of the leaf. The amount you use will depend on the size of the grape leaf and how full you like it to be. Fold the edges of the leaf in toward the center and then roll the leaf up from the broad bottom to the top. Repeat until you have used up all the leaves or stuffing.

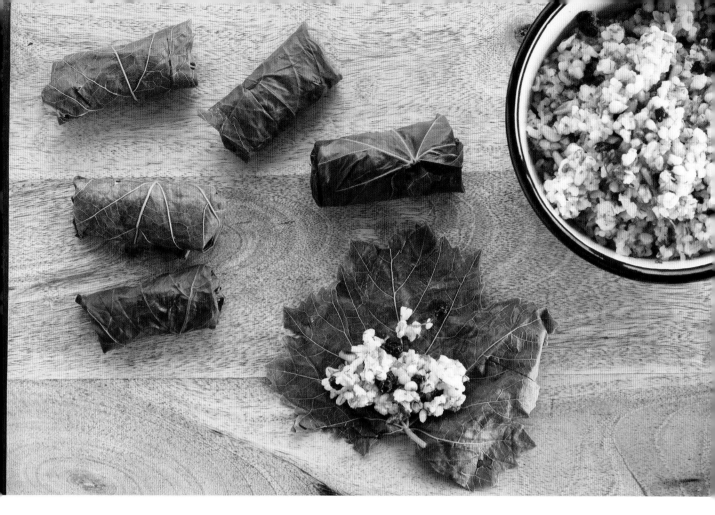

7. If you are using fresh grape leaves, you will need to steam the dolmas. Place them in a saucepan, nestling them together so that they do not unfold as they steam. The dolmas can be stacked if necessary. Add enough water to the pan to submerge half of the first layer of dolmas (usually about ½ inch of water will suffice). Add 2 tablespoons oil and 2 tablespoons lemon juice, cover, and set over medium-high heat. When the liquid comes to a boil, reduce the heat to low, and let steam until the grape leaves are tender and soft, about 20 minutes.

8. Garnish with fresh mint and serve with a little red wine vinegar for dipping. Most dolmas are served cold, but you can eat them hot if you like them that way! These can be made ahead and refrigerated until serving.

RICE SALAD

There is usually stuffing left over, which makes a tasty rice salad to serve as a side dish or main course. Sometimes I double the recipe so that I'm sure to have some leftovers. Feta cheese makes a great addition.

ROASTED EGGPLANT WITH CHICKPEAS, SPICY PEPPERS, AND MINT OIL

Cooling and soothing, the mint in this recipe balances the spice of the hot peppers. The advantage of using the mint as an infused oil is that it endows an essence of mint, without any of the green leafy taste that would accompany fresh mint . . . not that I don't personally love that green leafy taste! The mint oil is like a breath of summer, a reminder of the lightness and sense of freedom that accompanies sunshine and long days.

While this dish stands alone well, it is also nice served alongside couscous, rice, or some other grain.

⁘ YIELD: 4–6 SERVINGS ⁘

¾ cup dried chickpeas (about 1½ cups cooked)

2 medium eggplants, cut into 1-inch pieces (about 4 cups total; I do not peel)

3 tablespoons olive oil
    Salt and freshly ground black pepper

1 bell pepper, cut into 1-inch pieces

1–2 green chiles (like poblano or Anaheim), cut into ½-inch pieces, or 1 jalapeño pepper, seeded and minced

4 garlic cloves, thinly sliced

1 tablespoon minced fresh thyme or 1½ teaspoons dried

1 tablespoon fresh lemon juice

1 teaspoon ground paprika

¼ cup finely chopped fresh mint or homemade mint oil (see the note at right)

I. Soak the chickpeas overnight in enough water to cover them by 6 inches.

2. Strain the chickpeas from the soaking water. Combine them in a saucepan with enough water to cover by 2 to 3 inches. Bring to a boil, skim off any foam, reduce the heat, and cover; simmer, stirring often, until the chickpeas are tender, 35 to 50 minutes. Set aside to cool in their cooking liquid.

3. Preheat the broiler. Position the broiler rack about 6 inches from the heat source. Spread the eggplant on a baking sheet, drizzle with 1 tablespoon of the oil, and season generously with salt and black pepper. Broil for 15 to 20 minutes, until cooked through and slightly browned, stirring every few minutes. (If you do not have a broiler, you can bake the eggplant at 450°F/230°C; it may take a little longer.) Remove from the oven and transfer to a large serving bowl.

4. Spread the bell peppers, chiles, and garlic on the same baking sheet, drizzle with 1 table-spoon of the oil, and season generously with salt and black pepper. Broil for 10 minutes, stirring every few minutes. Remove from the oven and transfer to the serving bowl with the eggplant. Add the thyme and lemon juice and mix well.

5. Strain the chickpeas and spread them on the same baking sheet. Drizzle with the remaining 1 tablespoon oil and season with the paprika, salt, and black pepper. Roast for 5 to 7 minutes, stirring once or twice. Remove from the oven and transfer to the vegetable medley.

6. Season to taste with salt and serve, garnished with fresh mint or a drizzle of mint oil.

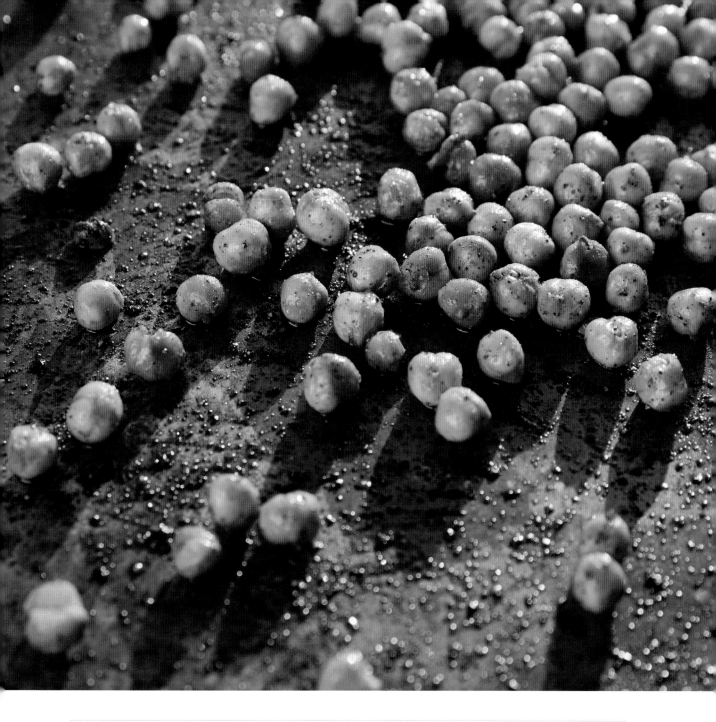

MAKING MINT OIL

To make mint oil, follow the instructions for Basil Oil on page 274, substituting any type
of fresh mint for the basil. Note that the mint oil is best when given 24 hours to steep.
Leftover mint oil can be used on anything that you would use olive oil for — just plan the flavors
accordingly. The last time I prepared mint oil, I used what was left in a salad dressing with
fresh garlic and champagne vinegar.

INDIVIDUALITY

It is common to talk about individuality in regard to our personality — our way of being and relating that distinguishes us from others and makes us unique. Sometimes embracing our individuality is empowering and exciting; it makes us feel good about ourselves. At other times it is challenging, making us feel insecure, self-conscious, or out of place. Particularly in a world where mass media and other social influences are pervasive, it is easy to see our individuality as positive or negative based on how it fits within larger cultural trends.

It's important to remember that the same level of individuality that we find in our personality is present in our body, and we must consider our own unique constitution when thinking about our individual health. When a new diet fad comes out or a new superfood appears on the scene, it's important to know that any dietary change or supplement might work for some people but not for others. That is because each of our bodies is different, and each of us has different needs. Something that works great for one person may not work at all for another. Some people will do well eating lots of fat, protein, and other sweet-tasting foods to nourish and ground them, while those same foods may make others sleepy, sluggish, and lethargic. Some people will be over-stimulated by too many pungent or bitter foods, while a generous supply of those flavors may be just the metabolic stimulation needed to get the sleepy, sluggish person off the couch! The same is true of other activities and inputs for the physical body. Different people need different amounts of sleep, water, and exercise. They are comfortable in different temperature ranges, they prefer different types of beds, and they need different kinds of walking shoes. All of these differences make us unique, and respecting these unique aspects of who we are carries the blueprint for our health and well-being.

Knowing this, you can understand why no advice applies indiscriminately to everyone. If the advice isn't designed specifically for you, it may not work for you. (And that means you can't assume everything I say in this book will apply to you!) Not to mention the fact that our needs change seasonally and through-out our lives, so what works for you at one point may not be appropriate

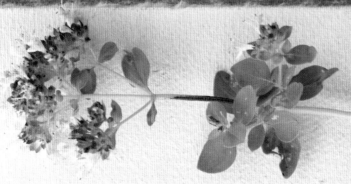

forever. So, once again, we are left to find our own individual approach to our wellness — to listen to our body and pay attention. Learning the language of our body is how we find health, allowing us to support our own unique needs.

One way to conceptualize this is to create a net of your own inner wisdom, informed by your observations of your body, that filters all the information that comes at you from society, the experts, mass media, advertisements, and so on. The net filters inputs — it throws out what doesn't feel right or make sense, holds on to things that feel true, and has a category for ideas that you might be unsure about but you're willing to try. When you try something new — a new food, a different exercise regimen, a new dietary program — you listen to your body for answers, each time gaining information that you can add to this language of your body that you are learning to speak.

As we develop and learn to embrace our own individuality, it can be hard not to compare ourselves to others. When watching what others eat, how they shop, and what they cook, we question ourselves, we judge ourselves, and still,

after all that effort, we are left without answers. Much of health these days is measured by appearance: our weight, our complexion, the shine of our hair, how much energy we seem to have. We have to remember that every part of our self is part of our unique individual nature. To be healthy, we don't have to be like anyone else; we only have to do a good job of being ourselves.

BASIL BITTERS

The bitter flavor, with its strong stimulating effect on the digestive system, is excellent for many digestive issues. The term *bitters* is used to describe an herbal extract or tincture of bitter plants. As a medicinal preparation, it introduces the bitter flavor and thus stimulates the metabolism. Bitters are commonly used in cocktails and other drinks, but they can also be included in the diet as a dietary supplement. In addition to helping to reduce cravings, herbal bitters are wonderful for relieving digestive distress, including cramping, gas, bloating, lack of appetite, acid reflux, heartburn, and indigestion.

◆ YIELD: ABOUT 1½ CUPS ◆

1 cup coarsely chopped fresh basil

½ cup coarsely chopped fresh dandelion root or ¼ cup dried

½ cup coarsely chopped fresh thyme or ¼ cup dried

¼ cup finely grated fresh orange or lemon zest or 2 tablespoons dried

2 tablespoons coriander seeds or fennel seeds

100-proof vodka

I. Pack the basil, dandelion root, thyme, orange zest, and coriander seeds into a clean pint jar. Add enough vodka to cover the mixture. Label and set aside to steep in a cool, dark place for 3 to 6 weeks. Check after 1 week to make sure the herbs are still submerged beneath the alcohol. If they are not, push them down with a spoon and/or add more alcohol.

2. At the end of the steeping period, strain the tincture through fine cheesecloth or cotton muslin. Pour some into a dropper bottle for use, and store the rest in a glass jar with a tight-fitting lid in a cool, dark place. The tincture will keep for 3 to 5 years.

USING BASIL BITTERS

Take 15 to 30 drops of basil bitters in a sip of room-temperature water 15 to 30 minutes before meals, one or two times a day or as needed, to stimulate digestion, encourage liver metabolism, and begin to reduce cravings. Take before meals for lower gastric issues like cramping, gas, bloating, and nervous indigestion, and after meals for upper gastric issues like heartburn, acid reflux, and indigestion. As a tonic, take seasonally for 1 to 3 months in spring or summer to support liver and digestive health and promote detoxification.

TURMERIC FIRE CIDER

Fire cider is a traditional herbal remedy with a long history of use in folk medicine. This infused vinegar combines spicy herbs that increase circulation and stimulate the metabolism with pungent, sour vinegar and sweet, soothing honey. It can be taken regularly as a tonic or used as needed to prevent or support recovery from a cold or flu, to clear upper and lower respiratory congestion, to increase circulation, and to enhance immunity. It is also a potent, warming digestive aid. Turmeric makes a flavorful addition; it supports liver function and digestion.

◆ YIELD: ABOUT 1½ CUPS ◆

½ cup chopped onion

½ cup chopped garlic

¼ cup grated fresh ginger

¼ cup grated horseradish root

¼ cup grated fresh turmeric root or 1 tablespoon plus 1 teaspoon ground dried turmeric

Cayenne pepper (I use half a medium fresh pepper or ¼ teaspoon ground dried cayenne)

Raw apple cider vinegar

2–4 tablespoons raw honey

1. Combine the onion, garlic, ginger, horseradish, turmeric, and cayenne to taste in a glass jar. Add enough vinegar to completely cover all the ingredients.

2. Cover the jar. Vinegar erodes metal, so use a plastic, glass, or cork lid when making infused vinegars, or put a piece of waxed paper between the lid and the liquid.

3. Set the mixture aside to steep in a cool, dark place for 4 weeks.

4. Strain out the herbs using a fine-mesh strainer or fine cheesecloth or cotton muslin.

5. Sweeten with honey to taste, shaking or stirring well to dissolve. Store at room temperature; it will keep for up to a year.

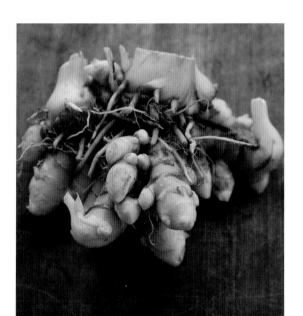

USING TURMERIC FIRE CIDER

As a general tonic, take 1 teaspoon to 1 tablespoon once or twice a day in a little water. For treating colds or flu, take 1 teaspoon every hour up to six times a day. Note that the heat of the fiery vinegar may aggravate acid reflux, heartburn, and indigestion.

TARRAGON-INFUSED VINEGAR

Herb-infused vinegars are one of my favorite ways to preserve and carry the bounty of fresh herbs from the growing season into the darker seasons of late fall and winter. It is easy in the summer months to take fresh herbs for granted and forget the magic inherent in picking them from the garden. But popping open a bottle of herb-infused vinegar from the refrigerator on a cold winter's day is like taking a breath of that fresh, warm garden air. The sweetness of these herbs lives on in their essence, infused as they may be in vinegars and other preparations. A member of the mystical and sacred artemisia family, tarragon has a special magic all its own, quietly blessing the garden with unassuming grace. It will just as gracefully infuse your vinegar with summer wonder and wait in the refrigerator until it is called upon.

◆ YIELD: 1½ CUPS ◆

1   cup packed coarsely chopped fresh tarragon

1½   cups raw apple cider vinegar

I. Pack the tarragon into a clean pint jar. Pour the vinegar over the tarragon, making sure that all the plant material is covered. If necessary, push the herbs down with a spoon.

2. Cover the jar. Vinegar erodes metal, so use a plastic, glass, or cork lid when making infused vinegars, or put a piece of waxed paper between the lid and the liquid.

3. Set the vinegar in a cool, dark place, and let steep for 2 to 3 weeks.

4. Strain out the herbs through a fine-mesh strainer or fine cheesecloth or cotton muslin. At this point I like to transfer the vinegar into an old vinegar bottle. These bottles usually have a nonmetal lid and are friendlier for pouring and daily use. Store the vinegar in the refrigerator, where it will keep for 1 year.

NOTE: You can substitute any culinary herb(s) for the tarragon in this recipe.

USING TARRAGON VINEGAR

Tarragon-infused vinegar has an earthy, anise-like flavor that complements fish and white meats, eggs, cheeses, fruits, root vegetables, greens, and other vegetables like asparagus, artichoke, and tomato. It's lovely in salad dressings. The flavor of the tarragon softens and complements the vinegar, making both more versatile.

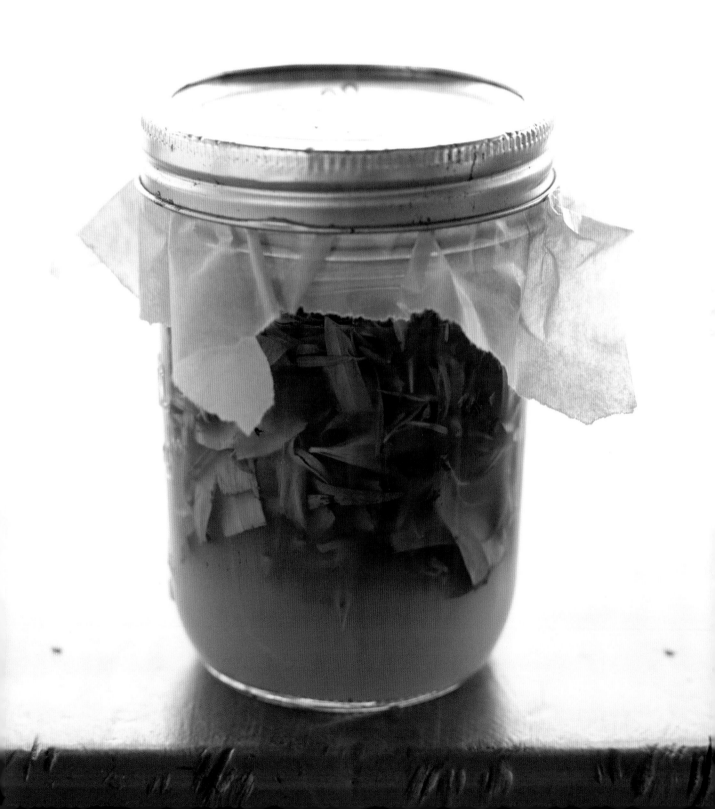

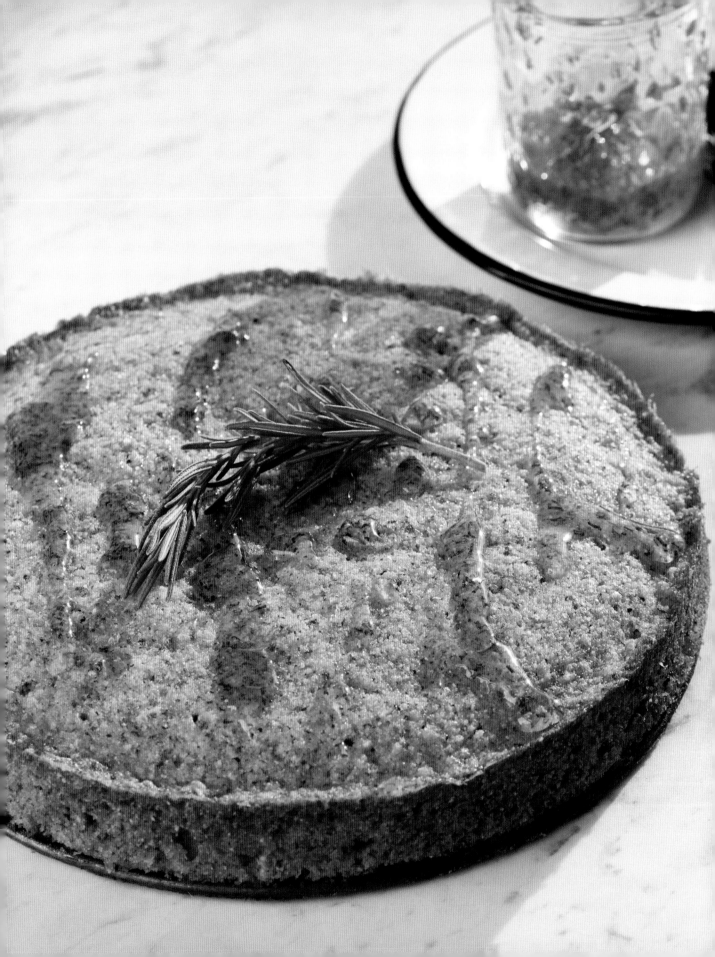

HAZELNUT CORNMEAL CAKE
WITH ROSEMARY HONEY

We are hardwired to want to eat delicious treats. Unfortunately, there is so much poor-quality food out there that when it comes to eating sweet treats, many people either blindly eat too much or spend more time avoiding and trying to resist temptation than they do enjoying the good-quality options. There is nothing wrong with enjoying a dessert or a sweet treat. In fact, hanging out at the dinner table for long enough to eat dessert after a meal would be a good thing for most people! Instead of spending energy thinking about all the sweet treats you don't believe you should nibble, try putting that energy into making and enjoying a homemade dessert every now and again.

◆ YIELD: 8 SERVINGS ◆

1¼   cups raw hazelnuts

¾   cup (1½ sticks) unsalted butter, softened

¾   cup unrefined cane sugar

1   cup cornmeal

4   eggs

1   teaspoon vanilla extract

Zest of 1 lemon, finely grated

1   teaspoon baking powder

½   teaspoon salt

ROSEMARY HONEY TOPPING

¼   cup honey

2   tablespoons finely chopped fresh rosemary or 1 tablespoon dried

1. Soak the hazelnuts in enough water to cover them by 2 inches for at least 4 hours, and up to 12 hours. Drain, then put the hazelnuts in a food processor and grind until they create a coarse flour.

2. Preheat the oven to 325°F (170°C). Grease a 9-inch round pan.

3. Combine the butter and sugar in a large bowl and mix well with an electric mixer. Add the homemade hazelnut flour, along with the cornmeal, eggs, vanilla, and lemon zest, and mix well. Then add the baking powder and salt and mix well.

4. Pour the batter into the prepared pan. Bake for 45 to 50 minutes, or until a toothpick inserted into the middle comes out clean. Allow to cool completely and then remove from the pan.

5. While the cake is baking, prepare the rosemary honey topping: Combine the honey and rosemary in the top of a double boiler. Bring an inch or two of water in the lower pan to a boil, then reduce the heat to low and let the honey and rosemary infuse until the mixture gives off a rich, earthy aroma, 15 to 20 minutes. (You can substitute other herb-infused honeys if you like; lavender and sage are two of my other favorites. For detailed instructions on making herb-infused honey, see page 66.)

6. Slice the cake, plate, and top each slice with a drizzle of rosemary honey. It is best when the honey is warm. If you prepare this cake in advance, drizzle the warm honey over the entire cake at once and place a sprig of fresh rosemary on top.

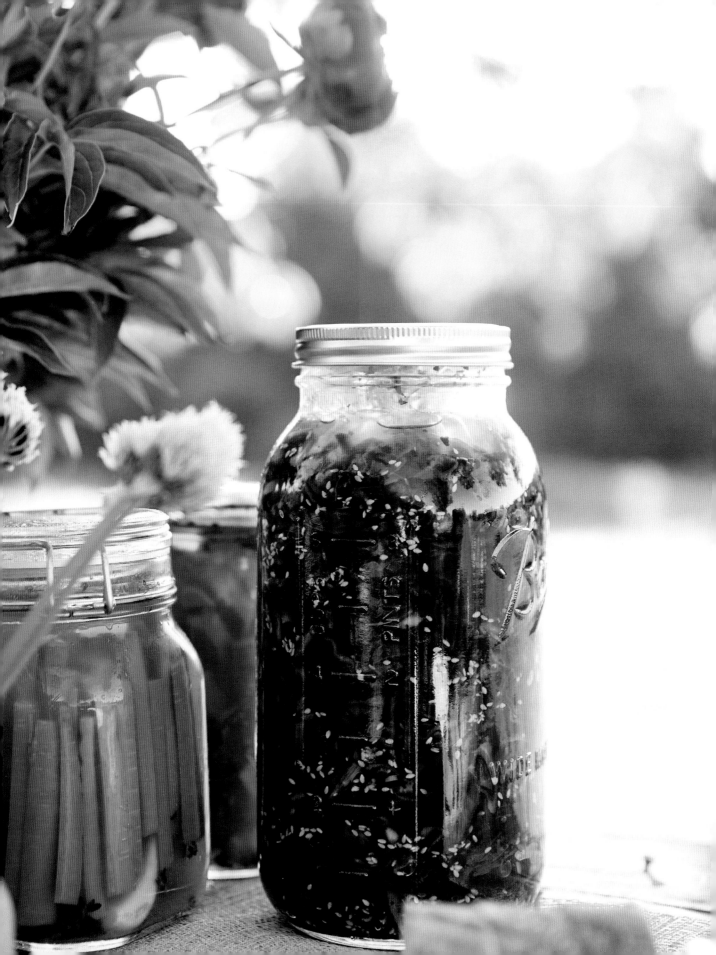

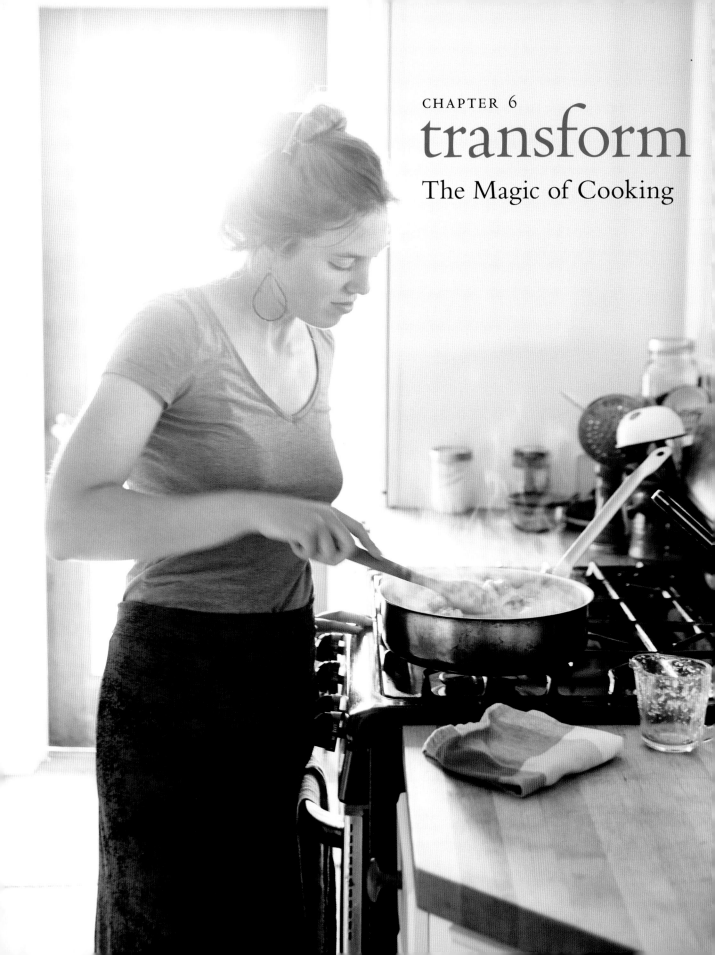

CHAPTER 6

transform

The Magic of Cooking

IN THE FOOD-SCIENCE ERA we live in, we think of nutrition very linearly, assessing a food's value based solely on the nutrients it contains. But this cultural obsession with assessing worth — "this food is good for us and that one is bad for us" — based on a food's constituents, and ignoring any other criteria, overlooks many aspects of what makes food nutritious, including where that food came from, the sustainability of its production, how old or fresh it is, how it is prepared, and how it is consumed. These questions are important ones.

Many of our ancestors survived well on diets that were not very diverse, with some eating only a few different types of foods their whole lives. But the foods they ate were carefully prepared for maximum nutritional benefit. They were also highly valued and respected, because food — always a challenge to obtain — was seen as sacred. The processes that surrounded the acquisition and preparation of food were as important as the foods themselves. Rituals celebrating sacrifice, harvest, and abundance were all common.

Cooking itself is a ritual of transformation. Cooking transforms food into more easily digestible parts and pieces, breaking down the cell walls of vegetables to make the minerals more bioavailable, breaking down the collagen in muscles, cartilage, and connective tissues into easy-to-digest gelatin, and denaturing proteins to make them easier for the body to absorb. Cooking with heat is one of the most common ways to transform food, since the heat can break food down and render it more digestible, but there are many other ways as well. Drying and freezing also break down the cell walls of plant material, giving greater access to the nutrients inside. If you have ever prepared tea from fresh and dried plants, you can see this process in action. The tea made from the dried plant is a rich, dark color, indicating the presence of vitamins and minerals that are more easily extracted by the hot water because the cell walls were already broken down through the drying process. Make a tea from a fresh plant, and it will be clear and light; although lovely and aromatic, it will not have as many vitamins and minerals as a tea made from the same plant dried, because the cell walls are intact and the minerals and vitamins remain locked inside the plant's fibrous body.

As you can see from the tea example, the nutrients a food contains are of little importance if our preparation techniques do not maximize the benefits of those nutrients and make them bioavailable. And there are a host of transformative cooking techniques, beyond using heat, that "predigest" food and make it more nutritious for us. Juicing breaks down cell walls of fibrous plant material, creating a juice rich in bioavailable nutrients. Marinating meat creates enzymatic reactions that make meat more tender and more digestible. Marinating vegetables or tossing a salad with dressing softens the vegetables and helps break down the cell walls — like so many cooking practices, it makes food not only taste better but also more nutritious. Fermentation is also a wonderful transformer of food, making nutrients more bioavailable and also creating entirely new nutrients. All of these methods of cooking make it easier for the greatest transformative process of all — the human digestive system — to successfully function and thrive.

Transforming the seasonal bounty into storable forms is also an important kitchen process. We can transform a field of tomatoes that will rot within weeks into bags of frozen tomatoes or jars of canned tomatoes. We can transform a cabbage into a batch of lactofermented sauerkraut that will last all winter in a crock in the basement. In a broad sense, preserving food is about using leftovers. Not only can we use up leftovers from a previous meal, we can use the leftovers of a bumper crop and a full, lush, productive season. Using leftovers in all forms is transformative — taking advantage of what we have and allowing it to be reused in a new context. It is also respectful, acknowledging the value of all living things and all nourishment. Last night I steamed spinach with grated garlic and ginger. This morning I sautéed the leftovers, cracked a few eggs over it, and finished it off with some freshly grated Parmesan. The possibilities are boundless. If you have a lot of apples you can sauce them, cider them, pie them, pickle them, dry them, chutney them, and eat them. Transforming leftovers into new creations keeps us flexible and helps us use our creative faculties. You never know what will inspire you to make something delicious. A photo in a cookbook, a craving, a bunch of cilantro, a ripe tomato, or some leftover spinach: anything can become a culinary masterpiece if you bring the magic and creativity of transformation to it.

Cooking, marinating, growing, harvesting, fermenting, and preserving all teach us about the value of process. Processes of transformation

Cooking itself is a ritual of transformation.

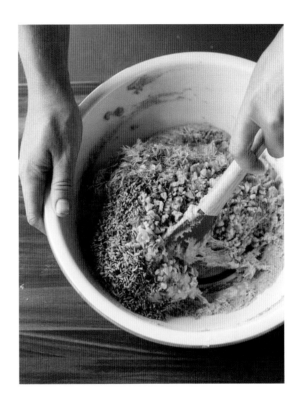

teach us to create and problem-solve, to follow our instincts and learn from them, to accept our mistakes and grow from them. All aspects of our lives can benefit from transformative processes. When we work through something, we knead it out like bread dough, watch as it rises, smell it while it bakes. Our circumstances and relationships in life don't change overnight — they change over time, they rise and fall, bake and burn, smell good and smell sour. Becoming an active participant in the processes of transformation in the kitchen can help us embrace the slow, melodic processes of change, struggle, love, challenge, and joy.

PARSLEY AND TOMATO STEAMED EGGS

The best days start with a slow transition from the world of sleeping and dreaming to the world of waking life. When I can, I like to linger in that soft, gentle place, giving myself time to enjoy the peace and observe the contrast it can have with the everyday pace of things. It can also be a time with greater access to your consciousness and creative inspiration. This recipe emerged from such a place. Wandering into the kitchen one morning, I just knew that this dish would be the perfect thing for breakfast. Perhaps it was the tomato on the counter, the crisp, fresh onions in the fridge, or the sweet, salty smell of parsley that often haunts my dreams. This recipe presents yet another opportunity to transform seasonal bounty into a celebration for the senses.

✦ YIELD: 1 SERVING ✦

1 tablespoon olive oil

1 small onion, sliced into ¼-inch-thick half-moons

1 cup coarsely chopped fresh parsley

2 garlic cloves, chopped

1 medium tomato, chopped, with the juice (about 1 cup)

Salt and freshly ground black pepper

2 eggs

Grated Parmesan cheese, for garnish (optional)

I. Warm the oil in a skillet over medium heat. Add the onion and sauté until translucent, 4 to 5 minutes. Stir in the parsley and garlic, and cook, stirring often, until the parsley is soft and bright green, about 1 minute. Add the tomato, season with salt and pepper, and cook, stirring frequently, until the juice is hot and sizzling, about 1 minute.

2. Spread the mixture evenly across the pan. Crack the eggs over the bed of tomatoes and season lightly with salt and pepper. Reduce the heat to low, cover, and cook until the whites turn opaque and are cooked through, 4 to 5 minutes (or longer for a more solid yolk). If you like a runny yolk, you will have to watch carefully to catch the eggs at that perfect moment when the whites are just cooked but the yolks are still moist.

3. Serve the eggs hot, garnished with Parmesan, if desired.

VARIATIONS
You can add other summer veggies to this dish, including squash, zucchini, green beans, and bell peppers, or greens.

ALMOND-WASABI PESTO

I often make pesto by first grinding together the nuts, garlic, and cheese before adding aromatic greens such as arugula, parsley, oregano, or basil. One time my partner, Casey, and I were making a huge amount of pesto and we started running low on nuts. We pulled out some wasabi-roasted almonds and made a batch of pesto with them. The smell was so exotic and appealing, and while the pesto was good, we both agreed that it had been even better before we added the greens. The idea was born for a wasabi and almond spread — a pesto, if you will, without the leafy herbs. It's amazingly delicious served with crackers, bread, or veggies.

◆ YIELD: 4-6 SERVINGS AS AN APPETIZER ◆

1   cup raw almonds
    Unrefined salt
3   garlic cloves
¾–1 teaspoon wasabi powder
3   tablespoons olive oil
2   tablespoons grated Parmesan cheese
    (optional)

I. Soak the almonds in enough water to cover them, mixed with ⅛ teaspoon salt, for 6 to 8 hours or overnight. After soaking, drain the soaking water and rinse the almonds.

2. Place the almonds in a food processor with the garlic, wasabi powder, oil, and Parmesan, if using. (If you're skipping the Parmesan, add an extra dash of salt and drizzle of oil.) Blend until the nuts and garlic break down, but before the mixture forms a paste. Taste, then add salt and more wasabi powder as desired. (It is important to add the seasonings at this phase so that they get mixed in well.)

3. Blend the mixture until it forms a paste; it will almost form into a dough in the food processor. Serve at room temperature. Store any leftovers in the refrigerator, where they will keep for 5 days.

LACTOFERMENTED DILLY BEANS

When I was growing up, my friend Sophie's mom used to make dilly beans. Since my mom always made cucumber pickles, I remember the moment I ate my first dilly bean as an eye-opener. Not only did I love it, but I realized that anything could be pickled! Sophie and I mostly spent our time together outside, barefoot, building forts, eating wood sorrel, getting muddy, and playing with her many cats. At the end of such epic playdates, we would venture inside, both thirsty and hungry, and dilly beans hit the spot. Those childhood dilly beans were vinegar pickled; here is my lactofermented version, just as satisfying and refreshing all these years later.

◆ YIELD: 1 QUART ◆

¾ pound green beans

1 head garlic, cloves separated and peeled

1 teaspoon whole black peppercorns

1 handful fresh dill (leaves, stems, or flower umbels) or 1–2 tablespoons dill seeds

FOR THE BRINE

2 cups nonchlorinated water

1 tablespoon noniodized salt

1. You can remove and compost the stems of the green beans if you want, but you don't have to; during the fermentation process, they soften to the point that you can eat them. Cut any large garlic cloves in half lengthwise.

2. Place the garlic, peppercorns, and dill in the bottom of a clean widemouthed 1-quart mason jar. Pack the green beans into the jar, leaving at least ¾ inch of headroom at the top of the jar.

3. Prepare the brine: Warm ¼ cup of the water, add the salt, and stir until dissolved. Stir that salty water into the rest of the water.

4. Pour enough brine over the vegetables to cover them by ¼ to ½ inch. (You should have enough brine, but make more if you need to.) Put the lid on the jar and set aside to ferment at room temperature. I leave my fermenting beans on the counter by the sink to make the next step easier.

5. As the fermentation process progresses, gas will form inside the jar. Without taking the lid off, loosen the lid of the jar to release pressure. I do this over the sink, as sometimes the jar contents will bubble up and some of the brine can leak out. Leave the lid loosened until the bubbles stop, secure the lid and let the jar ferment for another day. Do this daily for the first week.

6. At the end of the week, remove the lid completely to make sure the brine still covers the green beans by ½ inch; any beans exposed to air may mold. Add more brine as needed and tighten the lid back on the jar.

7. Set the jar aside in a cool, dark spot to ferment for 4 weeks. Check them every week to make sure there is still sufficient brine covering the beans and to release any pressure. It is common for a powdery-looking film, called kahm yeast, to form on the surface of the brine. You may also see spots of mold, which will usually form in a thicker layer and may look hairy or textured. As long as the growth is on the surface of the ferment and hasn't penetrated the vegetables themselves, you can simply use a clean spoon to scrape off the yeast or mold, and it's perfectly safe to continue to ferment or to eat the vegetables.

8. Begin to taste the green beans after 3 weeks. They should be sour, salty and softer than when raw, but still crunchy. If they are not very sour or if they still taste or seem raw, they have not fermented long enough; replace the lid and give them another 1 to 2 weeks. The speed of fermentation will vary depending on the ambient temperature. They will ferment faster in warmer temperatures and slower in cooler temperatures.

9. When you like the taste, store the jar in the refrigerator, where the beans will keep for 6 months. Once they are refrigerated, the beans do not have to be submerged beneath the brine; the cold will keep it from spoiling.

FERMENTATION: THE GREAT TRANSFORMER

For me, fermentation is one of the most magical of all kitchen transformations: it makes already existing nutrients more bioavailable, even as it creates new nutrients. Take sauerkraut as an example. There is the famous story of European sailors bringing sauerkraut with them on long voyages to prevent scurvy, a condition resulting from a deficiency in vitamin C. Cabbage has vitamin C in it, but fermented cabbage has even more because the fermentation process boosts the vitamin C content, and it also produces some B vitamins. The natural preservatives produced by the fermentation process meant that the sauerkraut would keep for the duration of the voyage.

Another great benefit of fermentation is probiotics. The same bacteria that are responsible for the fermentation process support our own digestive processes. When you eat fermented foods, you're making a positive contribution to your gut flora (positively transforming your inner ecosystem). Healthy gut flora helps support immunity, reduce excessive inflammation, improve skin health, and can reduce allergies. There is even a connection between the health of our gut flora and our mental and emotional health and brain chemistry. This makes eating fermented foods an important part of any holistic protocol for relieving depression or anxiety.

RED PEPPER AND FETA AMUSE-BOUCHE

When I moved to the Bay Area to go to college, I got to know my mom's cousin, Chris, who lived in Aptos County just a few hours south. She had us to her farm, where she prepared a delicious meal of fresh, simple food, cooked just right. I remember watching her cook this very dish. I peered over her shoulder inquisitively and intently as she gently placed the peppers in the pan, rotated them, and flipped them. She explained the importance of cooking the peppers over such low heat, saying, "I want the sugars to caramelize." Caramelization — the slow, steady transformation of sugars that brings out the sweetness and rich flavor in all kinds of vegetables — is one of the many cooking techniques that highlight the inherent goodness of food. I thank Chris for this recipe and the many other ways that she has inspired me over the years.

◆ YIELD: 4 SERVINGS AS AN APPETIZER ◆

2 large red bell peppers

1–2 tablespoons olive oil

2 tablespoons finely chopped garlic

2 tablespoons finely chopped fresh parsley

Salt and freshly ground black pepper

3–4 ounces feta cheese, thinly sliced

I. Cut about ½ inch from the tip and tail of the bell peppers and remove the seeds. Slice the peppers in half lengthwise and then cut each half into thirds or quarters, making relatively flat slices.

2. Warm the oil in a skillet over low heat. Add the peppers and cook over low heat for 10 to 15 minutes on each side. This long, slow cooking allows the sugars in the peppers to caramelize. Try not to let the peppers burn or even brown too much. If they start to brown or stick, reduce the heat and add more oil if necessary. Flipping them periodically also helps slow the cooking process. When they are done, the peppers should be cooked just enough to be soft and sweet throughout, but al dente enough to hold their shape.

3. Transfer the pepper slices to a plate and toss with the garlic, parsley, and a pinch of salt and black pepper. Don't use too much salt, as the feta is salty. Arrange the peppers faceup on the plate, placing any bits of parsley and garlic left on the plate onto the pepper slices. Top each pepper with a thin slice of feta. Serve warm or at room temperature.

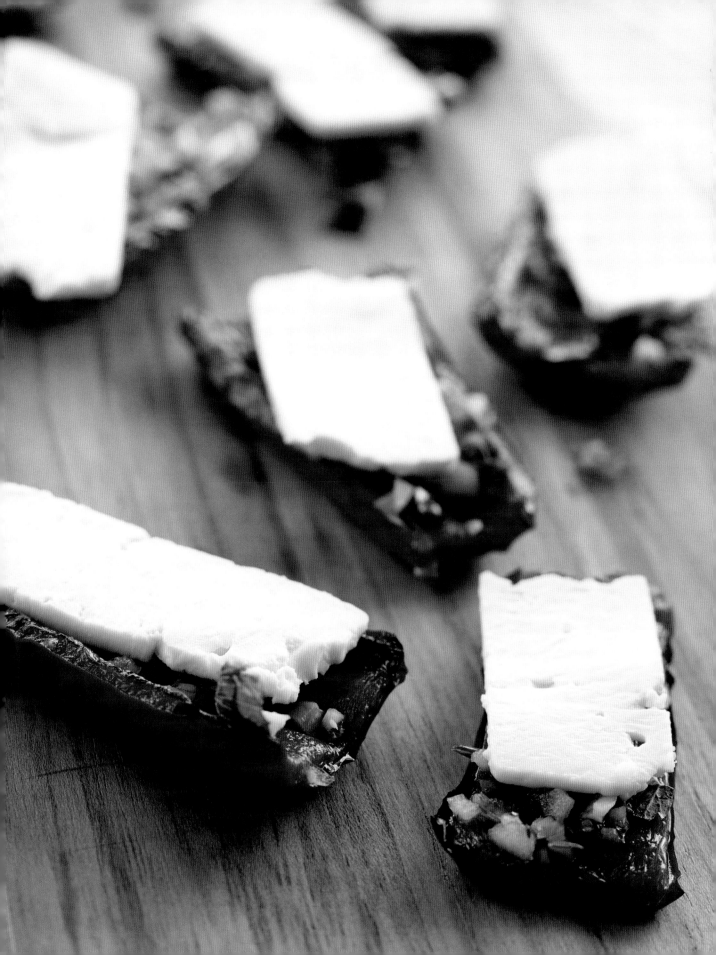

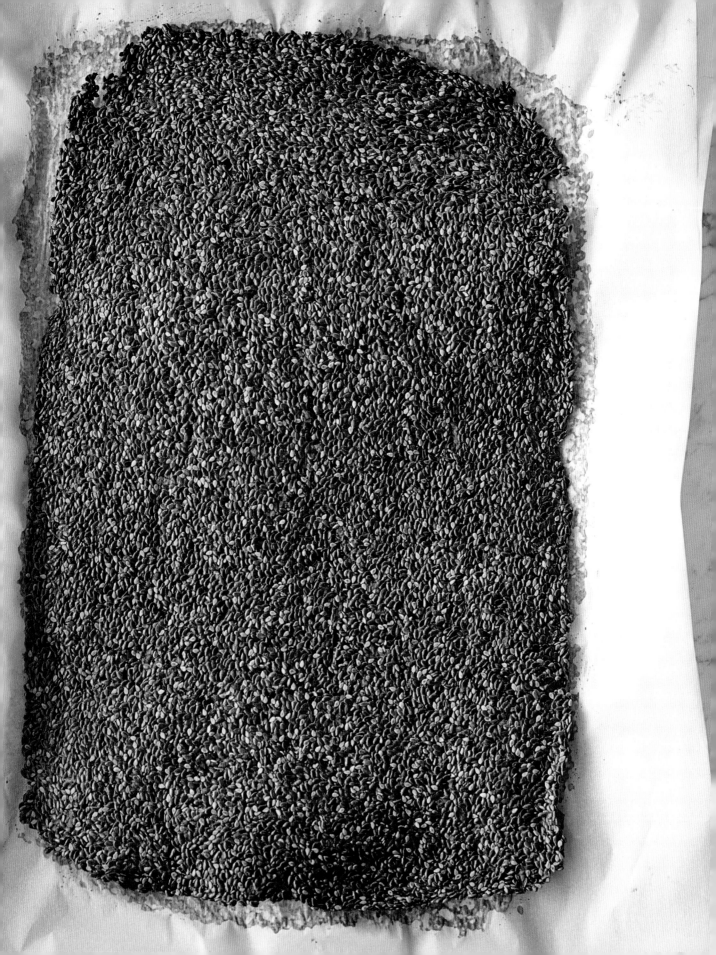

HERBED FLAX CRACKERS

I originally learned how to make flax crackers by soaking the seeds in the whey left over from cheese making. Recently, while reading *Fermented Vegetables* by Kirsten and Christopher Shockey, I stumbled across a recipe that uses leftover pickle or kraut brine in flax crackers. I quickly began using brine in place of the whey, alongside herbs, flaxseeds, and sesame seeds. The brine adds the most delicious flavor: sour and salty and imbued with the goodness of the herbs, spices, and probiotic bacteria from the ferment.

You can prepare these crackers in a food dehydrator or bake them in the oven. Dehydrating will preserve the heat-sensitive enzymes and vitamins that baking destroys. However, baked crackers still contain great nutrition and are easier to digest than most commercial crackers.

◆ YIELD: ABOUT ¾ POUND ◆

2 cups flaxseeds

½ cup sesame seeds

¼ cup finely chopped fresh herbs or 2 tablespoons dried

1–1½ cups leftover fermentation brine (see the list below)

1–1½ cups water

1. Combine the flaxseeds, sesame seeds, and herbs in a bowl. Add 2½ cups of liquid, made up of brine and water, and mix well. Cover with a clean cloth and set aside to ferment for 10 to 16 hours. After sitting for a few hours, the mixture will form into a thick goop (from the flaxseeds).

2. Preheat the oven to 400°F (200°C) and line two baking sheets with parchment paper.

3. Give the goop a good stir, then spread it about ⅛ inch thick on the baking sheets. Bake for 20 to 25 minutes, until the crackers are crispy on top.

4. Remove from the oven and flip the cracker, parchment and all, on the baking sheet. Try to peel the parchment paper away. If it does not separate easily from the cracker sheet, return to the oven to cook for another 5 minutes or so, and then try again. Once you've successfully peeled off the parchment, bake the crackers for another 5 to 15 minutes, until the crackers are completely crispy. They should easily snap into pieces. If you have to tear them to separate them and there is moisture around the seeds in the cross section, they are not done; return them to the oven for another 5 to 10 minutes. Be careful here — they burn quickly! If you have not spread the goop evenly on the tray, one side of the cracker sheet may be done before the other. In this case, break off the crispy half and return the other half to the oven to continue baking.

5. Store the crackers in an airtight container, where they will keep for 7 to 10 days.

BRINES

When picking a brine for making your crackers, remember that the flavor of the ferment will influence the flavor of the cracker. Recipes in this book that can be a source of brine for these crackers are

- Deep-Sea Purple Kraut, page 83
- Lactofermented Dilly Beans, page 196
- Pickled Daikon with Cilantro and Lime Zest, page 170
- Thyme and Jalapeño Pickled Carrots, page 109
- Vital Roots Kimchi, page 116

THYME-INFUSED POLENTA
WITH PARMESAN

Polenta is one of those comforting staple foods that is absolutely delicious and incredibly easy to make. Once you get the technique down, you can whip up polenta on the fly and flavor it with anything. While a classic polenta is simple, with butter or olive oil, herbs, and maybe some cheese, you can add just about anything you want. It makes a lovely side dish, especially with main dishes that have some juice or gravy for soaking up, like Braised Beef Shanks with Gremolata (page 91) or Roasted Tomatoes with Basil and Olive Oil (page 232). It can be served hot, in a porridge-like form, or cooled (it will solidify) and then sliced.

⬥ YIELD: 4 SERVINGS AS A SIDE DISH ⬥

4 cups water

1 teaspoon salt, plus more to taste

A few twists of freshly ground pepper

4–6 sprigs fresh thyme

1 cup polenta or grits

1–2 teaspoons finely chopped fresh thyme

½ cup freshly grated Parmesan cheese

2 tablespoons butter

1. Combine the water, salt, pepper, and thyme sprigs in a saucepan and bring to a boil. Slowly whisk in the polenta (slow is key for avoiding lumps). Continue to whisk until it returns to a simmer. Reduce the heat to low and simmer gently, stirring often, until the mixture thickens, about 20 minutes.

2. Stir in the chopped thyme, Parmesan, and butter. Season to taste with additional salt. Remove the thyme sprigs before serving.

LEFTOVERS

Polenta hardens as it cools. If you want to serve leftover polenta in porridge form, heat it in a pan over low heat with a little water, stirring it to break apart the clumps as it softens. You can also slice hardened polenta and bake it on a greased baking sheet at 350°F (180°C) for about 10 minutes, or sauté it in a pan with butter, olive oil, ghee, or lard. I look forward to thin slices of leftover polenta sautéed in olive oil and garlic and served with eggs for breakfast.

BONE BROTH

Bone broth is rich in minerals, gelatin, amino acids, and healthy fats. It is excellent for the digestive, musculoskeletal, immune, and endocrine systems. The cooking process transforms bones (something that humans could not otherwise even chew, much less extract nutrients from) into one of the most nutritious and easy-to-digest foods that I know of. A lot of us think of bones as leftovers to be tossed out with the trash, but the cooking process elevates them to royalty. Adding something acidic to your broth, like vinegar, citrus juice, or wine, helps extract minerals from the bones as the broth cooks. The longer the broth cooks, the better. I recommend you prepare your broth in a slow cooker, where it can simmer for days. But you can use a soup pot on your stovetop also.

Bone broth can serve as a wonderful base for medicinal herbs. Immune-boosting herbs like shiitake and maitake mushrooms and astragalus root or mineral-rich herbs such as nettle and seaweed can be added at the beginning, with the bones, to enjoy the long, slow cooking process. Tender aromatic herbs such as the thyme, rosemary, and parsley can be added in the last few hours so that their aromatic oils don't evaporate during the long cooking process. Also consider keeping vegetable scraps in the freezer to add to your stock with the bones for extra flavor and nutrition.

♦ YIELD: 3-4 QUARTS ♦

2 pounds bones (lamb, beef, chicken, fish; see note)

¼ cup apple cider vinegar

1 gallon water, or whatever amount your slow cooker will hold

4–6 sprigs fresh parsley (about ¼ cup)

4–6 sprigs fresh thyme or 1 tablespoon dried

2 sprigs fresh rosemary or 1 tablespoon dried

2 sprigs fresh sage or 1 tablespoon dried

1 bay leaf

I. Combine the bones and vinegar in a slow cooker with enough water to cover by at least an inch. Cook on high until the liquid begins to simmer, then reduce the heat to low and cook for at least 48 hours and up to 72 hours — the longer the better. As the broth cooks, the water level will reduce; add hot water as needed to keep the level of the water above the bones. Don't worry if the bones float to the top of the broth; that's different than there not being enough liquid to cover them.

2. When the broth is 2 to 3 hours away from being done, add the parsley, thyme, rosemary, sage, and bay leaf.

3. When it is done cooking, turn off the heat and let cool slightly. Put a colander over a soup pot and pour the contents of the broth through the strainer. The broth will end up in the pot below, and the bones and herbs will remain in the colander.

4. Let the broth cool completely before transferring to containers and storing in the refrigerator or freezer. It will keep in the fridge for up to 1 week and in the freezer for up to 6 months.

NOTE: You can get bones at any butcher or fishmonger. You can also use bone scraps from meats you have cooked and eaten, including chicken carcasses and lamb, beef, or pork bones.

COCONUT FISH CHOWDER

It's a cold February night and I'm home alone, sitting on the floor by the woodstove with fish chowder. I served myself a shallow bowl so the chunks of fish and corn shoulder up out of the broth. I'm warm and content, sipping the slightly spicy, slightly sour broth between sweet bites of last summer's corn and soft pieces of wild-caught cod. I think of my grandfather, growing up on a small island off the coast of Maine. I know his family didn't eat coconut milk, but they certainly ate a lot of fish. Casually influenced by ingredients from other parts of the world, this meal of mine feels comforting, the way that making and sharing an old family recipe might bring some sense of hope that things both change and stay the same.

◆ YIELD: 4-6 SERVINGS ◆

2 tablespoons coconut oil

1 large white onion, finely chopped

3 cups sweet corn, fresh or frozen

1 jalapeño pepper, finely chopped (seeds removed, if you like, to tame the heat)

   Salt and freshly ground black pepper

3–4 cups water

1 pound white fish (cod, haddock, halibut, sole, et cetera)

1 (14-ounce) can coconut milk

   Juice of ½–1 lime

1 cup chopped cilantro

I. Heat the oil in a soup pot over medium heat. Add the onion and sauté until translucent, 3 to 5 minutes. Add the corn and jalapeño and season with salt and pepper. Sauté for 1 to 2 minutes, then add 3 cups of the water. Bring to a simmer and let cook gently, uncovered, until the corn is tender, about 5 minutes.

2. Add the fish. You do not need to cut it up; it will flake apart into perfectly bite-size pieces as it cooks. Stir often while the soup returns to a low simmer. The fish fillet will begin to break apart as you stir, indicating that it is starting to cook through. Cook until its color changes from translucent/clear to white/opaque, 5 to 15 minutes, depending on the thickness of the fillet.

3. When the fish is just cooked through, add the coconut milk and a tablespoon or so of the lime juice. If the soup seems too thick, thin with a bit more water. Season to taste with additional lime juice, salt, and pepper. Stir in the cilantro just before serving.

CILANTRO WITH SEAFOOD

Eating cilantro with fish is a sustainable way to help the body process heavy metals and other toxins that may be found in wild-caught fish. The cilantro acts as a natural chelator, binding with heavy metals and helping to pull them out of the body. We see here, once again, the way that food preparation techniques can serve as powerful tools of transformation.

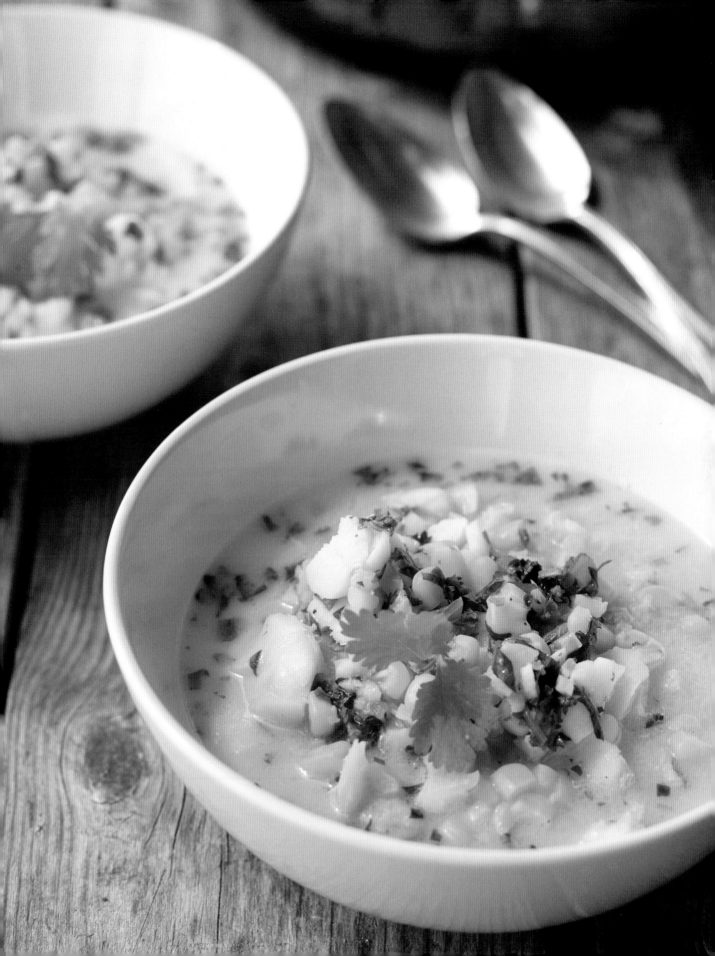

HOMEMADE SAUSAGE

The tradition of sausage derives from our ancestors' effort to use all parts of an animal, both for nutritional purposes and out of respect for the animal. Sausage is made from bits of ground scrap meat and fat mixed generously with herbs and spices. It is traditionally prepared in a casing made from the intestinal lining of an animal, which keeps it fresh and is easier to store. While sausage links are an important part of our culinary heritage, they add an extra step that these patties avoid. If you feel inspired, I encourage you to give making your own links a try. Preparing your own ground sausage allows you to experiment with different combinations of herbs and spices. And it can remind us modern humans that every little bit counts in our transformation of food to sustenance.

◆ YIELD: 1 POUND ◆

1   pound ground pork

2   tablespoons fresh oregano or 1 tablespoon dried

1   tablespoon fresh thyme or 2 teaspoons dried

1   teaspoon ground coriander

1   teaspoon fennel seeds, whole or ground

¼   teaspoon freshly ground black pepper

¼   teaspoon salt

⅛   teaspoon red pepper flakes (optional)

1. Combine the pork in a bowl with the oregano, thyme, coriander, fennel seeds, black pepper, salt, and pepper flakes, if using. Mix with a spoon or your hands until the spices and meat are well combined.

2. Heat a skillet over medium heat. Add a small spoonful of the sausage mixture and cook until cooked through; this should take just a few minutes, depending on the size of your spoonful. Taste the cooked sausage, then season the remaining raw sausage mixture as desired and mix well.

3. Form the sausage mixture into patties about ½ inch thick and 2 to 3 inches in diameter.

4. Cook the patties in the skillet over medium heat until the outside is browned and the center is cooked through (pink, but no longer bloody), 2 to 3 minutes on each side. Serve hot.

BEYOND PATTIES

This mixture can also be cooked as ground meat, without forming patties.
Cook in a skillet over medium heat, allowing it to brown as it cooks, breaking it into medium-size chunks. Cooked this way, the sausage is a great base for soups, stews, stir-fries, and tomato sauce. It also makes a tasty addition to quiche or a topping on a pizza.

OREGANO-CRUSTED CHICKEN

This recipe works well for any cut of chicken, with the fresh oregano offering a rich, earthy flavor. You can use bone-in or boneless legs or thighs, or the breast, whole or sliced into strips. You can even use this herb combination as the rub on a whole chicken and roast it in the oven. I usually make this dish in early summer, when fresh oregano is plentiful. It is good served hot or cold, so it lends itself well to picnics, yard parties, and leftovers. I usually grill the chicken pieces so that the edges get crispy and browned, or I roast them in a hot oven, finishing them under the broiler to help crisp up their oregano crust. You can also pan-fry them in ghee or lard over high heat.

+ YIELD: 4 SERVINGS +

½ cup chopped fresh oregano

½ cup chopped scallions

3–5 garlic cloves, finely chopped or pressed

2 tablespoons olive oil

Salt and freshly ground black pepper

2 pounds boneless chicken or 3–4 pounds bone-in chicken, with the skin

Ground paprika, for garnish

Squeeze of lemon, for garnish (optional)

1. Combine the oregano, scallions, garlic, oil, and a healthy pinch of salt and pepper in a mixing bowl and mix well. Add the chicken pieces and toss until they are evenly coated with the herb mixture. Add more oil if needed to get the herbs to stick.

2. Preheat a grill, or preheat the oven to 375°F (190°C). Grill the chicken or roast it on a baking sheet and finish it off under the broiler for a few minutes to brown the tops. The length of the cooking time will depend on the cut of chicken and the thickness; boneless meat will cook faster, while bone-in meat will take longer. Chicken is done when it reaches 165°F (75°C) in the thickest part, all the juices run clear, and the meat is firm to the touch.

3. Serve hot, garnished with paprika for color and with a squeeze of lemon, if desired.

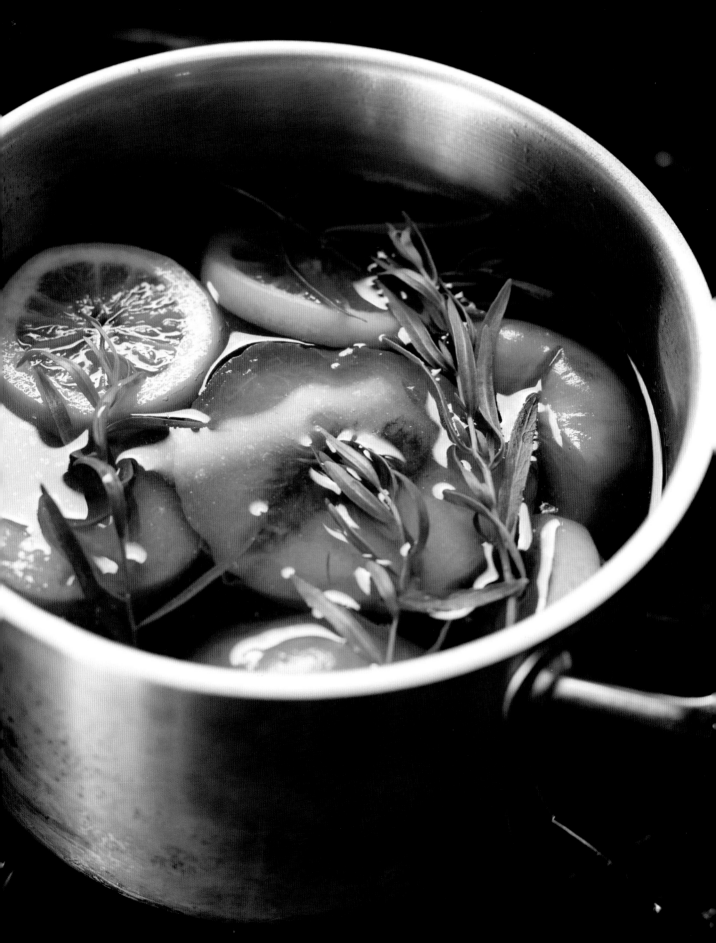

POACHED PEACHES WITH TARRAGON

Nothing feels closer to eating pure sunshine than biting into a ripe, juicy peach on a summer's day. When the air is hot and sticky, and food begins to feel heavy and unappetizing, the peach appears as a welcome respite, its relief cool and sensual. Tarragon's vibrant aromatics are softer and sweeter than those of other culinary herbs (think of the sharper aroma of mint, oregano, thyme, and lavender). This gentleness lends itself well to the soft sweetness of ripe fruit. Allowing the tarragon to steep like tea during the last step of this recipe captures the herb's subtle essences. This dish makes a fabulous after-dinner digestive aid, not to mention a satisfying dessert, and it can stand alone as an afternoon snack or part of a breakfast spread. Consider serving it with oatmeal, biscuits, soft whipped cream, yogurt, or ice cream.

⋆ YIELD: 4 SERVINGS ⋆

4	cups water
¼–½	cup unrefined cane sugar
½	lemon, sliced into ¼-inch-thick rounds
2	tablespoons brandy
1–1½	pounds peaches, cut in half and pitted
4–5	sprigs fresh tarragon or 1 tablespoon dried

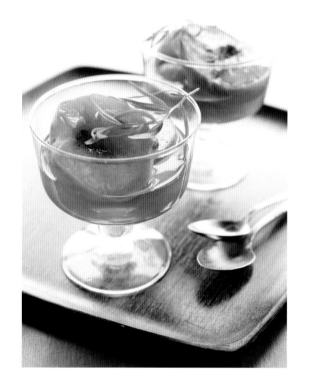

1. Combine the water, sugar (more if you want sweetness, less if you prefer tartness), lemon slices, and brandy in a medium saucepan over medium heat. Heat gently, stirring, until the sugar is dissolved.

2. Add the peaches and bring to a simmer. Let simmer until the peaches are soft, at least 5 minutes. Then remove the peaches with a slotted spoon and set aside. I prefer to leave the skins on, but if you don't care for them, they slip right off after being cooked.

3. Continue simmering the poaching liquid until it has reduced by about half, 10 to 15 minutes. Turn off the heat, return the peaches to the pan, add the tarragon, and let sit with the lid on for 10 minutes.

4. Serve the peaches warm, with a scoop of their poaching liquid.

NUMB?

Large amounts of tarragon can make your mouth feel numb. So don't be alarmed if you experience a numb sensation on the tongue during or after eating this dish.

SAGE AND ORANGE PEEL THROAT SOOTHER TEA

Sage is a fabulous antibacterial, and its pungent, bitter, aromatic compounds stimulate metabolism and activate the immune system. It lends itself well to treating common ailments, including colds and the flu, sore throats, stomach bugs and indigestion, tonsillitis, and mouth sores. The addition of honey to this tea makes it especially soothing in cases of a sore or inflamed throat, and it balances the flavor of the bitter for those who are sensitive.

◆ YIELD: 3 CUPS ◆

3   cups boiling water

¼   cup fresh sage or 2 tablespoons dried

1   tablespoon grated or chopped orange zest
    Honey (optional)

Combine the sage and orange peel in a teapot or jar and pour the boiling water over them. Cover with a lid and let steep for 5 to 15 minutes. Strain and sweeten with honey to taste, if desired. Drink ½ cup, hot, every 1 to 2 hours to soothe a sore throat or symptoms of a head cold.

CITRUS PEEL

Citrus peels have a wonderful, uplifting aroma — great for dispelling depression, invigorating the mind, and uplifting the spirits. The oils in the peel are antimicrobial, lending themselves well to kitchen cleaning projects and teas for colds and flu, like this one here. The inner white pith is a gentle bitter and digestive aid, excellent for gas, bloating, constipation, poor digestion of fats and oils, and lack of appetite. Use the fresh zest or entire peel in cooking, or use it fresh or dried in a soup stock or to make a tea. Enjoy the aromatherapy by putting leftover citrus peel in a pot of water on the stove or woodstove and letting the oils evaporate into the air as it simmers, disinfecting and enlivening.

MINT TISANE

Serving a fresh, hot mint tisane after a meal provides a good excuse to linger at the table, chat, digest, and relax. The tisane itself soothes digestion and settles the stomach. Mint tisane also makes an excellent refresher served iced on a hot day.

◆ YIELD: 3 CUPS ◆

½–1 cup fresh mint, any variety

3 cups just boiling water

Put the mint in a teapot or jar and pour the boiling water over it. Cover with a lid and let steep for 5 to 10 minutes. Strain and serve hot.

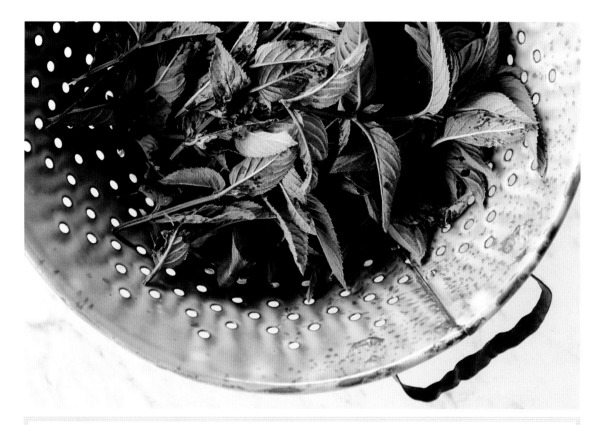

TISANES

A tisane is simply an herbal tea. The word has been used to differentiate between teas made from the tea plant (black tea, green tea, white tea, et cetera) and those made from other herbs. For no reason other than my own preference and habit, I use the word *tisane* mostly to describe hot water infusions of fresh, aromatic herbs — the name sounds rather elegant and elevates the appeal — but technically you can call any water-based preparation of herbs a tisane. Fresh herbs create a subtle and very gentle tisane that captures the aromatic qualities of the herbs in a light, smooth base. Experiment with using any of the common aromatic culinary herbs to make your own tisanes.

ROSE-MERRY-BERRY SYRUP

The rose has long been associated with beauty and the heart — not the anatomical organ, although rose's sour astringency does support cardiovascular tone, but the heart as the emotional home of the human spirit. With its iconic soft scent that soothes even the hardest of days, it helps us find comfort in the simple beauty of life.

Hawthorn berries and blueberries are both loaded with antioxidants, which help the body combat free radicals that can damage the cardiovascular system. Metaphorically, you can think of free radicals as those nagging, irritating feelings and self-critiques that get in the way of our truly loving ourselves and finding beauty in ourselves just as we are. Rosemary is a tonic for the cardiovascular system that gently stimulates circulation. Emotionally, it helps balance fear, encouraging us to be flexible and to get in touch with the courage that lives deep within us all.

◆ YIELD: ABOUT 3 CUPS ◆

4   cups water

1   cup fresh or frozen blueberries

1   cup fresh or ½ cup dried hawthorn berries

½   cup fresh rosemary or ¼ cup dried

½   cup fresh rose petals or ¼ cup dried

1   cup raw honey

I. Combine the water, blueberries, hawthorn berries, rosemary, and rose petals in a saucepan and bring to a simmer over medium heat. Reduce the heat to low and simmer gently, uncovered, until the volume of liquid has reduced by about half, 30 to 45 minutes. Sometimes I estimate the drop in volume by watching the ring that forms inside the pan; other times I use a chopstick to measure and mark the water level as it is cooking. The volume does not have to be exact, so don't worry too much about measuring.

2. Remove from the heat and let cool slightly, then strain through a fine-mesh strainer or fine cheesecloth or cotton muslin. Pour the liquid into a measuring container. If the volume is less than 2 cups, add water to bring it up to 2 cups. Add the honey and stir until completely dissolved.

3. Store the syrup in a glass jar, labeled with the contents and date, in the refrigerator, where it will keep for 3 to 6 months — if you don't devour it completely before then. If mold forms on the surface of the syrup or along the edges of the jar, this is just because of exposure to oxygen. You can simply scrape this surface mold off, transfer the syrup to a clean jar, and continue to use it (the smaller the jar, the less exposure to oxygen and the less likely it is to form mold).

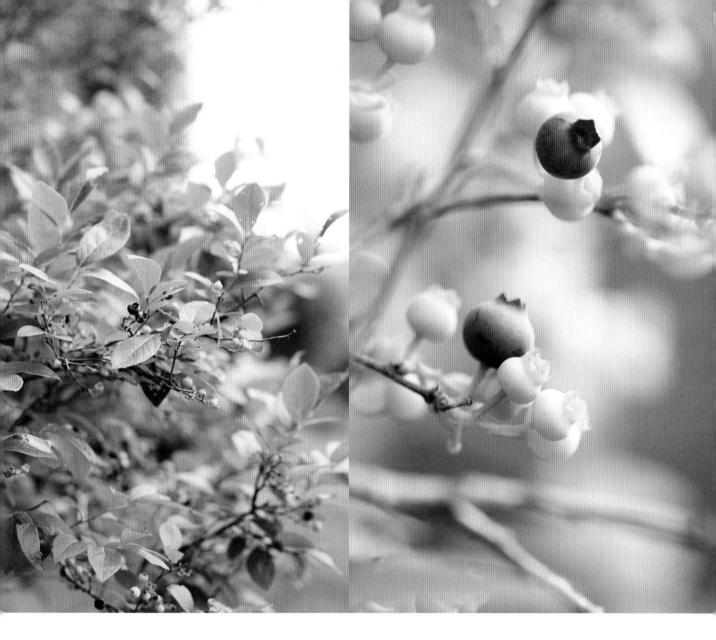

USING YOUR SYRUP

Use Rose-merry-berry Syrup liberally to flavor water, tea, cocktails, and sparkling water. It's lovely in dressings or marinades, or on yogurt, oatmeal, ice cream, or other desserts. And it's delicious — you may not be able to stop yourself from eating it by the spoonful. To use the syrup as a tonic to strengthen the cardiovascular system and support the heart spirit, take 1 to 2 tablespoons per day for 3 to 6 months.

If you prefer a less sweet syrup, instead of 1 cup of honey, use ½ cup honey plus ¼ to ½ cup herb-infused vinegar (to taste). See the recipe for Tarragon-Infused Vinegar (page 186) as an example.

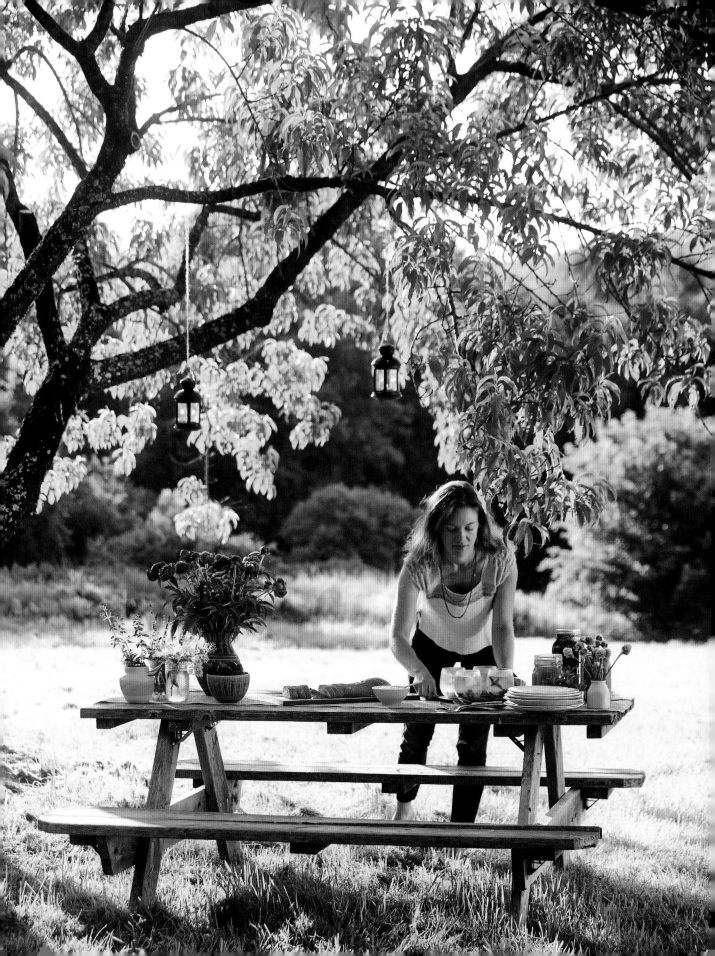

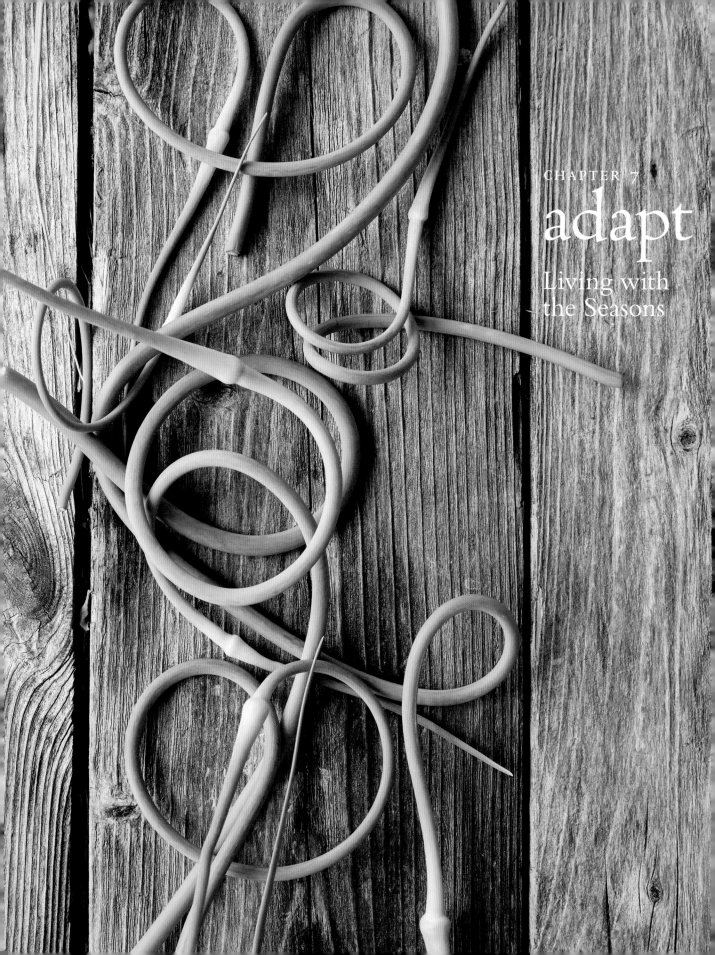

adapt

Living with
the Seasons

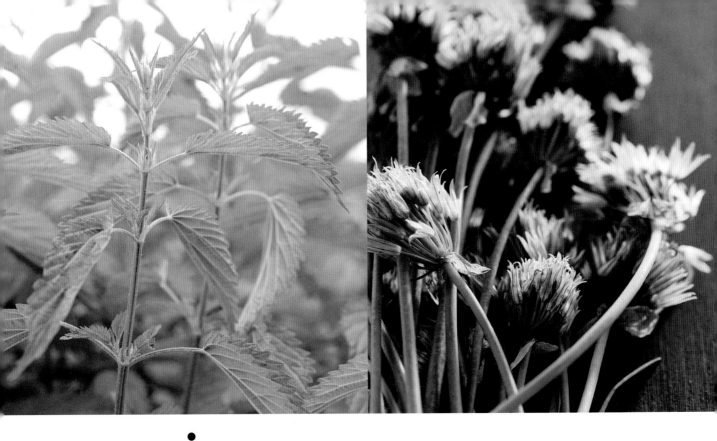

spring

SPRING IS THE DAWN OF THE YEAR. There is a great awakening in spring: the senses come alive to the smells, sounds, and sights of the world as they emerge from the restful hibernation of winter. Days grow longer, rains come, seeds germinate — it is a time of beginnings, growth, and expansion. Spring is the time to take the first steps, to start projects and set out to accomplish goals. Our first steps may not always seem closely tied to long-term end results. "Spring-cleaning" the house, for example, may not seem like it is helping you get a new job or finish last year's projects, but it sets the stage and makes space for your accomplishments to thrive in the days and months to come.

In spring, we can support our body by waking up the metabolism with foods and herbs that gently stimulate digestion and support the liver. You can think of this as spring-cleaning the body, helping to get things moving and clearing cobwebs to prepare for productivity in the seasons ahead. The body's metabolism naturally increases in the springtime as days lengthen and we become more active. An active and healthy metabolism provides energy and inspiration for mind, body, and spirit — just the energy we need for spring's beginnings.

Nature provides an abundance of fresh foods in spring that nourish the body, kick-start the metabolism, and support gentle cleansing. The first plants to appear in spring are tender green herbs and weeds: dandelion, nettle, violet, garlic mustard, chickweed, sorrel, plantain, and more, depending on where you live. These young greens are rich in minerals and fiber, providing valuable nutrition to the body after a winter of eating

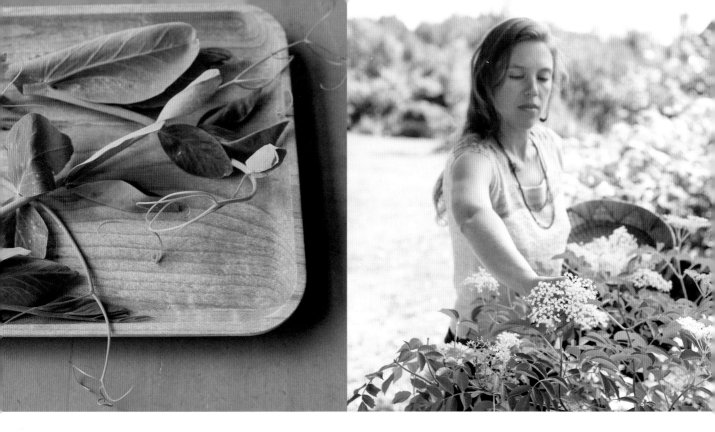

food that has been stored or shipped from warmer climates. They are also alive with flavor. Many, in fact, have a bitter flavor that stimulates the liver and digestive metabolism, helps balance blood sugar, and increases the appetite.

While wild greens are particularly dense with nutrition and bold flavors, cultivated greens are also an important part of the spring diet. From sweet overwintered greens to hearty cold-germinating crops, spinach, kale, collards, lettuce, arugula, parsley, and anything else you can get your hands on are wonderful for remineralizing and jump-starting the metabolism.

Sour is another important flavor for spring, stimulating liver metabolism and the release of bile from the liver and gallbladder, cleansing the tissues, and improving our absorption of minerals. Consider adding a squeeze of lemon or other citrus to your water or to your greens. You can also enjoy sour herbs such as hibiscus or rose hips as teas. Or try fermented foods: yogurt, kefir, sauerkraut, lactofermented pickles, and kvass are all great sour foods to incorporate into your diet in spring to help wake up and nourish the body.

Spring is a transition season, with great variations in the weather and in your body's needs. The body craves smooth transitions, and you can help your body ease into spring by tuning in and listening to your instincts. Incorporate fresh, vibrant foods and raw salads into your diet as you crave them, but don't hesitate to make a hearty stew on a rainy day. Soak up the sun when it is out, but remember to bundle up when the air is cool or the wind blows. Taking care to help the body transition smoothly allows you to preserve your energy for the many beginnings you are germinating at the dawn of your new year.

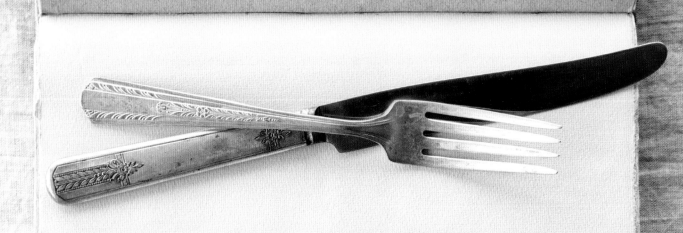

DOING YOUR BEST

Doing the best we can and accepting and embracing it as good enough is an important way to nourish ourselves and to learn to be adaptable. Negative emotions eat away at us and drain our energy. When we can accept our choices and see them as good enough and healthy enough under the circumstances or for their own reasons, we free ourselves of the judgment and guilt that could result instead.

Accepting that we are doing the best we can also gives us permission to exist within our means, with less pressure to live up to an ideal. There are a lot of food ideals out there — eat local, eat organic, eat pastured animal products, grow your own food, make your own food, preserve your own food, and on and on. We might struggle with attaining these ideals for many reasons: cost, access, time, energy. Financial pressure is a real source of stress for the body and mind. Buying food we can't afford because it lives up to an ideal or worrying that we are not eating healthy because we cannot afford the "right" option does more harm to the body than good. When we make decisions from a holistic place that takes into account all aspects of our well-being, we are doing our best. If you can't afford certain food choices, embrace the gift of what you *can* afford. If you're traveling and faced with only less-than-perfect food choices, make the best choice you can and eat it with appreciation.

We live in an imperfect world. We have to constantly weigh our decisions against the reality of what exists and the reality of what makes sense for us as individuals. So give yourself permission: do the best you can, and trust that it is good enough.

POACHED EGGS WITH BÉARNAISE

When spring came around the first full year I had chickens, I began to anticipate an abundance of eggs for my kitchen, yet instead there seemed to be fewer and fewer eggs in the coop. Completely free range, the chickens roamed the yard as they pleased, foraging for bugs and grubs and eating grass. After finding an egg in the woodpile one day, I began to suspect there might be more eggs hidden elsewhere. I smiled, thinking about how perfectly timed the traditional spring Easter egg hunt is for finding eggs in all the small places. Indeed, it turned out my chickens were laying prolifically — everywhere *but* the coop.

Spring is a time of great fertility and plenty, marking the beginnings of life, growth, and ideas. The egg — tangible, abundant, nourishing, and complete — is certainly worth hunting for.

◆ YIELD: 4 SERVINGS ◆

FOR THE BÉARNAISE SAUCE

- ½ cup plus 1 tablespoon butter
- 1 shallot, finely minced

  Salt and freshly ground black pepper
- 2 tablespoons white wine vinegar
- 3 egg yolks
- 2 teaspoons water
- 1–2 tablespoons finely minced fresh tarragon

FOR THE POACHED EGGS

- 1 tablespoon white vinegar
- 4–8 eggs

  Salt and freshly ground pepper

1. Prepare the béarnaise sauce: Melt 1 tablespoon of the butter in a small skillet over low heat. Add the shallot and sauté until translucent, 3 to 5 minutes. Sprinkle with salt and pepper, add the white wine vinegar, and cook, stirring often, until the shallots are tender and the vinegar has evaporated, 3 to 5 minutes.

2. While the shallot is cooking, melt the remaining ½ cup butter in a pan over low heat and transfer into a measuring cup that will allow for easy pouring.

3. Set a large pot of water over high heat to bring to a boil.

4. While the water is heating, combine the egg yolks in a blender with the water. Put the lid on and blend at the lowest setting. Once the mixture is creamy, remove the lid and, with the blender still running at its lowest speed, slowly drizzle in the melted butter.

5. When the butter is thoroughly combined, add the sautéed shallot and the tarragon, and blend until just combined. Season to taste with salt and set aside in a warm place until you're ready to serve.

6. When the pot of water reaches a rolling boil, you're ready to poach the eggs. Stir the white vinegar into the boiling water, then reduce the heat to keep the water at a simmer. Carefully crack each egg into the water. Simmer for 1½ to 2 minutes for a lightly poached egg, or 2 to 3 minutes for a medium poached egg. Remove from the water with a slotted spoon, let any excess water drain away, and lightly season with salt and pepper.

7. Dress each egg with 1 to 2 tablespoons of the béarnaise and serve immediately; the egg will continue to cook as it cools.

SERVING SUGGESTION: I like to serve the eggs on a bed of steamed asparagus or spinach or, during the summer months, with a grilled tomato.

WILD HERB AND GREEN GARLIC SOUP

Foraging for wild greens takes focus, patience, and determination. If you are rushing, foraging is a pain and a bore; if you are relaxed, it is full of joy, giving you the space to appreciate the moment, to enjoy the sounds around you and let your mind wander a little. Spring is so often a time of intense doing: raking the yard, readying the garden, spring-cleaning the house, making plans, going places, seeing people. All the activity is inspiring, but it can be overwhelming. Taking time to settle into the task at hand offers fresh perspective and helps clear the mind. It helps you reconnect to your inner inspiration — a welcome respite and important balance to such action-packed days.

◆ YIELD: 4 SERVINGS ◆

4   tablespoons butter

2   cups chopped green garlic (3–4, including the bulbs and green tops) or 4 cloves cured garlic

2   cups chopped potatoes, in ½-inch cubes (I leave the skins on)

1   cup chopped onion (about 1 medium onion)

    Salt and freshly ground black pepper

2   cups chicken stock, vegetable stock, or water

2   cups whole milk, heavy cream, or a combination

6–8 ounces wild herbs, chopped (about 6–8 packed cups)

    Crème fraîche or sour cream, for garnish (optional)

1. Melt the butter in a soup pot over low heat. Add the garlic, potatoes, and onion, and sauté, stirring often, until the potatoes have begun to soften at the edges, about 10 minutes. Sprinkle with salt and pepper.

2. Add the stock and milk. Increase the heat to medium, bring just to a simmer, then reduce the heat and simmer until the potatoes are soft, 10 to 15 minutes. Add the greens and boil gently, uncovered, until the greens are just tender but still have their vibrant green color, 3 to 5 minutes.

3. Remove from the heat. Purée with an immersion blender or in a blender. (Always be careful when puréeing hot liquids in a blender. Never fill the container more than one-third full to avoid the risk of the lid blowing off.) Serve hot, garnished with crème fraîche or sour cream.

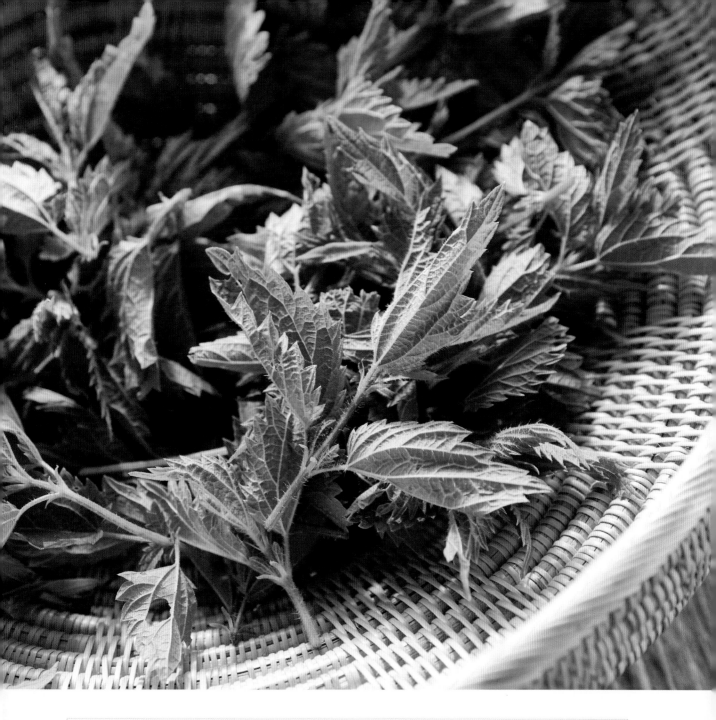

WILD HERBS AND GREENS

There is no limit to the greens you can use in this soup. Just make sure you have
correctly identified whichever plants you are harvesting. This soup will be different every time,
depending on the greens you use; adjust the quantity of each depending on how much
you like the flavor. Some of my favorite wild greens include garlic mustard, nettle, lamb's quarters,
dandelion, wild sorrel, mallow, violet, and watercress.

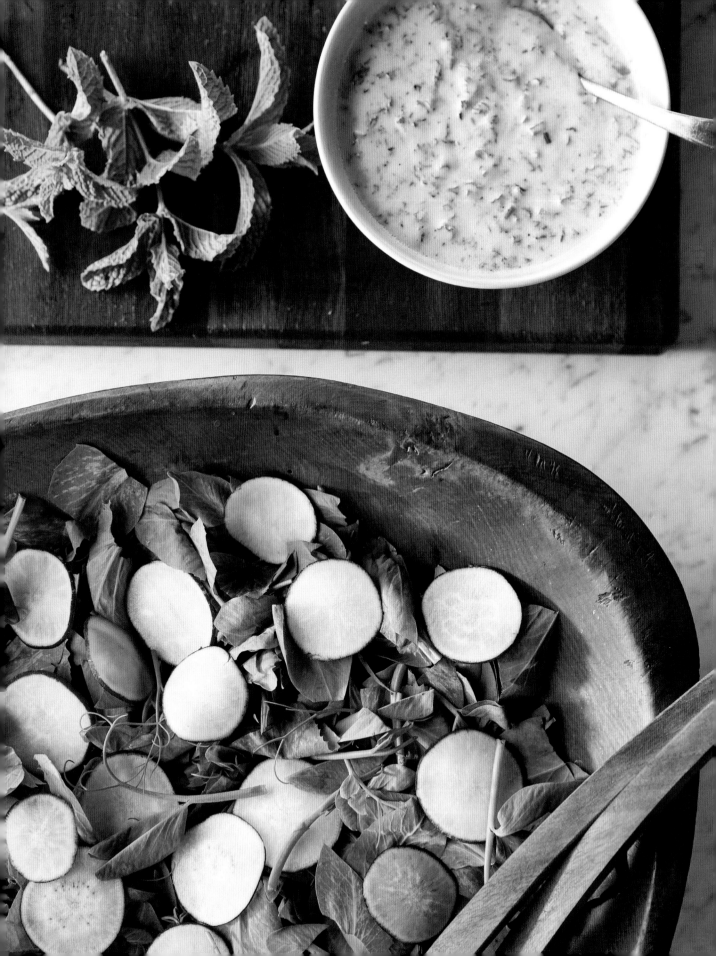

PEA GREENS AND RADISH SALAD WITH YOGURT MINT DRESSING

Climbing, curling, crawling . . . peas, like other plants that climb, are full of remarkable determination. If they don't have anything to climb up they keep growing anyways, sometimes even twisting together, using one another for support. It's their nature, and with or without structure they follow that instinct to twist and climb and ramble. There is a very springlike energy in their frantic quest forward: even though they may not know exactly where they are going, they never lose sight of that drive to move ever onward.

Like many spring foods, pea greens offer us that most tender first growth, the new quality that we look forward to and savor because it happens only once a year. For something so determined, these baby greens are remarkably tender.

◆ MAKES 4 SERVINGS ◆

½ pound pea greens, tough stems removed, roughly chopped

½ pound red radishes, thinly sliced

Fresh whole mint leaves, for garnish

FOR THE DRESSING

½ cup plain yogurt

¼ cup olive oil

¼ cup finely chopped chives or scallions

¼ cup finely chopped fresh mint

1 tablespoon raw apple cider vinegar

Salt and freshly ground black pepper

I. Put the pea greens in a bowl and arrange the radish slices on top.

2. Prepare the dressing: Combine the yogurt, oil, chives, mint, vinegar, and salt and pepper to taste in a jar or bowl and shake or mix well. If the dressing is too thick, add a little water (up to 1 tablespoon) to thin it.

3. Drizzle the dressing over the salad and toss well. Garnish with mint leaves. Any extra dressing can be stored in the refrigerator, where it will keep for up to 5 days. It goes well with other salads, steamed vegetables, and grains.

LEMON ROASTED ASPARAGUS
WITH BAKED GOAT CHEESE

The part of the asparagus we eat is the young, tender plant shoot — and if eating the most tender, freshest part of a plant's growth was not exotic enough, the short season enhances asparagus's delectability. They are worth looking forward to all year and indulging in fully when in season. Roasting asparagus spears is one of the easiest ways to prepare them and to maintain their fresh flavor and crisp texture. I often crave goat cheese in the spring; the soft texture and sour, tangy flavor is an excellent complement to the juicy, sweet asparagus. This duo makes a nice light meal served alongside crispy bread with olive oil or lettuce with vinaigrette. It can also be served as a first course or as a side dish.

◆ YIELD: 4 SERVINGS ◆

2   tablespoons finely chopped chives

2   tablespoons finely chopped fresh oregano

2   tablespoons finely chopped fresh thyme

2   tablespoons finely chopped pecans or walnuts

2   tablespoons plus 2 teaspoons olive oil

8   ounces soft goat cheese
    Salt

1   pound asparagus, tougher stems snapped off

1   teaspoon fresh lemon juice

I.   Preheat the oven to 375°F (190°C).

2.   Combine the chives, oregano, thyme, and pecans in a shallow dish and mix well. Pour 2 tablespoons of the oil into a shallow bowl.

3.   If the goat cheese is not already in a log, roll it into a log 1½ to 2 inches in diameter and flatten the ends. Slice the cheese into ½- to ¾-inch-thick disks, making 8 total pieces. If they crumble or break apart, gently press them back together. One at a time, dip the cheese disks into the oil, then gently press them into the herb mixture, thoroughly coating all sides, and place them on a baking sheet. When you're done, sprinkle the cheese disks with salt.

4.   Place the asparagus on a separate baking sheet. Drizzle with the remaining 2 teaspoons oil and the lemon juice, add a sprinkle of salt, and roll them around on the sheet until they are well coated.

5.   Put the sheet of asparagus in the oven to bake. After 5 minutes, add the sheet of cheese. Bake for 5 to 6 minutes longer, until the asparagus is bright green and cooked through but still has a nice crunch and the cheese begins to sizzle and the center is soft.

6.   Let cool for 3 to 5 minutes and then use a spatula to carefully remove the disks from the baking sheet. Arrange on a platter with the asparagus and serve immediately.

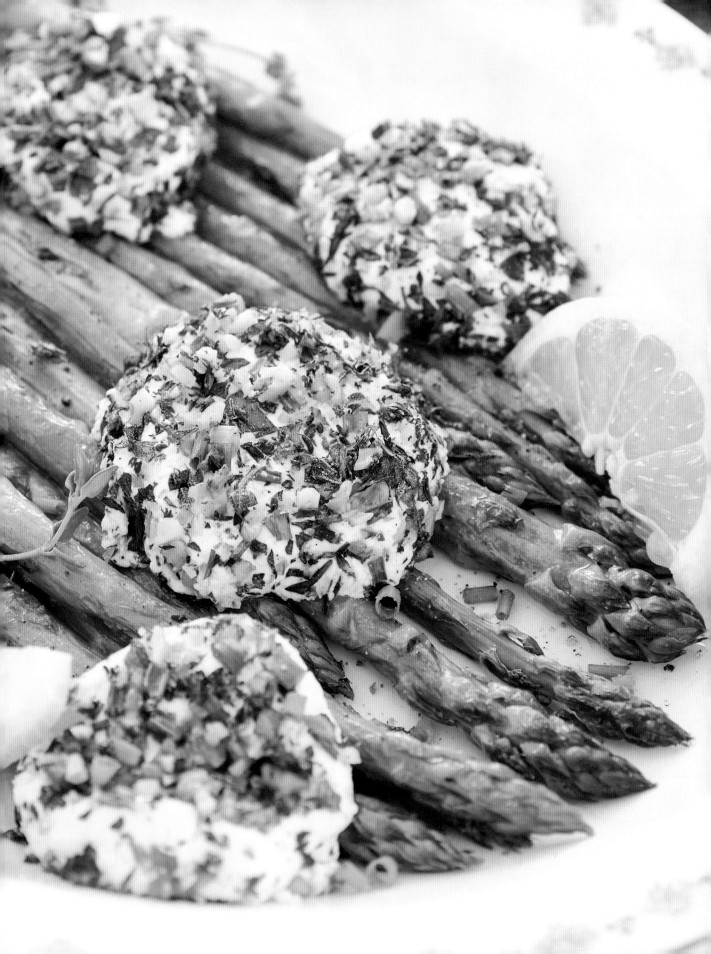

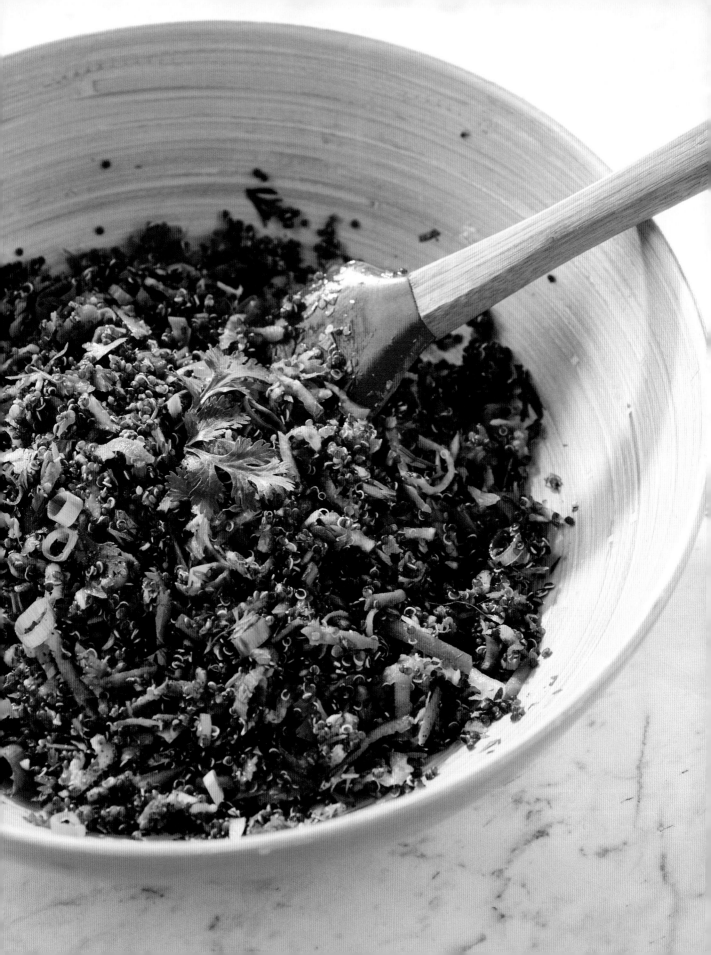

RED QUINOA SALAD WITH RADISH AND CARROT

With the rebirth of spring comes an abundance of social gatherings, as we emerge from the dark and reconnect with each other — picnics, potlucks, meals with friends, casual fare on the porch. For those moments, the perfect spring-inspired dish is easy to prepare, versatile, and delicious served cold. Cilantro and radish both love cool, sunny spring days and provide a lively, refreshing flavor. After soaking the quinoa overnight, you hardly have to cook it, which reduces the salad's preparation time significantly. I first made this dish for my brother's annual outdoor potluck birthday bash. The lawn was radiant with the neon green growth of early spring, friends and family enjoyed lively conversations, the wind gently rustled the trees, and bits of color from flowering trees painted the horizon — the day was alive with the energy of the new season.

◆ YIELD: 4 SERVINGS ◆

1½	cups uncooked red quinoa
1	tablespoon raw apple cider vinegar
1	cup grated carrot (1 large or 2 small)
1	cup grated radish or hakurei turnip (about ⅓ pound)
	Juice of 1 lime
½	cup finely chopped chives or scallions
¼	cup finely grated fresh ginger (2–3 inches)
⅛–¼	cup finely grated garlic (3–4 cloves)
2	tablespoons sesame oil
2	tablespoons tamari
½–¾	cup chopped cilantro
	Salt and freshly ground black pepper

I. Soak the quinoa with the vinegar and enough water to cover by 2 inches for 12 to 24 hours. I usually start soaking the quinoa the night before I prepare the dish; that way I can cook it anytime the next day.

2. Strain the quinoa from its soaking water, rinse in cold water, and combine in a saucepan with enough water to cover by 3 inches. Bring to a boil, then reduce the heat and simmer, uncovered, for 5 minutes. Turn off the heat, cover, and let cool for 10 to 15 minutes. Strain the quinoa through a fine-mesh strainer and place in a bowl to cool completely.

3. Meanwhile, combine the carrot and radish with the lime juice in a large bowl and mix well. Add the chives, ginger, garlic, oil, and tamari, and mix well. Once the quinoa has cooled, add it to the bowl along with the cilantro. Mix well, season with salt and pepper to taste, and serve.

LAVENDER AND DANDELION FLOWER MUFFINS

As ubiquitous as dandelions are, their flowers do not have a long season. Vibrant green grass carpeted with bright yellow flowers so sunny that they boast a golden halo are an iconic spring landscape here in New England. It's an image that can't help but inspire a daydream of children happily racing about, picking flowers to make a dandelion chain, and laughing as they collapse to the ground, filled with pure joy at being finally sprung from the house after a long winter. It doesn't matter that the flowers quickly wilt — the joy and laughter of spring remain long after the blossoms have passed.

◆ YIELD: ABOUT 10 MUFFINS ◆

2¼	cups flour (I use a combination of white and wheat spelt)
2	teaspoons baking powder
1	teaspoon baking soda
1	teaspoon ground cinnamon
½	teaspoon salt
½	cup (1 stick) butter, melted
2	eggs, lightly beaten
¾	cup milk
½–¾	cup honey (depending on how sweet you like your muffins)
1	teaspoon vanilla extract
2	cups loosely packed dandelion flower petals (base and green leaves removed)
2	tablespoons dried lavender flowers
½	cup chopped nuts (optional)

1. Preheat the oven to 400°F (200°C). Generously grease 10 cups in a muffin pan.

2. Combine the flour, baking powder, baking soda, cinnamon, and salt in a large bowl and mix well.

3. Combine the butter, eggs, milk, honey, and vanilla in a separate bowl and whisk together. Add to the dry ingredients and mix until just combined. Add the dandelion petals, lavender flowers, and nuts, if using, and stir until just combined.

4. Fill the prepared muffin cups to the top with batter. Bake for 14 to 17 minutes, or until a toothpick inserted into the center comes out clean.

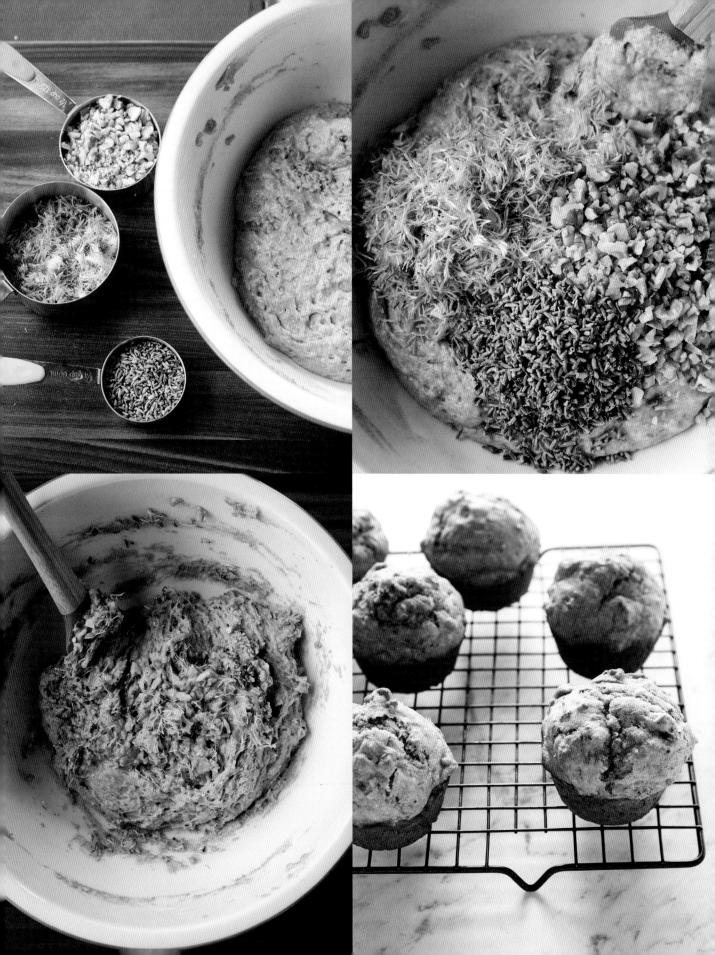

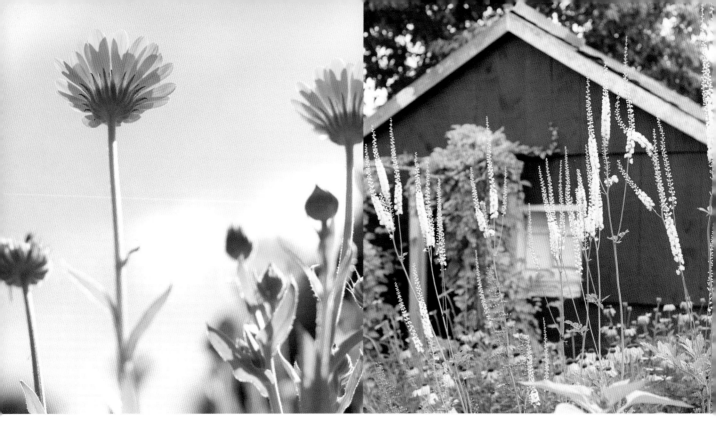

summer

SUMMER HAS TWO DISTINCT QUALITIES.
One is the sense of utter calm and contentment born from abundance. The other is
the frenetic sense of urgency that is inspired
by such rapid growth. Summer is a time of
expansion and plenty. Everything is powerful.
The sun is hot, the air is warm, the storms are
loud and assertive, plants grow and bloom,
animals bustle, abundance surrounds. With
that bounty comes feelings of security: it feels
safe and easy to relax and bask in the joy of
food and life that surrounds us. At the same
time, all that activity inspires activity within
us, encouraging us to go to the neighborhood
potluck and then plan our own, to go on
vacation, take a road trip, play at the beach,
take long walks in the woods, work in the
garden, go swimming, and watch the sunset
with a picnic dinner. It can be exciting, overwhelming, inspiring, playful, relaxed, busy,
energetic, and exhausting all at the same time.

Living with grace in the summertime is
about learning to balance these many qualities. It is a call to find calm and contentment
amid great growth, activity, and expansion.
It is an invitation to have fun and experience
joy and also to find the quiet, introspective,
meditative quality that accompanies the
energy of the busy bee. When you are in the
yard or garden, for example, thinking about
all the things you have to do, remember to
look up and watch the wind rustle the leaves
of the trees. As you go through your summer,
however busy it may be, remember to take
the time to acknowledge and enjoy all the
beauty that surrounds us. Summer is a time of

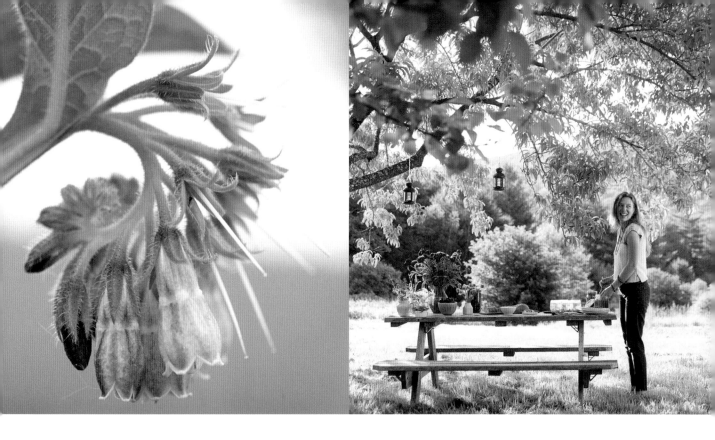

immense joy; as the saying goes, don't forget to "stop and smell the roses."

When it is hot out, eating hot food and heating up the house by cooking often feel unappealing. Not coincidentally, summer provides bountiful crisp, colorful vegetables and juicy, ripe fruits. Green salads, grain salads, or other cold dishes are all good choices, as are smoothies and fresh fruit and vegetable juices. Look to cooling foods and herbs, like cucumbers, cilantro, mint, and melons, for their marked cooling and hydrating effects.

While cooling foods are appropriate for summer, so are spicy dishes, which are often featured heavily in the cuisines of hot climates. This is because spicy food makes you sweat. Sweating releases heat from the core of the body and cools you as it evaporates from your skin.

There are many summer-appropriate recipes speckled throughout this book. Consider Cilantro Lemonade (page 129) to cool you off on a hot summer day, or Cucumber Raita with Dill and Black Mustard Seeds (page 115) to complement a summer picnic, or a spicy dish such as Roasted Eggplant with Chickpeas, Spicy Peppers, and Mint Oil (page 180). When the garden is overflowing with summer's bounty, you might try Ratatouille (page 87) or Red Pepper and Feta Amuse-Bouche (page 198). When late summer begins to feel like fall and root vegetables and squashes are on the horizon, you might seek comfort in some parsley pesto (page 77). And of course, in the spirit of summer, don't forget to put some of that busy bee energy into a few of your own experiments in the kitchen!

ROASTED TOMATOES with BASIL AND OLIVE OIL

Summer provides a bounty of fresh food that is delicious all on its own, with little help from the cook. In this time of ready abundance, it doesn't take that much work to put good food on the table. And that frees us up to spend more time outside, enjoying the season and growing food, for example. It also frees us to spend time in our kitchen pickling and preserving the harvest for the seasons ahead . . . or just relaxing! These roasted tomatoes are a great example of the way that a simple food preparation technique can enhance the flavor of fresh food without distracting you from its inherently delicious nature.

◆ YIELD: 4 SERVINGS ◆

- 4 perfectly ripe tomatoes
- 1–2 tablespoons olive oil
- Salt and freshly ground black pepper
- 1 handful basil leaves (about ¼ cup)

1. Preheat the broiler. Position the upper oven rack so it sits 6 to 8 inches from the heat source.

2. Slice the tomatoes in half along the equator (in the center, between the top and bottom). Drizzle about 1 teaspoon of the oil on a baking sheet. Place the tomatoes, cut side up, on the baking sheet. Generously season each with salt and pepper and a drizzle of oil. Broil the tomatoes for 5 to 7 minutes, until the tomatoes look tender and the tops are sizzling.

3. While the tomatoes are roasting, cut the basil. Stack the leaves on top of one another and roll them into a cylinder, then finely chop into thin strips. Remove the tomatoes from the oven, transfer to a serving platter, and garnish with the basil and another drizzle of oil. Serve immediately.

VARIATIONS

These roasted tomatoes are excellent fresh from the oven, but they also store well in the refrigerator for a few days. You can reheat them and serve with poached eggs or slice them and add to sandwiches, salads, or grain, pasta, or bean dishes.
The tomatoes are also good with grated Parmesan cheese sprinkled on top before they're roasted.

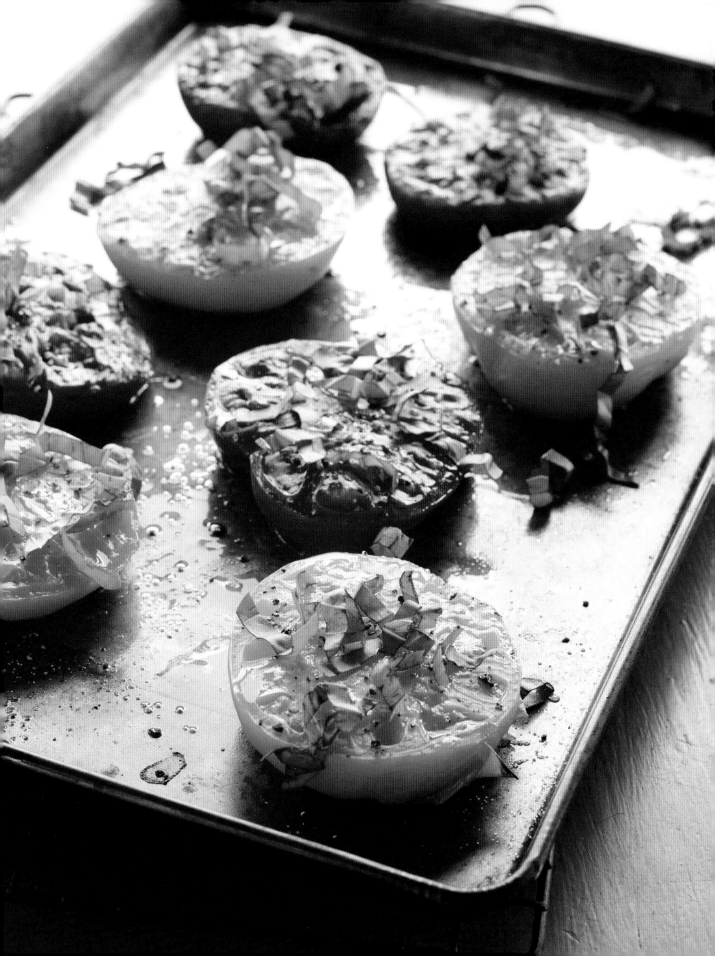

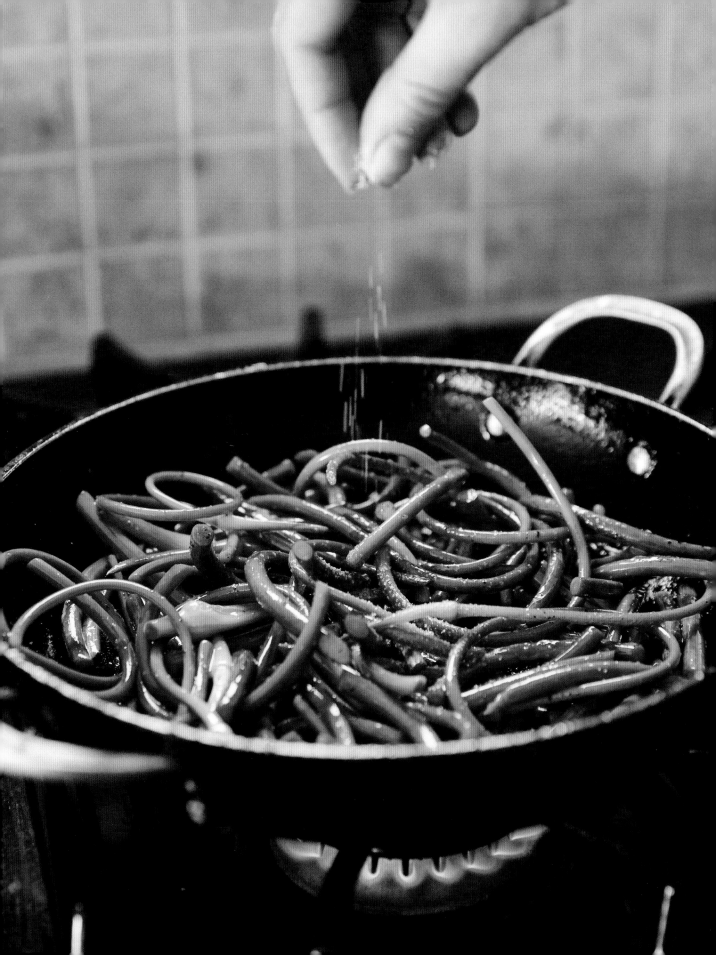

GARLIC SCAPES IN WHITE WINE

Garlic scape season is an abundant one. But there is only so much scape pesto, steamed scapes, roasted scapes, grilled scapes, sautéed scapes, scape salad dressing . . . you get the idea . . . a person can eat! While I love these curly wonders, I also sometimes scratch my head, pondering what else I could possibly do with them. When my freezer is full of pesto and I'm sick of everything else, this is one trick up my sleeve.

For those who don't struggle with the issue of scape mania, consider growing your own garlic to join the fun. You can also often find garlic scapes for sale at farmers' markets. See Garlicky Braised Lamb (page 286) for another scape use.

◆ YIELD: 4 SERVINGS AS A SIDE DISH ◆

2 tablespoons olive oil

½ pound garlic scapes, chopped into 4-inch pieces

Salt and freshly ground black pepper

½ cup dry white wine

I. Heat the oil in a large skillet over medium heat. When the oil is hot, add the scapes and sauté, stirring often, until the scapes are bright green, 3 to 5 minutes. Season generously with salt and pepper, then add the wine and immediately cover. Let the scapes cook, stirring occasionally, until tender, 5 to 8 minutes.

2. Once the scapes are tender, remove the lid and turn up the heat. Cook, stirring continually, until the scapes brown slightly and the remaining wine has evaporated. The sugars in the scapes may caramelize a little; this is a good thing, so just keep stirring. Serve hot.

MISO PEANUT SAUCE

With a little flock of hens in the backyard and a partner who owns a farm, I usually have ample eggs and veggies. During the summer months I try to keep rice wrappers around. These thin sheets of pressed, dried rice can be rehydrated and used to wrap a spring roll. Many a time, when there is no other plan for dinner, we lay out bowls of thinly sliced or grated veggies, aromatic herbs, scrambled eggs, peanut sauce, and other spring roll fixings, and then we each stuff our own rolls, right at the table. This is one of the sauces I make for these meals. It can be put in a spring roll, served on the side as a dipping sauce, cooked into a stir-fry, or tossed with steamed vegetables or rice noodles. It makes a satisfying accompaniment to a light summer meal.

For the best-tasting sauce, use a natural peanut butter without additives. The ingredients should be nothing more than peanuts, with maybe a little salt.

◆ YIELD: ABOUT 1 CUP ◆

2	cups packed cilantro
½	cup natural peanut butter
½	cup water
2	tablespoons sesame oil
2	tablespoons unsweetened rice wine vinegar or raw apple cider vinegar
2	tablespoons tamari
2	tablespoons chopped fresh ginger
2–3	garlic cloves
1	tablespoon naturally fermented, unpasteurized miso (I like brown rice miso)
⅛	teaspoon cayenne pepper
	Salt (optional)

Combine the cilantro, peanut butter, water, oil, vinegar, tamari, ginger, garlic, miso, and cayenne in a food processor and blend until smooth. Taste for salt before serving; depending on how salty your miso paste is, you may want to add a pinch.

KITCHEN NOTES

If you want the sauce to be thinner, more like a dipping sauce, just add more water. Serve garnished with cilantro, fresh green onions, or chives. The sauce goes very well with mint; consider adding mint to your spring roll toppings or garnishing with mint oil (follow the instructions for Basil Oil on page 274, substituting fresh mint for the basil and letting the oil steep for 24 hours). Store any leftover sauce in the refrigerator, where it will keep for up to 5 days. This recipe makes about 1 cup, which I usually find serves 4 people as a sauce or condiment and dresses 8 ounces of pasta.

SPICY BLACK BEAN SALAD

Picnics are one of my favorite summer activities. Long, warm days lend themselves well to a leisurely meal outside. All you need is a basket, bag, or box for your supplies and food that is good served at room temperature. A picnic blanket can be a nice touch, but even that isn't necessary. You can picnic almost anywhere: in the backyard, along a riverbank, at the edge of a pond or swimming hole, under a sunset, or in the park. The simple act of packing a meal and heading outside can feel like vacation. A picnic makes it easy to get lost — lost in conversation, in tasty food, in the landscape, and in the joy and playfulness of summer. This spicy salad is a great, flavorful accompaniment for any summer picnic. I like to dice the veggies into very small pieces, so that you get all the flavors in every bite!

◆ YIELD: 2 SERVINGS AS A MAIN COURSE OR 4 SERVINGS AS A SIDE DISH ◆

1   cup dried black beans

1   cup chopped cilantro

1   cup corn kernels (see the note below)

¾   cup diced cucumber or cucamelon

¾   cup diced bell pepper (red, orange, or yellow)

¾   cup cherry tomatoes, halved or quartered

½   cup finely chopped red onion

2   tablespoons finely chopped garlic

1   tablespoon finely chopped jalapeño pepper

2   teaspoons ground cumin

1   teaspoon ground coriander

1   teaspoon ground turmeric

3   tablespoons olive oil, plus more as needed

2   tablespoons fresh lime juice

    Salt

I. Soak the beans in enough water to cover by 6 inches for 8 to 12 hours.

2. Drain the beans and transfer to a saucepan with enough water to cover by 2 inches. Bring to a boil. Skim any foam off the top, then reduce the heat and simmer gently, covered, stirring every 10 minutes, until the beans are soft through, 50 to 60 minutes. Add more water as needed to keep the beans covered by a couple inches. Let the beans cool for 10 to 15 minutes in their cooking liquid and then drain and let cool completely.

3. Combine the beans with the cilantro, corn, cucumber, bell pepper, tomatoes, onion, garlic, and jalapeño, and toss to combine. Add the cumin, coriander, turmeric, oil, lime juice, and a generous pinch of salt and toss again. Add more oil as needed to moisten.

CORN: COOKED, RAW, OR FROZEN

Leftover cooked corn on the cob is perfect for this recipe; just cut it off the cob and it is ready to use. If you have uncooked corn, cut it off the cob raw and sauté it in olive oil over medium heat until it is just cooked through, 3 to 5 minutes. It should be bright yellow and sweet but still crunchy, with a good "pop." You can use frozen corn if that is all you have, but I think fresh is better. If you're using frozen corn, thaw it completely and drain it well before adding it to the salad.

HERBES DE PROVENCE

Herbes de Provence is a blend of herbs that originates from the southeastern Provence region of France. The herbs can vary, but the character of the blend is marked by the anise-like flavors of tarragon and fennel and the floral notes of lavender. The blend can be used on fish, meats, and grilled vegetables. I think it also makes a nice tea.

◆ YIELD: 2 TABLESPOONS ◆

1   teaspoon dried marjoram or oregano

1   teaspoon dried summer or winter savory

1   teaspoon dried tarragon

1   teaspoon dried thyme

1   teaspoon dried rosemary

½   teaspoon dried lavender flowers

½   teaspoon ground fennel seeds

Combine the herbs in a bowl, adjusting the proportions to suit your own palate. Mix well and store in an airtight container in a cool, dark spot. The blend should keep for up to a year.

YOUR HERBAL PANTRY

If you have a surfeit of herbs during the summer months, consider drying some of them to use in an herbes de Provence mix later on. See page 57 for details on how to dry herbs. You can also experiment with making other herbal blends to use in cooking or for teas.

HERBAL BALSAMIC VINAIGRETTE

Salads are a summer staple at my house. It's so easy to combine whatever greens, weeds, veggies, and herbs I can take from the garden with whatever cheeses, nuts, leftover grains or beans, and meat or fish I have on hand in the fridge. Hefty salads are an easy, satisfying lunch on a hot summer day, and having dressing on hand makes them more convenient, delicious, and digestible. This dressing is perfect for the growing season — it takes advantage of the fresh herbs flourishing in the garden and brings the warmth and delightful aromatic essence of summer straight to your plate.

◆ YIELD: 1½ CUPS ◆

1   cup olive oil

3   tablespoons balsamic vinegar

1   teaspoon Dijon mustard

1   teaspoon raw honey

2   tablespoons chopped chives or chive blossoms

2   tablespoons fresh oregano

2   tablespoons fresh tarragon

2   tablespoons fresh thyme

1–2   garlic cloves, roughly chopped

Salt and freshly ground black pepper

Combine the oil, vinegar, mustard, and honey with the chives, oregano, tarragon, thyme, garlic, and a pinch of salt and pepper in a blender and blend until smooth. Add more vinegar or mustard if you like a dressing with a more pungent flavor. Store in the refrigerator, where the dressing will keep for 2 to 3 weeks.

GARDEN TEA

Teas like this one, made with whatever fresh herbs are available, are wonderful in spring and summer, when herbs grow with enthusiasm. Stimulating, pungent, bitter, aromatic herbs like these support metabolic processes, including the digestion and assimilation of nutrients, and encourage gentle clearing and cleansing just when the body needs it.

◆ YIELD: 4 CUPS ◆

1   handful fresh herbs (oregano, marjoram, mint, rosemary, sage, lavender, lemon balm, or any combination)

4   cups boiling water

Combine the herbs in a teapot or jar and pour the boiling water over them. Cover with a lid and let steep for 5 to 15 minutes. Strain and enjoy hot or at room temperature.

SAUTÉED BLUEBERRIES
WITH LAVENDER ESSENCE AND WHIPPED CREAM

When it comes to fresh fruit, less is usually more. This is almost like a blueberry soup — a simple and honest celebration of the berry. The berries are gently warmed, just to coax out the juices, and subtly complemented with aromatic lavender and creamy butter. The best part is watching the whipped cream dissolve softly into the beautiful purple berries, making marbled patterns in varying shades of blue and purple. This makes a great afternoon snack, breakfast, or dessert.

◆ YIELD: 4 SERVINGS ◆

1	tablespoon fresh or dried lavender flowers
¼	cup boiling water
3	cups fresh blueberries
1	tablespoon unsalted butter
2–4	tablespoons raw honey
1	cup heavy cream

I. Put the lavender flowers in a teapot or jar and pour the boiling water over them. Cover with a lid and let steep for 10 minutes, then strain into a saucepan.

2. Add the blueberries, butter, and honey to taste to the lavender infusion. Heat over medium heat until the berries soften and release their juices, 5 to 6 minutes.

3. While the berries are cooking, whip the cream until it forms soft peaks. Serve the berries hot, in bowls, with generous dollops of the whipped cream.

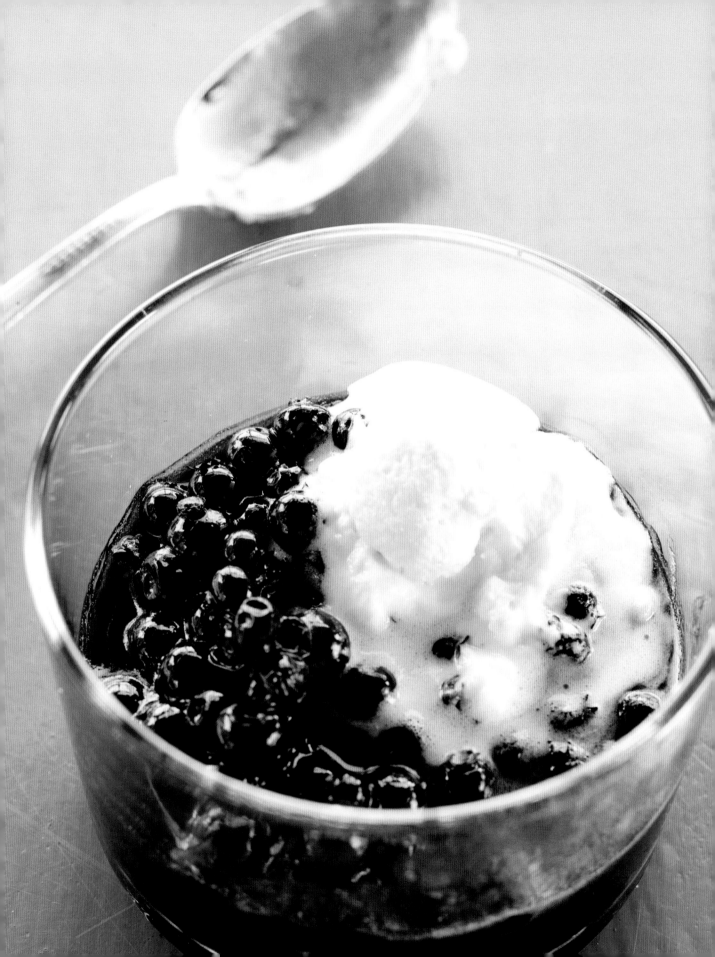

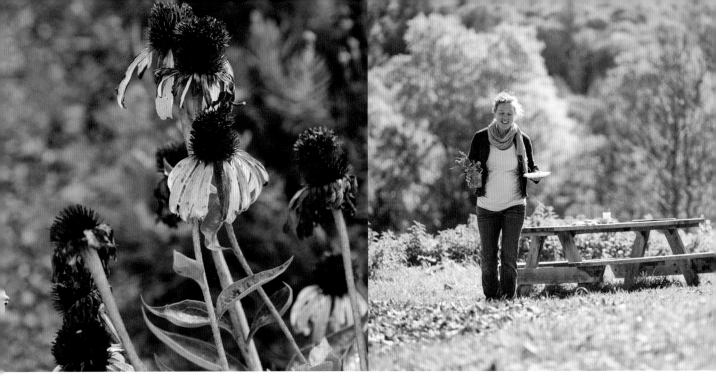

fall

LIKE SPRING, FALL IS A TRANSITION SEASON, marking the time between the warmest and the coldest, the brightest and the darkest seasons of the year. Whereas in spring we prepare for the outward and expansive qualities of summer, in fall we begin to prepare for the quieter, more contracted space of winter. Making our way from the abundance of summer into the solitude of winter can be a challenge. Fall is the time for soaking up the last of the season's warmth and color. It is also a time to practice letting go.

After trees and flowers bloom and fruit ripens, there is rotting. The great process of decomposition and decay begins in fall. As we let go of the rich life that characterizes every nook and cranny of the summer world, we watch days get shorter and colder, we watch weather patterns change, we watch leaves and plants pass and fall and begin to decompose, and we watch animals gather and store. It is a reminder that change is both inevitable and beautiful and that all life ends to be reborn in another form: in spring, seeds will sprout in the organic material of last fall's fallen leaves.

In our lives, we can learn lessons about trusting process and seeing the evolution and forward growth that transition can bring. Fall can be an important time to reassess your values — to shed layers, to practice letting go of things, people, or patterns that don't serve you, and to make space to be who you truly are in the quiet internal moments to come. This could look like cleaning out your closet and getting rid of old clothes, or saying no to too many social activities or obligations at work. Letting go might even look like giving yourself permission to relax on the couch with a good book instead of cleaning the house. It is a time to let go of what you don't need —

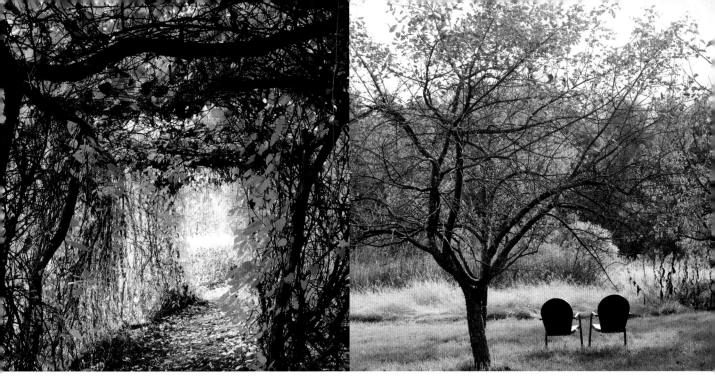

and maybe even some of the things you *think* you do need — in order to reserve and preserve the bounty that already exists inside you. You will need that bounty of the soul in the dark months to come.

Fall provides plentiful orange, yellow, and red foods: pumpkins, squashes, sweet potatoes, carrots, beets, corn. These are the storage crops, the foods that have traditionally sustained agriculturalists through the doldrums of winter. They are also the last gifts of the sun. Their rich, warm colors serve as mementos of the joy and warmth provided by those nourishing, life-sustaining golden rays. These foods are heavy, sweet, rich in calories, and full of vitamins and minerals. According to traditional Chinese medicine, it is these foods that build and strengthen the blood and build deep energy reserves, preparing the body for the winter months ahead.

Fall is a time to transition to warmer foods: roasted root vegetables, stewed meats and vegetables, and soaked and slow-cooked grains. Salads here and there can freshen up a meal, as can fermented foods, pesto, and other condiments. But as the season progresses, days get shorter, and temperatures drop, it is important to eat more cooked foods, the kinds of foods that leave you feeling satisfied and warm inside.

You might also consider bringing the beauty and warmth of fall's colors into your home. Dry a few cobs of corn to decorate the wall or the front door, make a table arrangement with fallen leaves or dried flowers, or string hot peppers or fallen leaves from thread and hang them on the wall. Make space for these colors to glow and radiate in your home, so that they can fill even the darkest of winter days with warmth and color.

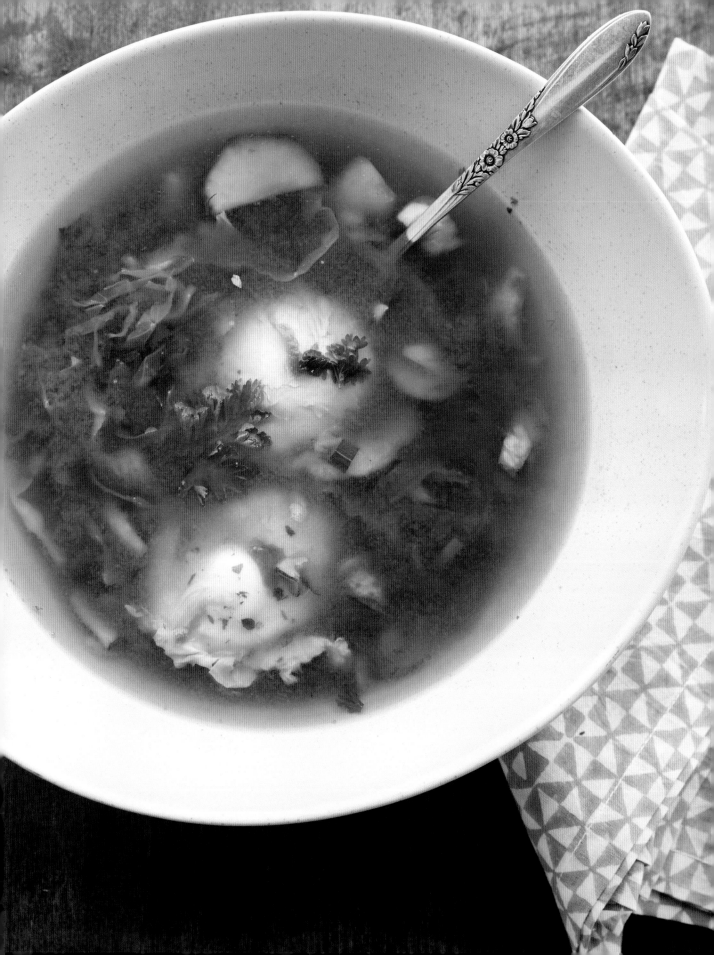

BREAKFAST FOR CHAMPIONS

Breakfast is an important meal, yet mornings can be a busy time. Many quick breakfast foods are highly processed and rich in simple carbohydrates and sugars that give short-term energy without providing fuel for later. In contrast, a breakfast that has good fats and protein, in a form that doesn't take a lot of energy for the body to process and absorb, will leave you feeling immediately energized *and* offer fuel for the day ahead. This simple breakfast is a breakfast for champions, offering all the nutrition you need in a form that is easy to digest and assimilate. While it is quick to make, it does require that you sit down to eat it, which in itself sets an intentional and well-grounded tone for the day.

✦ YIELD: 1 SERVING ✦

2 cups water, vegetable broth, or Bone Broth (page 203)

2 tablespoons chopped fresh herbs of your choice (parsley, cilantro, garlic, thyme, oregano, chives, et cetera)

¼ teaspoon apple cider vinegar or white vinegar

2 tablespoons chopped fermented vegetables (try Vital Roots Kimchi, page 116; Deep-Sea Purple Kraut, page 83; or Pickled Daikon with Cilantro and Lime Zest, page 170)

1 tablespoon miso paste

2 eggs

1. Combine the water in a small saucepan with the fresh herbs and vinegar and bring to a gentle boil. While the water is heating, put the fermented vegetables and miso paste in a serving bowl.

2. When the broth reaches a gentle boil, gently crack each egg into the saucepan. Cook at a gentle simmer until the eggs are cooked to your liking, 1 to 3 minutes for a medium yolk or 4 to 5 minutes for a well-done yolk. I like a runny yolk, so I cook the eggs just until the whites are cooked through, about 1½ to 2 minutes.

3. Spoon the cooked eggs and their broth into the serving bowl. Break up the miso with a spoon and gently stir until it has dissolved.

NOTE: This recipe calls for just 2 cups of liquid for poaching the eggs because that's the amount of broth that I like to eat with my soup. For this amount of liquid you will need to use a small saucepan (5 to 6 inches in diameter) so that the liquid is deep enough for poaching the eggs. If you use a larger pan, you will need more liquid.

BAKED SWEET POTATO WITH SESAME-PEANUT AIOLI

Dips, dressings, and other condiments make any meal or snack exciting. Aioli, in particular, offers the wonderful benefits of healthy fats and egg yolk. When I first started making aioli, I was working as a nanny and cook for a family in Oakland. I whipped up aioli one day with the kids and they loved it. We steamed asparagus to eat with our "special dip," but I soon discovered that they loved anything and everything with it. I expanded our repertoire to other dips and condiments, which they also adored, but aioli remained their favorite. This sesame-peanut version is a true winner: it makes your taste buds explode with delight. Be sure to add enough salt to complement the slightly bitter flavor of the sesame.

◆ YIELD: 4 SERVINGS ◆

4   medium sweet potatoes

1   tablespoon olive oil

1   tablespoon fresh thyme or 2 teaspoons dried
    Salt and freshly ground black pepper

FOR THE AIOLI

2   egg yolks

¼   cup toasted sesame oil

½   cup sesame oil

2   tablespoons chopped roasted peanuts

1   small garlic clove, very finely minced
    (about ¼ teaspoon)

⅛–¼   teaspoon salt

I. Preheat the oven to 375°F (190°C).

2. Slice the sweet potatoes into rectangular pieces about ½ inch square and 3 inches long (I don't peel them). Toss in a mixing bowl with the oil and thyme, and season generously with salt and pepper. Place on a baking sheet and roast for about 45 minutes, stirring every 10 to 15 minutes, until the sweet potatoes are tender but crisp and caramelized on the edges.

3. While the sweet potatoes are roasting, prepare the aioli: Put the yolks in a bowl and add just one drop of cold water. Combine the two types of sesame oil in a measuring cup with a pouring spout. With a whisk, beat the yolk rapidly and slowly, and then slowly begin to add the oil in a steady, thin stream. It may be useful here to have a helper so that one person can hold the bowl steady and whisk and the other can gently pour the oil into the bowl. If a helper is not available, wedge the bowl in place (between cutting boards or in a large dishcloth) to keep it steady as you whisk. As you add the oil, the aioli will begin to form a mayonnaise-like texture.

4. Stir the peanuts and garlic into the aioli, along with the salt. Let sit for 10 to 15 minutes so the garlic flavor has a chance to infuse.

5. Serve the sweet potato wedges with the aioli as a dip.

PEANUTS

I like to use roasted, unsalted peanuts in my aioli. If the peanuts are not roasted when you buy them, roast them yourself before chopping them. Simply heat them in a skillet over medium heat, stirring often, until they are lightly browned. If you only have salted peanuts, you can use them; just leave the salt out of the aioli.

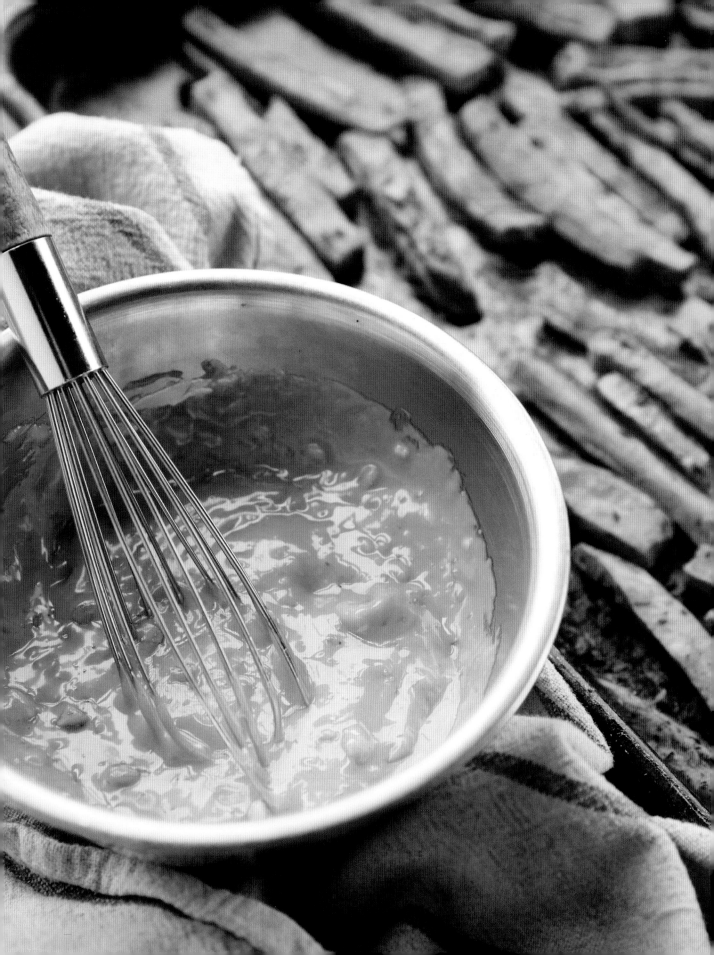

LEEK AND GORGONZOLA CUSTARD

The onion family has an offering for every season of the year. In spring, green onions and chives offer a welcome invigorating pungency that seems to match the urgency of the season. In fall, leeks' soothing, sweet, and satisfying flavor helps us relax and let go. The storage onion awaits us in the darkness of winter, steady, solid, and dependable. I look forward to leeks all year long. I love to slice them into rounds and use them in soups and other dishes, where they soak up the flavor of the broth around them and offer satisfying texture. Custard, so smooth and creamy, shares the comforting quality inherent to soups. Its texture complements the soft, gentle offering of the leeks and cream alongside the Gorgonzola, which, pungent and strong, challenges it all.

◆ YIELD: 6 SERVINGS AS A SIDE DISH ◆

2 tablespoons butter

3 cups diced leeks (2 medium/large leeks or 4–5 small ones)

2 teaspoons fresh thyme or 1 teaspoon dried

Pinch of ground cinnamon

Salt and freshly ground black pepper

5 egg yolks

1 cup heavy cream

1 cup whole milk

3 tablespoons chopped fresh parsley

4–6 ounces Gorgonzola cheese, crumbled

I. Preheat the oven to 350°F (180°C). Butter a 2-quart casserole dish.

2. Melt the butter in a skillet over low heat. Add the leeks and sauté until aromatic, about 3 minutes. Add the thyme and cinnamon and season generously with salt and pepper. Sauté until the leeks are tender, 5 to 7 minutes. Let cool for a few minutes.

3. Whisk the yolks together in a bowl with the heavy cream and milk. Add the parsley, cheese, and leeks, and mix well.

4. Pour the mixture into the prepared casserole dish. Place the dish in a larger pan and pour enough warm water into the outer pan that it comes halfway up the sides of the inner casserole. Bake until the center is set. The cooking time will depend on the thickness of the custard. At 2 inches deep, it takes 65 to 85 minutes to bake.

5. Remove the custard from the water bath. Let it cool for 10 minutes before serving.

SERVING SUGGESTION: You can serve this custard as a dip, with crackers, toasted bread, and raw, roasted, or steamed vegetables. You can also bake the custard in small ramekins for individual servings; the ramekins will not take as long to cook as the larger casserole.

WHITE FISH WITH HERB BUTTER

Fall instincts urge us to gather, collect, store, and make. There is an urgency to enjoy the last of the seasonal bounty and also to preserve it. Herb compound butters are a celebration of the simple goodness of fresh herbs and butter. Not to mention they are a fabulous way to preserve fresh herbs into the colder months. See page 62 for more details. Throughout winter, while you and your garden are hibernating, cooking with these flavorful butters will bring a smile to your face. This recipe is just one example of the many ways that herb butters can be used in simple preparations to yield mouthwatering results.

◆ YIELD: 4 SERVINGS ◆

FOR THE HERB BUTTER

3 tablespoons finely chopped fresh herbs of your choice

4 tablespoons (½ stick) unsalted butter, softened

Salt

FOR THE FISH

2 pounds white fish (like haddock, cod, sole, or halibut)

Salt and freshly ground black pepper

Juice of 1 lemon

1. Preheat the broiler or a grill.

2. While the broiler or grill is heating, prepare the butter: Combine the herbs with the butter and mix well. Season with a few pinches of salt and set aside.

3. Prepare the fish: Season it generously with salt and pepper. If you're using a broiler, lightly butter a baking pan and place the fish, skin side down, in the pan. If you're cooking on a grill, you can skip the pan. Squeeze the lemon juice over the fish.

4. Broil the fish about 6 inches from the heat source, or grill it, until the fish is cooked through (the fish should flake and the center should be just opaque). The cooking time will depend on how thick the fish is. A 1-inch-thick piece of fish may take only 4 to 7 minutes, while a thicker piece may require 10 minutes or longer. I usually check after 5 minutes and every 2 minutes after that. You do not want to over-cook the fish. Keep in mind that it will continue to cook for a minute or two after you remove it from the oven or grill.

5. As soon as the fish is done, transfer it to a serving tray with its cooking juices and dollop the compound butter along the top.

HERB COMBINATIONS

Some of my favorite combinations of herbs for the compound butter in this dish include

- Thyme and lemon zest
- Chives, tarragon, and lavender
- Parsley and garlic

CHICORIES WITH WARM VINAIGRETTE

Salads, using the term broadly, serve as palate cleansers; they are refreshing and can offset heavier flavors in a meal. They are also often served before a meal, priming the appetite and stimulating digestion. The chicory family is the home to some of my favorite salad greens, including endive, frisée, escarole, radicchio, and dandelion greens. They are bitter, crunchy, and particularly beautiful. While these greens are often available throughout much of the growing season, they can withstand colder temperatures into late fall, and I often find myself craving them then.

I am not always interested in salad in the colder months simply because it's cold and the raw greens feel tough and out of place. This warm dressing remedies that. It softens the greens and allows us all the joy of salad in a seasonally satisfying form. It also works well on hearty lettuces and spinach.

◆ YIELD: 4 SERVINGS ◆

1 pound chicory greens (radicchio, endive, escarole, or frisée; spinach or hearty lettuces also work)

2 tablespoons butter

2 medium shallots, finely minced (about ¾–1 cup)

½ teaspoon fresh or dried thyme
Freshly ground black pepper

½ cup white wine

2 tablespoons white wine vinegar or sherry vinegar

¼ cup olive oil
Salt

I. Chop the greens into bite-size pieces, put in a serving bowl, and set aside.

2. Melt the butter in a skillet over low heat. Add the shallots, thyme, and a healthy grind of black pepper, and sauté until the shallots are tender, 3 to 5 minutes. Then add the wine and cook, stirring frequently, until it reduces by about half (you can turn the heat up here if needed). Remove from the heat, whisk in the vinegar and oil, and season with salt to taste.

3. Toss the warm dressing with the greens and serve immediately, garnished with freshly ground pepper.

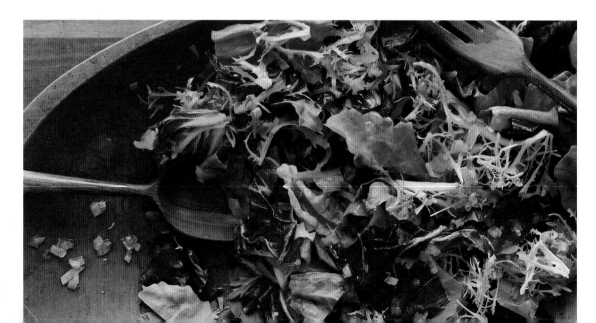

ROOT VEGETABLE PIE

There are two types of fall foods: those of the late-summer/early-fall season and those of the late-fall/close-to-winter season. Early fall holds on to the gifts of late summer, like tomatoes, eggplants, peppers, and basil. These foods retain the warmth of the sun in their flesh, nourishing our inner light in preparation for the dark season ahead. Late-fall storage crops contain the same light, but with a new quality: they are grounded, heavy, substantial, holding us close and wrapping us up as we approach what could be a bleak time of year.

This dish takes the shape of a rose — daring and inviting us to dig in, with an essence of the sweet satisfaction that good, simple food promises even in the darkest and coldest times.

⬥ YIELD: 4-6 SERVINGS ⬥

3½–4 pounds root vegetables (beets, turnips, potatoes, sweet potatoes, parsnips)

2 tablespoons olive oil

2–3 garlic cloves, mashed or finely minced

2 teaspoons fresh thyme or 1 teaspoon dried

⅛ teaspoon garam masala

Salt and freshly ground black pepper

2 tablespoons butter, olive oil, or coconut oil

I. Preheat the oven to 375°F (190°C).

2. Slice the root vegetables thinly, into rounds about ⅛ inch thick.

3. Toss the sliced roots in a large bowl with the oil, garlic, thyme, garam masala, and a healthy sprinkling of salt and pepper, making sure to separate the slices so they are evenly coated.

4. In a pie dish or similar size cast-iron pan, layer the root slices, first along the edges, then inward, packing them in as best you can and working your way in toward the center in a spiral. The roots will shrink as they cook, so make them fit snugly now.

5. Cover the pan and bake for 25 minutes. Then remove the cover, place thin slices of the butter along the top, sprinkle with salt and pepper, and return to the oven to bake, uncovered, for 15 to 20 minutes longer, until the roots are fully cooked and a little crispy on top.

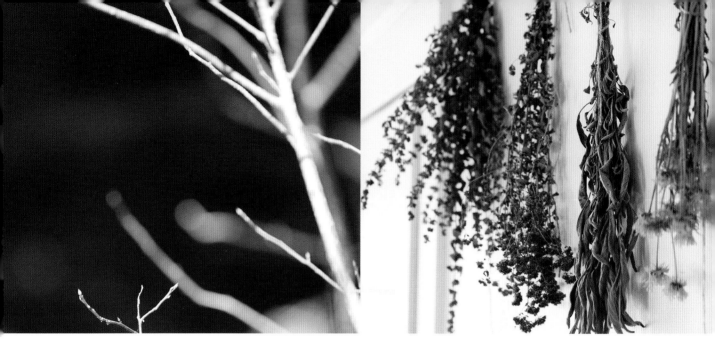

winter

WINTER IS MARKED BY DARKNESS. Less sunlight brings colder temperatures and muted colors. There is less action and less doing — shorter, colder days ask us to hibernate and rest. The slower, gentler pace provides an invitation to access our inner world, to drift into the deepest parts of our consciousness, to daydream and night dream, to rest, retreat, rejuvenate, restore, and reflect.

Winter's spirit is that of intuition, inner knowing, and reflection. Winter is the time to reflect on the year that has passed and think to the year ahead. It provides the quiet space we need to dream up our goals and intentions for the year to come. Spring, just on the horizon, provides the motivation needed to help those aspirations take root and grow.

During the darkness of winter, our body's inner metabolic fire slows. Digestion slows down, circulation slows down, and we may find ourselves feeling like we have less energy.

It is important to remember that this is just less energy of a certain type; we have limited fire energy — the energy of the sun — but the introspective, quiet, dark energy of the moon abounds and has much to teach us if we tune in and listen.

Finding health in winter requires that we respect and engage with the quiet energy of the season, while at the same time working to support our metabolic fire. In winter, our diets often turn to heavier foods: storage crops, meats, beans, and grains. These foods provide necessary nutrients and much-needed calories to keep the body warm. They are also very grounding and comforting. We need to be grounded and secure to access our inner world, so these foods help us connect with the energy of the season. They stand in contrast to the lighter, brighter foods of late spring, summer, and early fall, which match the outward, sunny, expansive quality of those seasons.

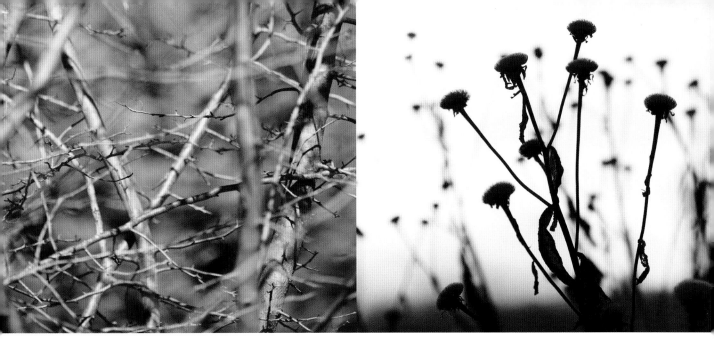

Preparing food in ways that improve its digestibility remains as important as ever. Roasting, braising, stewing, and other slow-cooking techniques popular during colder seasons improve digestibility, maximize nutrition, and warm body and soul, helping to counter the cold energy of the season and feeding our inner fire. Focus on warm drinks as well, including warm water, as cold drinks will cause further contraction and cold already exacerbated by the season around you.

In addition to avoiding foods that are cold in temperature, it can be helpful to avoid foods with cooling energy, including dairy, sugar, and tropical fruits like mango, papaya, and pineapple. These foods have a dampening effect on digestion that creates mucus in the system. If you do eat these foods, they should be warmed and/or spiced. For example, warm milk with cardamom, cinnamon, or nutmeg will be easier on digestion and less mucus-forming than a cold glass of milk or cold milk in a bowl of cereal. Spiced pumpkin pie is a more winter-appropriate sweet treat than cold chocolate mouse just out of the refrigerator. It's particularly important to avoid cold, mucus-forming foods if you are prone to respiratory congestion or if you are sick.

Often overlooked is the importance of spending time outdoors in winter. Being outside amid the quiet of winter's world connects us to its introspective, meditative qualities. Gentle outdoor exercise increases our metabolic fire, improves circulation, and helps us live in balance during a time when we may be naturally less active. Winter is the wisdom time, a time with great access to your own intuition and inner light. Let your vision of health and your inner compass guide you and burn brightly through winter and into the year to come.

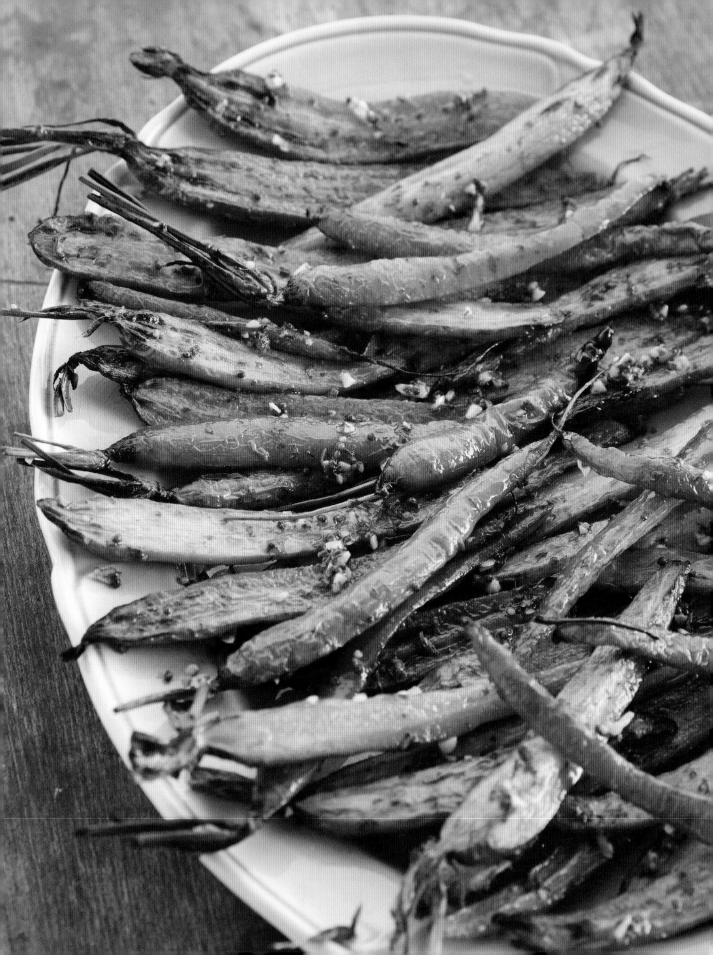

ROAST CARROTS WITH DIJON AND PARSLEY

A stocked pantry makes cooking easier and more fun. In summer, wild foods and a small kitchen garden complement pantry items well, but winter is the season to cherish the storage crops that hold up well in the basement or the bottom drawer of the refrigerator. Carrots are dependable, but no less exciting because of it. I appreciate their dependability, the subtle place they hold in soups, sauces, and mirepoix, where they are barely detectable, and how well they rise to the occasion of being featured on their own. Dijon, fresh garlic, and parsley liven up a midwinter's meal and complement the root's sweet, "carroty" flavor.

◆ YIELD: 4 SERVINGS AS A SIDE DISH ◆

1¼	pounds carrots
1–2	tablespoons olive oil
	Salt and freshly ground black pepper
3	tablespoons butter
2	tablespoons finely chopped fresh parsley
2	tablespoons whole-grain Dijon mustard
2–3	garlic cloves, minced

1. Preheat the oven to 400°F (200°C).

2. If the carrots are small, you can leave them whole or cut them in half or quarters lengthwise. If they are bigger, I like to slice them into ovals on a diagonal about ¼ inch thick.

3. Toss the carrots on a baking sheet with the oil, adding enough to coat, and season generously with salt and pepper. Roast for 15 minutes, stirring every few minutes, then reduce the heat to 350°F (180°C) and roast until cooked through and crispy on the edges. If the carrots are whole, this will take 20 to 25 minutes longer; if they are sliced, it may require only another 5 to 15 minutes.

4. While the carrots are roasting, melt the butter over low heat. Remove from the heat and let cool slightly, then whisk in the parsley, mustard, and garlic.

5. When the carrots are done, transfer them to a bowl and immediately toss them with the butter dressing. Add salt to taste. Serve hot.

HOT AND SOUR SOUP WITH TARRAGON VINEGAR

Just thinking about hot and sour soup makes my mouth water. It is the perfect way to start a meal, warming the digestive fire and stimulating the appetite. There is no reason to make it overly spicy; the subtle heat of the white pepper and the pungency of the vinegar, ginger, and raw garlic come together to offset the cold energy of the season by stimulating circulation and warming you from the inside out.

Hot and sour soup is great medicine for a head cold; it clears the sinuses, prevents further congestion, and stimulates the immune system. Adding the garlic at the very end helps preserve its antimicrobial and immune-stimulating actions.

◆ YIELD: 4 SERVINGS ◆

¼ cup dried black fungus mushrooms

1 cup boiling water

1 tablespoon sesame oil

1 cup chopped onion

2 cups sliced fresh mushrooms (crimini, shiitake, maitake)

1 (1-inch) piece fresh ginger, finely grated (1–2 tablespoons)

1 teaspoon ground white pepper

½–1 teaspoon red pepper flakes

2 tablespoons soy sauce or tamari

5 cups vegetable broth or Bone Broth (page 203)

¼ cup broken-up dried seaweed (alaria, digitata, nori, dulse, or a combination)

¼ cup plus 2 tablespoons Tarragon-Infused Vinegar (page 186)

2 tablespoons honey

3–5 garlic cloves, crushed or finely chopped

2 eggs, lightly beaten

3 tablespoons cornstarch (optional)

¼ cup cold water (optional)

Chopped scallions and cilantro, for garnish (optional)

I. Soak the dried mushrooms in 1 cup boiling water until they have softened and expanded, about 30 minutes. Drain, saving the soaking liquid for later use. Leave the mushrooms whole or slice them into bite-size pieces, as desired.

2. Heat the oil in a soup pot over medium heat. Add the onion and fresh mushrooms and sauté, stirring often, until the onions are translucent, about 5 minutes. Add the ginger, white pepper, and pepper flakes, and sauté until aromatic, 1 to 2 minutes. Then add the soy sauce and cook, stirring continuously, until it has been absorbed, 1 to 3 minutes.

3. Add the broth, the mushroom soaking liquid, the seaweed, and the rehydrated mushrooms. Bring to a simmer and cook until the mushrooms and seaweed are tender, about 15 minutes. Add the vinegar, honey, and garlic, and stir until the honey is dissolved. Taste for flavor, adding more soy sauce for salt, more vinegar for sour, and more honey for sweet, as you desire. To add more spice, you can add more pepper flakes, but keep in mind that their spicy flavor may take some time to infuse into the broth.

4. Slowly pour the beaten eggs into the hot broth. The eggs will cook almost instantly.

5. If you want to thicken the soup, mix the cornstarch and cold water together until the cornstarch has dissolved, breaking up any lumps. Add the cornstarch mixture to the hot broth at the very end, stirring continuously. The soup will continue to thicken until it returns to a simmer.

6. Serve hot, garnished with scallions and fresh cilantro, if desired.

VARIATIONS

Try adding other vegetables to the soup. Sometimes I like to add chopped sweet potato while the onions and mushrooms are sautéing, which makes the soup a little more filling and adds a nice sweetness that complements the spicy and pungent flavors in the broth. When I do this, I leave out the honey.

You can use any mushrooms here, and dried mushrooms work well in place of the fresh mushrooms. If you use additional dried mushrooms, soak them as described for the dried black fungus mushrooms in step 1, and use all that extra good soaking liquid in the soup, adjusting the amount of vegetable broth accordingly.

You can use any herb-infused vinegar in place of the tarragon vinegar.

HERB SALAD

In the winter I often eat fewer raw vegetables in favor of cooked roots and hearty greens. This is partly instinctual, arising from the body's desire for warming, nourishing, hearty foods, and partly the result of what is available in the colder months. When I find myself craving fresh greens and bold flavors — something to offset the heavier foods of the season — I go right for the herbs. Even in winter I can find generous bunches of bright-flavored, brilliantly green, hearty-looking cilantro, dill, and parsley at my local grocery store, and they make a wonderfully fresh base for this craving-quenching treat that will liven up any meal.

◆ YIELD: 4 SERVINGS ◆

⅓ cup pumpkin seeds

2 tablespoons sesame seeds

1 bunch fresh parsley, chopped into 1-inch pieces (1½–2 cups)

1 bunch cilantro, chopped into 1-inch pieces (about 1½ cups)

1 bunch fresh dill, chopped into 1-inch pieces (about 1 cup)

2 tablespoons finely chopped fresh thyme, oregano, mint, or sage

Salt and freshly ground black pepper

Juice of ½ lemon

1 teaspoon raw apple cider vinegar

¼ cup olive oil

I. Toast the pumpkin and sesame seeds in a small skillet over medium heat, stirring often, until the seeds begin to pop, 4 to 5 minutes. Set aside to cool.

2. Combine the parsley, cilantro, dill, and thyme (or whatever other herbs you're using) in a salad bowl. Sprinkle the toasted seeds over the herbs and season with salt and pepper. Sprinkle the lemon juice and vinegar over the salad, drizzle with the oil, and toss until well combined. Taste, adjust the seasonings as desired, and serve.

SALTING SALADS

Salt is a key ingredient in salads and salad dressings. The perfect amount balances acidity and brings out the flavor of the greens and the olive oil, or whatever oil you are using.

SHEPHERD'S PIE

Hearty foods are central to winter cuisine. They satisfy cravings, provide much-needed calories to help us stay warm, keep us grounded, and offer comfort. This recipe can be made with storage crops and frozen veggies from last summer's harvest. I use carrots and corn, but variations are endless. Make sure to season the meat and vegetables well, as that's where most of the flavor is. Ground beef makes an excellent substitute for the lamb, and you can always make a vegetarian version with extra veggies, mushrooms, or beans. This is a favorite in my family, so much so that my mom asked for it on her birthday last year . . . in May! Chilly weather calls us to these foods, no matter the season.

◆ YIELD: 8 SERVINGS ◆

1 tablespoon ghee (page 93) or olive oil

2 cups chopped onion

2 cups chopped carrots

2 tablespoons fresh oregano or marjoram or 2 teaspoons dried

1 tablespoon fresh thyme or 2 teaspoons dried

1 tablespoon ground paprika

2 teaspoons ground turmeric

1 bay leaf

3 cups corn kernels (fresh or frozen, thawed, and drained)

2 pounds ground lamb or beef

3–4 garlic cloves, minced

Salt and freshly ground black pepper

3–4 tablespoons grated Parmesan cheese

FOR THE MASHED POTATOES

3 pounds potatoes, red, white, or Yukon Gold, cut into 2-inch pieces (I leave the skins on)

1¼–1½ cups milk, cream, or half-and-half

4 tablespoons unsalted butter

Salt and freshly ground black pepper

1. Warm the ghee in a large skillet or saucepan over medium heat. Add the onions and sauté until translucent, about 5 minutes. Add the carrots and sauté for 2 minutes, then add the oregano, thyme, paprika, turmeric, and bay leaf. Sauté until the herbs are aromatic and the carrots begin to soften, 3 to 5 minutes. Add the corn, season generously with salt and pepper, and cook for 2 to 3 minutes.

2. Add the lamb. Cook until the meat is mostly cooked through, 5 to 7 minutes, stirring often and breaking up the meat into bite-size pieces. Because it will be cooked again in the oven, it is okay if the meat is still slightly pink inside. When it is done cooking, turn off the heat and stir in the garlic.

3. Prepare the mashed potatoes: Bring a large pot of water to a boil. Add the potatoes, return to a simmer, and cook until tender, 10 to 15 minutes. Drain off the water and return the potatoes to the pot. Mash with the milk, butter, and plenty of salt and pepper.

4. While the potatoes are cooking, preheat the oven to 375°F (190°C).

5. Pour the meat and vegetable mixture into a 9- by 13-inch casserole dish. Layer the potatoes over the meat and vegetables and smooth the top. Sprinkle with the Parmesan. Bake for 35 to 45 minutes, until it is bubbling and the top is golden.

BLACK BEAN AND SWEET POTATO CHILI

A big, hearty dish that is simple to make and satisfying to eat, chili allows you to feed a crowd or to store away some leftovers for the week. I find it a good way to put last season's frozen tomatoes to delicious use. It also handily accommodates any other frozen vegetables you might have stored away — corn, peppers, green beans, and greens all make great additions.

A bowl of steaming hot chili is great winter medicine — all its pungent spices stimulate immunity, increase circulation, and warm you up (you might even break a sweat!).

◆ YIELD: 5 SERVINGS ◆

½	cup dried black beans
2	tablespoons olive oil, lard, or ghee (page 93)
1	large onion, chopped (about 1 cup)
1	jalapeño pepper, finely chopped
3–4	garlic cloves, minced
2	tablespoons fresh oregano or 1 tablespoon dried
1	tablespoon chili powder
1	teaspoon ground cumin
1	teaspoon ground coriander
½	teaspoon ground cinnamon
1	bay leaf
1	pound ground beef or pork
	Salt
1	large sweet potato, cut into ½-inch cubes (about 2 cups)
2	cups diced tomatoes (fresh, frozen, or canned)
1	tablespoon unsweetened cocoa powder
1–1½	cups Bone Broth (page 203), vegetable broth, or water
2	cups packed spinach leaves (or other winter greens), in bite-size pieces
	Cilantro and sour cream, for garnish (optional)

1. Soak the beans in enough water to cover by 6 inches for 8 to 12 hours.

2. Drain the beans and transfer to a saucepan with enough water to cover by 2 inches. Bring to a boil. Skim any foam off the top, then reduce the heat and simmer gently, covered, stirring every 10 minutes, until the beans are soft through, 50 to 60 minutes. Add more water as needed to keep the beans covered by a couple of inches. Set the beans aside to cool in their cooking liquid.

3. Warm the oil in a pot over medium heat. Add the onion and sauté until translucent, about 5 minutes. Add the jalapeño, garlic, oregano, chili powder, cumin, coriander, cinnamon, and bay leaf, and cook, stirring continuously, until the herbs are aromatic, about 1 minute.

4. Add the beef, season generously with salt, and cook, stirring to break it up into bite-size pieces, until the meat is mostly cooked through, 5 to 7 minutes. Add the beans with their cooking liquid, along with the sweet potato, tomatoes, cocoa powder, and enough broth to cover all the ingredients by an inch or so. Bring to a simmer and simmer gently until the sweet potatoes are tender, about 15 minutes.

5. Add the spinach and simmer until it is wilted but still bright green, about 3 minutes. Season to taste with salt. Serve in bowls, garnished with fresh cilantro and sour cream, if desired.

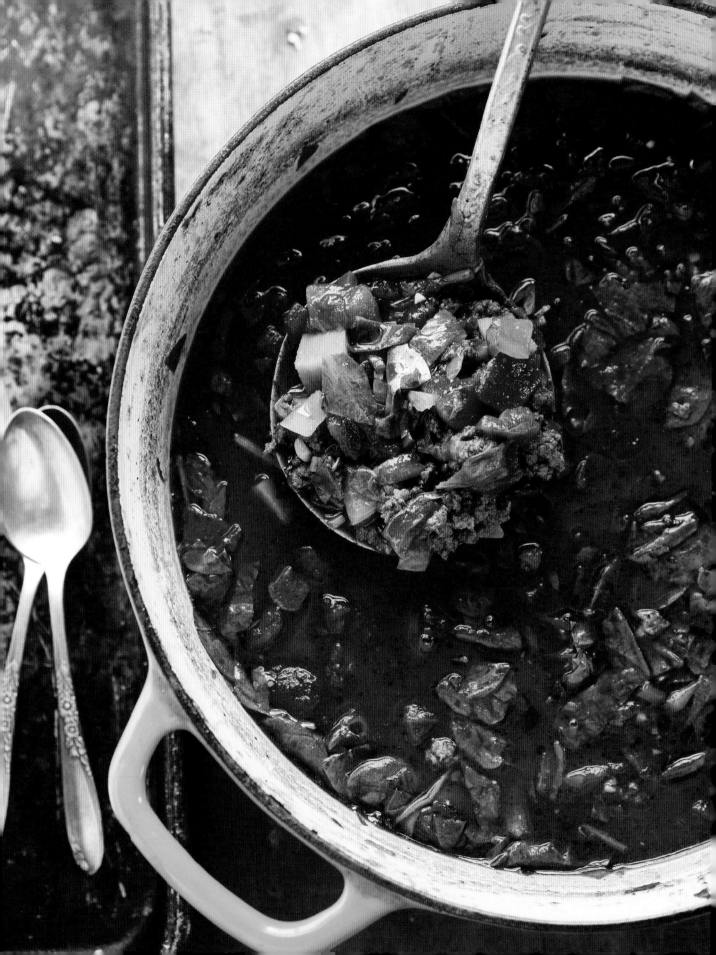

LEMON-THYME ROAST CHICKEN

Chicken is one of the few types of meat we roast whole, and it attracts a lot of attention because of it — it can make any meal feel like a special occasion. Afterward, you can use the bones to make Bone Broth (page 203) or Grandma's Chicken Soup (page 79), getting more than one meal and lots of nutrition from one place. The thyme, lemon, and garlic infuse the meat with flavor outside and inside, and they add great flavor to the gravy as well. Any leftover gravy can be used as the base of soups, stocks, cooked grains, or veggies. Roasting a chicken and making stock both fill a space with wonderful aromas, priming the appetite and creating a cozy, warm atmosphere on a cold winter day.

◆ YIELD: 4 OR MORE SERVINGS ◆

1 (3½- to 6-pound) whole chicken

1 head garlic, cloves separated and peeled

6–12 sprigs fresh thyme or 1 tablespoon dried
Salt and freshly ground black pepper

1 teaspoon olive oil or other fat

1 lemon

I. Preheat the oven to 375°F (190°C). Pat the chicken dry.

2. Chop two of the garlic cloves finely and cut the rest in half. If you're using fresh thyme, remove 1 tablespoon of leaves from the stems. Season the chicken generously with salt and pepper. Coat all sides of the chicken with the oil and then rub on the tablespoon of thyme leaves and the finely chopped garlic. Slice the lemon in half and squeeze half over each side of the chicken. Put the thyme stems with and without their leaves along with the rest of the garlic and the lemon peels into the cavity of the chicken.

3. Place the chicken breast side down on a baking sheet. Roast for 30 minutes. Then flip and cook breast side up until it reaches 165°F (75°C) in the thickest part and the juices run clear when you cut into the joint of the leg or wing with a knife. This method of cooking keeps the white meat moist but still allows the skin to crisp up in the end. The length of cooking time will depend on the size of the chicken. A 3½-pound chicken may only take 1 to 1¼ hours, while a 5- or 6-pound chicken may take up to 2 hours.

4. Remove the chicken from the oven and let rest for 15 to 20 minutes before carving and serving.

ONE-SHEET MEAL

When I'm roasting a chicken, I often surround it with chopped root vegetables to cook alongside the chicken and soak up the juices — it's a complete meal on a single baking sheet. Stir the veggies every so often as the chicken roasts to make sure they cook evenly and do not stick to the pan.

HERBAL MASALA CHAI

Warming spices such as cardamom, cinnamon, clove, nutmeg, black pepper, turmeric, cumin, and ginger (just to name a few!) are wonderful additions to the winter kitchen. These spices are carminative; they stimulate circulation to the digestive tract, warm the system, help ease tension, and support the body's breakdown and absorption of nutrients. In other words, they stimulate your inner metabolic fire! This stimulating action not only warms you up but also boosts circulation to the limbs, increases immune function, and reduces the congestion associated with colds and the flu.

Chai means "tea" in Hindi and *masala* means "blend." The tradition of masala chai as a blend of warming spices and black tea sweetened with milk and sugar originated in India, where the use of warming spices to support digestion is heavily integrated into cultural cuisine. This is my favorite version of masala chai; I make it without the black tea.

✦ YIELD: 4 CUPS ✦

4   cups water

2   tablespoons freshly grated ginger (preferable) or 1 teaspoon dried powdered ginger

1   tablespoon cinnamon chips or 1 cinnamon stick

1   tablespoon chopped fresh or dried orange peel

1   teaspoon cardamom pods

½   teaspoon whole black peppercorns

¼   teaspoon whole cloves

1   star anise pod

1   tablespoon black tea or 1 to 2 teabags (optional)

   Raw honey (optional)

   Whole milk or cream (optional)

   Ground cardamom or cinnamon (optional)

1. Pour the water into a medium saucepan. Add the ginger, cinnamon, orange peel, cardamom pods, pepper, cloves, and star anise. Cover and bring to a boil, then reduce the heat and let simmer for 10 to 15 minutes.

2. If you are using black tea, add it now. Return the lid to the pan and let steep for 3 to 5 minutes.

3. Strain and sweeten to taste with honey and milk, if using. Serve hot, garnished with a little ground cardamom or cinnamon, if desired.

WINTER TEAS

Hot herbal teas made from aromatic, bitter herbs act as great warming digestive aids in winter. They can take the place of, or supplement, other condiments and side dishes at meals or be drunk throughout the day. Many of our classic culinary herbs are antimicrobial, stimulate the immune system, and support the respiratory system, so they are excellent for fighting off wintertime colds and flus. The best examples include mint, thyme, oregano, basil, rosemary, and sage. Make sure to steep your herbal teas with a lid to keep the potent oils in the cup, and drink them hot to augment the medicinal benefits.

ELDERBERRY-THYME SYRUP

Elderberries provide a wonderful base for home remedies, particularly those for winter health. They are delicious, rich in flavonoids and vitamin C, and excellent for the immune system, with constituents that have been shown to be effective against many strains of influenza. The earthy flavor of the thyme complements the richness of the elderberry and the sweetness of the honey. Thyme and elderberry are both expectorants and help support the lungs. Thyme is also a powerful antibacterial and antifungal, working against infections throughout the body and particularly in the lungs. This syrup is a must-have for the winter health home pharmacy. Your biggest challenge will be keeping it around — it tastes so good you will want to use it all at once!

◆ YIELD: ABOUT 1½ CUPS ◆

½ cup fresh elderberries or ¼ cup dried

¼ cup fresh thyme or 2 tablespoons dried

1 teaspoon grated fresh ginger

2 cups water

½ cup raw honey

¼ cup brandy or apple cider vinegar

1. Combine the elderberries, half of the thyme, the ginger, and the water in a saucepan. Bring to a simmer, then reduce the heat and simmer, uncovered, until the volume of water has reduced by about half, 20 to 30 minutes. Sometimes I measure the drop in volume by watching the ring that forms inside the pan; other times I use a chopstick or some other implement to measure and mark the water levels as it is cooking. The volume does not have to be exact, so don't worry too much about measuring.

2. Remove from the heat, add the rest of the thyme, cover, and let steep for 15 minutes.

3. Strain through a fine-mesh strainer or fine cheesecloth or cotton muslin.

4. Pour the liquid into a glass pint jar. You should have about 1 cup of liquid if you used dried elderberries and 1 to 1¼ cups of liquid if you used fresh elderberries. If you are not left with at least 1 cup of liquid, simply add water to make up the difference.

5. Add the honey to the jar while the liquid is still hot. I like to use a canning jar with measuring increments on the side so that I can pour the honey right into the jar rather than using a measuring cup, which gets messy with honey. Shake or stir until the honey is dissolved, then add the brandy or vinegar. Store in the refrigerator. It will keep for up to 6 months if made with brandy, or up to 4 months if made with vinegar.

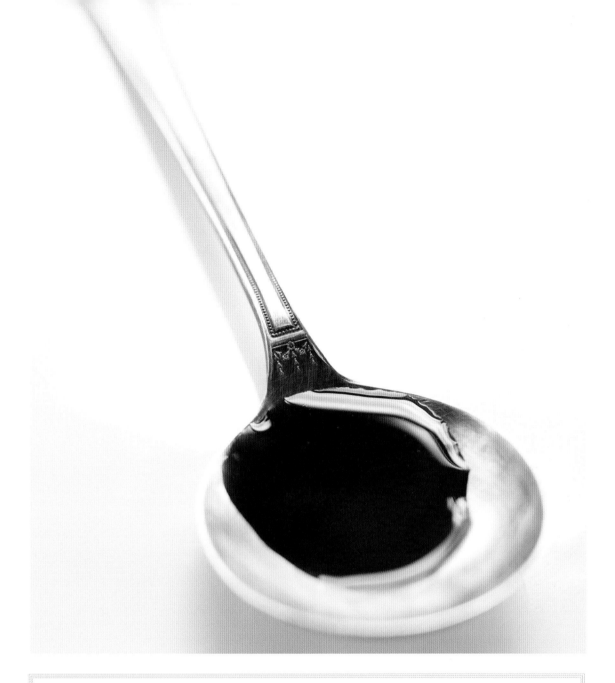

USING ELDERBERRY-THYME SYRUP

Take Elderberry-Thyme Syrup whenever you feel like you might be coming down with an illness, and continue to take it until all symptoms have cleared. Adults can take 1 tablespoon two or three times per day as needed to boost the immune system and support the respiratory system. Elderberry-Thyme Syrup is an excellent remedy for children. Children ages 5 to 10 can take 1 to 2 teaspoons, children aged 2 to 5 can take ½ to 1 teaspoon, and children aged 1 to 2 can take ¼ to ½ teaspoon. Children under 1 year of age should not be given this syrup, since it's generally recommended that they avoid honey.

Elderberry-Thyme Syrup can also be incorporated into the diet. Try putting some in your tea or other beverages, pouring it on pancakes, oatmeal, and other breakfast treats, or enjoying it by the spoonful.

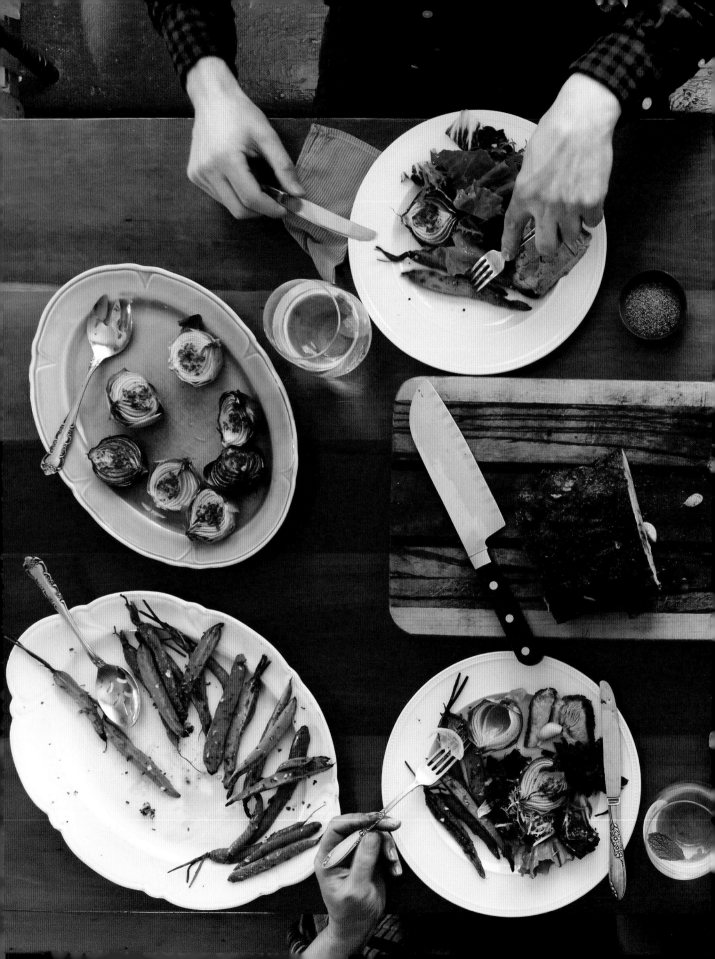

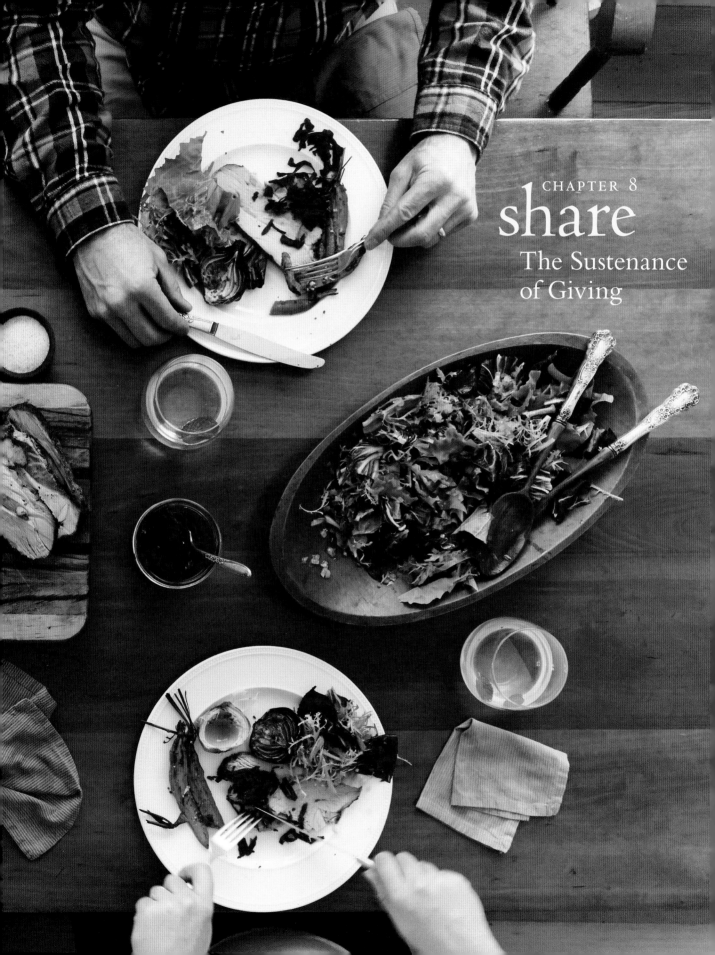

share

The Sustenance
of Giving

HUMAN BEINGS HAVE EVOLVED to find, raise, grow, cook, and eat food together. The instinct to share in sustaining one another is as real as our need to eat. However, daily rituals surrounding the sharing of food, such as communal preparation and enjoyment of meals, are not often prioritized in our modern culture. Food is often eaten alone or on the go, and the availability of processed, packaged, and preprepared food keeps us disconnected from the many important hands-on processes that help us feel that life is meaningful. While making time to prepare, share, and enjoy food with others may no longer be required to *feed* ourselves, it is an important part of what *nourishes* us — building community, creating bonds, and establishing connection to ourselves, others, and the larger ecosystem.

When I was growing up, my family always had dinner together. Sitting around the table was a place to unwind from the day's events, to catch up with one another, share stories, laugh, and enjoy food together. If you told my mom that something she'd made for dinner was good, she'd say, "That's because I made it with lots of love." No matter what she made, love was her secret ingredient — although she told us all about it, so I guess it wasn't so secret after all. . . . Secret or not, it was the glue that held us together, luring us in to sit down and enjoy one another's company, and our time at the table strengthened the bond.

When we feel relaxed, loved, and safe, we digest better and get more nutrition from our food. When we sit down to eat and enjoy food in the presence of good company, we derive more nourishment from the meal, both from the food itself and from our experiences in those moments of togetherness.

Sharing food with others creates an instinctual bond between us. As a society, as we have moved away from the rituals of preparing and eating food, we have lost some of that human connection. We have also lost some of the important skills of feeding large groups of people that allow celebrations around food to be commonplace and comfortable. Whether you are feeding friends and family, having people for dinner, or hosting an event, being able to feed people is a rewarding gift. And it will help you appreciate even more those times when other people feed and provide for you. One-pot meals, roasts, casseroles, soups, and other dishes that can be prepared ahead make it easy to feed large groups. It can also be wonderful to get everyone involved in making the food. Getting together with friends to "make dinner" is one of my favorite and most common social activities; nothing feels more satisfying than sharing good food and good company.

Eating is a call to celebrate. We celebrate the bounty of the food itself, the hands that grew and prepared it, the occasion to be together, and our ability to indulge our senses and enjoy ourselves. Eating deserves to be a ritual affair, done with intention, appreciation, love, and respect. It connects us to ourselves and others, yes, but it also stands to connect us to the larger processes of our ecosystem that provide the food that sustains us.

Food provides an invitation to share in the rhythms of the earth. Each time we eat, we are receiving a gift that the earth has shared with us. All food is some form of life: All plants are alive before they are picked and processed. All meat comes from a living being. All cheese, yogurt, eggs, and so on come from a living source. When our bodies die, when we compost our food scraps, when leaves fall and plants decay, we all become food for other organisms and new life. Within this web, there is no life without sharing.

True integration with this web of life, with our larger ecosystem, comes with appreciation. When the culinary experience begins with fresh, whole foods, it is easy to see the beauty of the world and to be amazed by it — to stand in wonder and appreciation for the natural sweetness of a berry, the creaminess of milk, or the aroma of basil. When we eat packaged, processed foods, it can be harder to find the same kind of appreciation. Because this food is so far removed from its origins, eating it does not serve as a reminder that we share this earth with that great web of life. It feeds us, yes, but it does not feed our sense of connection with the natural world.

Throughout history, the most significant way that humans have acknowledged the immense gift of food from the earth, from animals, and from other hands is by saying grace — an acknowledgment of gratitude, respect, appreciation, and wonder for the gift of food we are about to receive. Practices of gratitude do not have to be long or ornate, nor do they have to be formal or religious. They can be silent and personal or communal and public. Through this simple gesture, by acknowledging the beauty of what is being shared with us, we honor our place in the web.

Food gives us all the tools to reconnect, by allowing us to find meaning, and share, in the web of belonging.

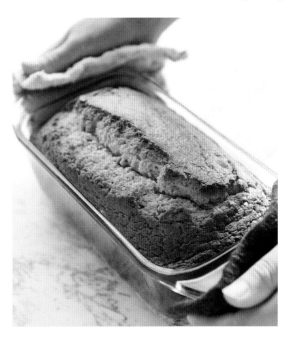

In the words of the late philosopher and poet John O'Donohue, "[People in] our times are desperate for meaning and belonging." Many of us do not have strong ties to community, family, culture, or place. This makes engaging with the processes of nature and the earth even more challenging. It can also make it more challenging to find the inspiration to share with others and ourselves. Food gives us all the tools to reconnect, by allowing us to find meaning, and share, in the web of belonging.

May you share generously and receive graciously.

PROSCIUTTO-WRAPPED DATES with SAGE

Food has the ability to mark time and experience. Each summer I look forward to ripe tomatoes and sun-kissed basil. I admire the wildflowers as they bloom and pass throughout summer and into autumn. In winter I love watching the wind blow and the snow fall, only to gratefully see it melt and the mud flow again come spring.

The first time I tested this recipe, I made it for my college roommate and her partner on their annual summer trip back east. It is always a special and joyous time of "catching up" and basking in the light of each other's company. I can easily conjure an image of all of us sitting in the kitchen, reaching for these little treats from the pan. When I shut my eyes, I see smiles, hear laughter, and even smell the prosciutto frying in the pan.

◆ YIELD: 4 SERVINGS AS AN APPETIZER ◆

⅓ cup soft goat cheese

2 tablespoons finely chopped fresh sage

10 dates, cut in half, pits removed

⅛–¼ pound thinly sliced prosciutto (4–6 slices)

I. Combine the cheese and sage in a small bowl and mix well. Generously stuff the cheese mixture into the date halves; each date half should get about a teaspoon. Slice the prosciutto into 20 approximately equal pieces, and wrap each slice around one of the stuffed date halves.

2. Heat a skillet over medium heat. Once it's hot, place the prosciutto-wrapped dates in the pan and cook, rotating occasionally, until browned, 3 to 5 minutes. Serve hot — I usually serve them right from the pan.

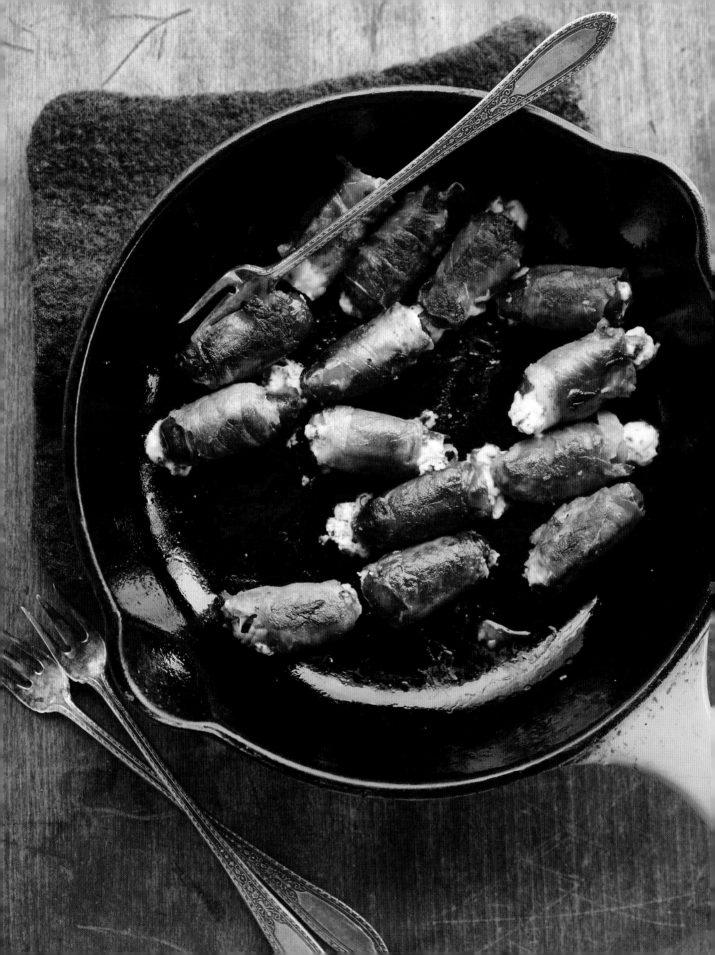

WHITE BEAN SPREAD WITH ROSEMARY AND MELLOWED GARLIC

When you roast garlic, the sharp-tasting sulfur compounds break down and the sugars caramelize, giving the garlic a sweetness that you might only catch a glimmer of in its raw form. While roasting is usually a dry process, slowly cooking garlic in olive oil is an easy and efficient way for the home cook to get the results of roasting, and it imparts a wonderful flavor to the oil. Of course, you can also roast garlic in the oven, either in its skin or peeled on a baking dish with a dash of oil. Make extra and smear it on toast or use it in Wilted Dandelion Greens with Garlic Confit (page 173) or Crispy Sage and Roasted Garlic Risotto (page 144). If you miss the pungency of raw garlic in this spread, you can always add a little bit.

◆ YIELD: 4-6 SERVINGS AS AN APPETIZER ◆

¾ cup dried cannellini or navy beans (enough to make 1–1½ cups cooked)

½ cup olive oil, plus extra for garnish

1 head garlic, cloves separated, peeled, and sliced ¼ inch thick

¼ cup fresh rosemary or 2 tablespoons dried

1 teaspoon balsamic vinegar or balsamic reduction

Salt and freshly ground black pepper

1. Soak the beans for at least 8 hours, and up to overnight, in enough water to cover them by 6 inches.

2. Drain the beans and transfer to a saucepan with enough water to cover them by 2 inches. Bring to a boil, skim any foam off the top, and reduce the heat to low. Let simmer, covered, stirring every 10 minutes, until the beans are soft through, 45 to 60 minutes. Add more water as needed to keep the beans covered.

3. While the beans are cooking, combine the oil and garlic pieces in a small pan or skillet. Heat over low heat, stirring every few minutes, until the garlic is golden brown and soft all the way through, 10 to 15 minutes once the oil gets hot. If at any point the oil gets too hot and sputters or begins to brown the garlic too quickly, take the pan off the heat and let it cool for a moment before returning it to the stovetop.

4. When the beans are done, drain them. Put them in a food processor with the oil and garlic, rosemary, vinegar, ½ teaspoon salt, and a few pinches of pepper. Blend until smooth. Season to taste with salt. Serve garnished with a drizzle of oil and, if you have it, a sprig of rosemary.

BLACK OLIVE AND PARSLEY TAPENADE

Olives are one of my favorite foods. Beauties of the Mediterranean, these flavorful and nutritious fruits can be pressed to make oil or cured to offer delightful sour and salty flavors. In fact, the cuisines of this region are full of assertive, vibrant, fresh flavors, including copious aromatic herbs, a wide range of citrus fruits, and deliciously salty cheeses. I love bringing these flavor profiles into my kitchen, gaining inspiration from their tastes as well as their place in cultural traditions from near and far. Cooking is like this — a creative hodgepodge of the senses, informed by a shared cultural experience that is somehow always larger than you are. And while I mostly eat food grown close to home, I am so grateful for the ways in which specialties from regions around the world share in my cooking experience.

◆ YIELD: 4-6 SERVINGS AS AN APPETIZER ◆

¾ cup pitted kalamata or other black olives

¼ cup pitted green olives

½ cup fresh parsley

1–2 garlic cloves

2 tablespoons olive oil

½ teaspoon ground paprika

Generous pinch of freshly ground black pepper

Combine the olives, parsley, garlic, oil, paprika, and pepper in a food processor and blend until the mixture reaches the desired consistency. I like my tapenade blended enough to hold the consistency of a spread while still having some texture; you may prefer a more smooth spread.

SERVING SUGGESTION: When I'm serving a crowd, I like to garnish the tapenade with paprika and olive oil and serve it with fresh bread, crackers, or raw or roasted vegetables. Tapenade also goes great alongside eggs, chicken, fish, pasta, and vegetable dishes (such as grilled zucchini or roasted cauliflower), and you can even use it in salad dressings. For variation, you can try adding anchovies or capers, traditional additions to the spread.

BASIL OIL

Making a wide and wonderful range of condiments, like herbal oils, pestos, and herb-infused vinegars, is one of the best ways to preserve and share the bounty of the harvest. When the growing season presents an abundance of herbs and other fresh foods, as it usually does, you can make condiments such as these, bursting with flavor and nutrients, and store them away for seasons when you have less. This basil oil is a true summer treat, uniquely aromatic and peppery. It can be used for cooking, added to salads, drizzled on tomatoes or other veggies, applied as a garnish on any prepared dish, or used on its own as a dipping sauce.

◆ YIELD: 1 CUP ◆

8 cups water

¼ cup sea salt

2 cups ice cubes (about a tray's worth, give or take)

2 cups packed fresh basil leaves and stems

1 cup olive oil

I. Bring 4 cups of the water to a boil with the salt. While the water is heating, prepare an ice-water bath with the remaining 4 cups water and the ice cubes. Separate the basil leaves from the stems and set each aside.

2. When the water is boiling, add the basil leaves and blanch for 60 seconds. Remove with a slotted spoon and put into the ice bath for 15 to 20 seconds, stirring to cool. Remove with a slotted spoon and set on a dishcloth or paper towels to dry.

3. Blanch the basil stems in a similar manner until tender, 2 to 3 minutes. Remove with a slotted spoon to the ice-water bath, stir and let cool for 20 to 30 seconds, and then remove with a slotted spoon and set aside on the dishcloth or paper towels with the leaves.

4. Pat the leaves and stems dry. Combine them with the oil in a food processor and blend. Transfer this slurry to a container, cover, and let sit for 12 to 24 hours in the refrigerator. The next day, strain the oil through fine cheesecloth, cotton muslin, or paper towels. Store in the refrigerator, where it will keep for up to a month (though it is often more flavorful when it is fresh).

NOTE: You can follow this recipe to make any fresh herb oil. Just substitute whatever herb you have for the basil. See page 64 for other methods of making herb-infused oils.

QUICK FIX

I have skipped the 12- to 24-hour steeping period before.
The oil is not as rich if you skip this step, but it is still delicious, so if you are in a rush,
you can consider eliminating or shortening the steeping time.

WARM POTATO SALAD
WITH CILANTRO
AND SOFT-BOILED EGG

It's a warm evening in late August and the sun has that restful quality that makes you feel like you've had a satisfying day. Two of my friends from high school are over for a visit. We sit on the porch with tea and a big bowl of warm potato salad full of the fresh taste of cilantro and tomatoes. We talk and laugh and eat, our cheeks rosy, maybe with warmth, maybe with joy. There is something to savor here — the reminder of good friends who feel like family and the fleeting enjoyment of the harvest's treats.

◆ YIELD: 4 SERVINGS ◆

4 large or 5 medium Yukon Gold potatoes, with their skins, cut into ½-inch cubes

3 eggs

2 tablespoons olive oil

1 tablespoon freshly squeezed lemon juice

½ cup finely chopped scallions

Salt and freshly ground black pepper

1 cup chopped ripe tomato, in ½-inch chunks (1 large or 2 small tomatoes)

1 cup packed whole cilantro leaves, stems removed

I. Place the potatoes in a medium saucepan, cover with water, and bring to a boil. Boil gently over medium heat until the potatoes are about half cooked, about 5 minutes. Add the eggs in their shells and cook until they are soft-boiled, 6 minutes for medium eggs and 7 minutes for large ones. Remove the eggs from the pan and set aside to cool. Check the potatoes: they should be cooked through but not mushy. Once cooked to your liking, strain them from their cooking water.

2. Place the potatoes in a large mixing bowl with the oil, lemon juice, and scallions. Sprinkle with salt and freshly ground pepper, and mix well. With the shells on, cut the eggs in half along the equator and use a teaspoon to scoop the insides into the bowl with the potatoes. Add the tomato (first draining off any juice) and cilantro and mix. If the salad is too dry, add more oil or a bit of the tomato juice. Season to taste with salt and pepper, mix well, and serve warm.

SOFT-BOILING EGGS

Soft-boiled eggs can be finicky, and cooking times vary with the size of the egg. For this recipe, I like the yolk to be custardy but not solid. If you feel your eggs turned out too soft or too hard, make a note of it and change it up next time. No matter how your eggs cook, the salad will be delicious, so don't feel you have to start over if they do not turn out how you were expecting the first time.

RED GRAPE CHIMICHURRI
WITH DILL AND OREGANO

Chimichurri is an herb-based condiment from Argentina. It caught my eye, or should I say my taste buds, because of its acid content; it usually calls for a splash of vinegar, which makes it light and fresh. The acidity grants it the ability to pair with many complex flavors, and this inspired me to put it alongside the sweetness of fruit. While this recipe is by no means a traditional chimichurri, I am certainly borrowing ideas from the traditional, which is some combination of parsley, garlic, olive oil, vinegar, oregano, and sometimes spicy peppers. Chimichurri is often served with grilled meat and offers great medicine to those eating, brightening up the flavor and the digestive processes. This more unconventional version can be served as a condiment with grilled meat or seafood, alongside grain or bean dishes, with crepes, or as an accompaniment to a cheese spread.

◆ YIELD: 4 SERVINGS AS A CONDIMENT ◆

1 cup red grapes

2 tablespoons finely chopped fresh oregano

1 tablespoon coarsely chopped capers

1 tablespoon finely chopped fresh dill

1 tablespoon finely chopped fresh mint

2 tablespoons olive oil

2 teaspoons white wine vinegar

Pinch of salt

I. Cut the grapes into a small dice (cutting each grape into quarters or sixths works well, depending on the size of the grape), doing your best not to smash them.

2. Combine the chopped grapes with the oregano, capers, dill, mint, oil, vinegar, and salt in a small bowl and mix well. Set aside to let the flavors marry for 20 to 60 minutes before serving.

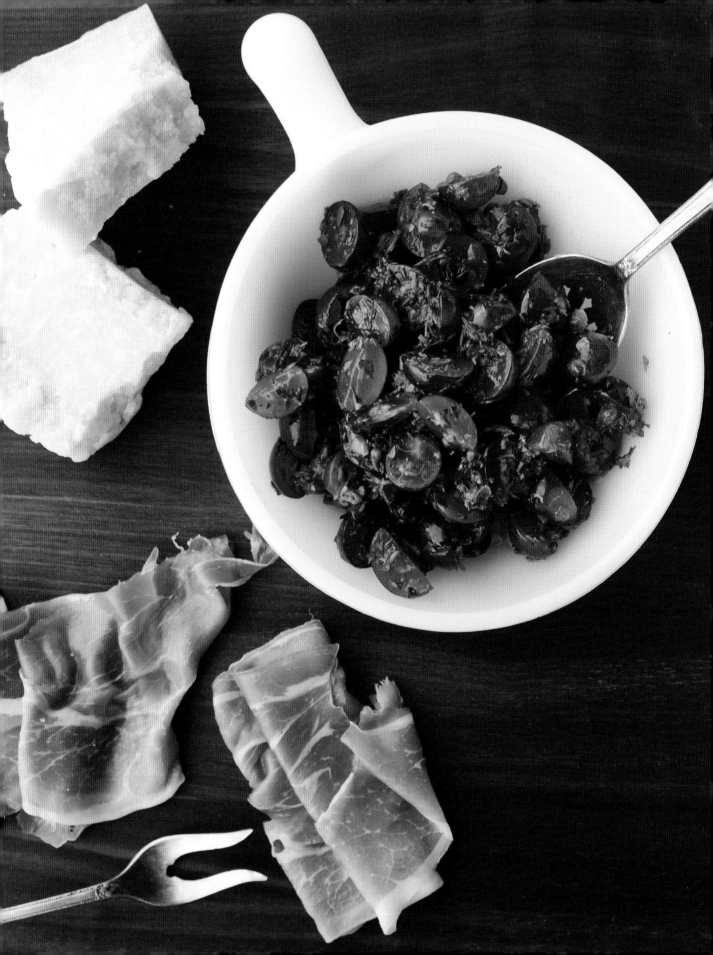

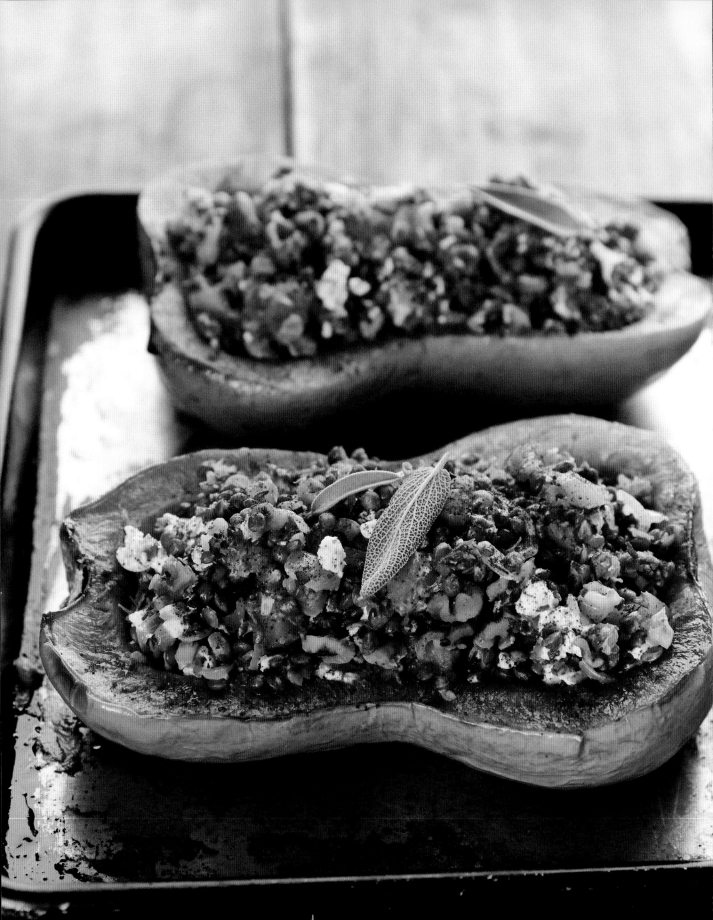

BUTTERNUT SQUASH STUFFED WITH FRENCH LENTILS AND WALNUTS

Squash is a fabulous storage crop that offers filling, sweet, comforting fall and winter fare. When it is the season, nothing makes me happier than the smell of hearty foods roasting in the oven and the bounty that greets me at the table. This stuffed squash works well alongside an invigorating dish like Chicories with Warm Vinaigrette (page 250), Spinach and Grapefruit Salad with Toasted Pumpkin Seeds (page 107; try using the squash seeds!), Apple and Parsley Salad (page 176), or Deep-Sea Purple Kraut (page 83).

◆ YIELD: 6-8 SERVINGS ◆

FOR THE FILLING

- 1 cup dried French lentils
- 1 cup walnuts
- 2 tablespoons olive oil
- 2 cups chopped onion (2 medium onions or 3 small)
- ¼ cup fresh sage or 2 teaspoons dried
- 2 tablespoons fresh thyme or 1 teaspoon dried
- 1 tablespoon fresh rosemary or 2 teaspoons dried
- 1 cup crumbled goat cheese

  Paprika and fresh sage leaves, for garnish (optional)

FOR THE SQUASH

- 2 butternut squashes, 2½–3 pounds each

  Olive oil

  Salt and freshly ground black pepper

I. Begin the filling: Soak the lentils in enough water to cover by 6 inches for 6 to 10 hours. Soak the walnuts in enough water to cover by 1 inch for 6 to 10 hours. Then drain both. Coarsely chop the walnuts.

2. Preheat the oven to 375°F (190°C).

3. Prepare the squash: Cut the squashes in half lengthwise and remove the seeds (consider saving them to roast). Rub the inside of the squash with oil and season with salt and pepper. Set the squashes facedown on a baking sheet. Roast for 40 to 55 minutes, depending on the size and shape of the squash, until the thickest part is just fork-tender. (If you cook it too long, the squash meat will start to separate from the skins, which will make it a little harder to serve.)

4. Meanwhile, continue the filling: Combine the lentils in a saucepan with enough water to cover by 1 inch. Bring to a boil, skim any foam off the top, then reduce the heat and simmer for 2 to 3 minutes. Turn off the heat, let sit for 15 minutes, and then drain; this "steeping" will help the lentils absorb water and continue to cook without getting mushy or falling apart.

5. Warm the 2 tablespoons oil in a large skillet over medium heat. Add the onion and sauté until soft, about 5 minutes. Add the sage, thyme, rosemary, and chopped walnuts, and cook until the fresh sage leaves turn bright green and aromatic or until the dried herbs are aromatic and tender, 1 to 3 minutes. Remove from the heat.

6. Drain any liquid from the roasting pan and turn the squash halves faceup. Scoop a bit of the squash from the neck to create more room for the stuffing. Dice that bit of cooked squash coarsely — it will be very soft, but cutting it will help make mixing it into the stuffing easier.

7. Combine the lentils with the onion mixture, and season generously with salt and pepper. Stir in the diced cooked squash and cheese until just combined. Spoon the stuffing into the squash. Bake, uncovered, for 15 minutes, or until the stuffing is hot through. (If you like, the squash can be stuffed ahead of time and baked just before serving.) Garnish with paprika and fresh sage leaves, if desired.

8. Serve hot. I like to let people eat it right out of the skin, although sometimes the skin is tender enough to eat too.

SQUASH SEEDS

Squash seeds are rich in minerals, including zinc, and can be roasted to make a great snack. Start by separating the seeds from the pulp, although don't worry about being too perfect here; small amounts of leftover pulp will cook down as the seeds roast. Spread the seeds on a baking sheet and season with some salt and pepper. Roast at 375°F (190°C) for 10 to 20 minutes, stirring a few times, until they are golden brown and crunchy. Sometimes, when they are done, they start popping in the oven! I toast mine while I am baking the squash or right after, when the oven is still hot. Just like roasting a chicken and using the bones to make broth, roasting squash seeds to eat later optimizes the plant's nutritional offerings, helps make the seeds storable for later consumption, and is a sign of your respect and appreciation for nature's bounty.

BEET HEARTS

Beets are incredible blood builders, full of vitamins and minerals that nourish and strengthen the blood, increase energy, and restore vitality. When you taste them, you feel the earthy nutrition exploding from every bite. Blood is our life force, and our heart is the muscle that helps move it. The heart is also a symbol of love. Love is the lifeblood of our emotions, the fuel that fires our ability to connect and share with ourselves, others, and nature in a way that makes life feel meaningful. This dish helps us nourish our blood and that love in our hearts. I made it once for Valentine's Day — spur-of-the-moment cutting vegetables into hearts! But really, every day deserves to be recognized for the love we are blessed with; share it with the loves of your life, including yourself.

◆ YIELD: 2 SERVINGS ◆

3 small to medium beets

2 tablespoons ghee (page 93) or butter

1 tablespoon fresh thyme or 2 teaspoons dried
　 Salt

1. Trim off the tip and tail of the beets. Cut a little extra from the tail end; this will make it easier to make the heart shape. Place each beet cut side down on the cutting board. Now to cut the heart shape: Cut a small triangular wedge from one side. Trace an imaginary line from the point of the triangle to the other side of the beet and make a mark at this point. Making this mark the point of your second triangle, cut the round edges off the side of the beet, starting at the mark. I usually only cut off about a 1-inch-long piece from each side of the mark. This will give you a very thick, somewhat angular "heart-shaped" beet. Turn the trimmed beet on its side and cut into thin heart-shaped slices. I usually cut the scraps into thin slices as well; there will be enough hearts to dominate with the scraps filling in.

2. Heat the ghee in a skillet over low heat. Add the sliced beets and thyme and sauté over low heat, stirring every few minutes, until the beets are cooked through and caramelized, about 40 minutes. When they're a few minutes away from being done, scatter a pinch of salt over the beets. Serve hot.

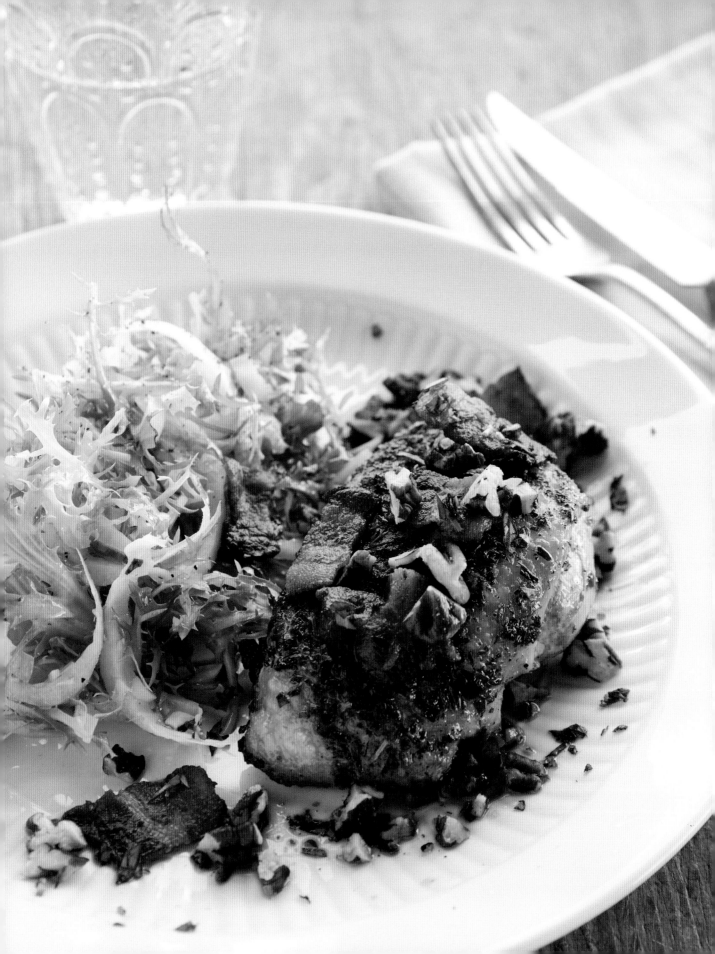

SEARED DUCK WITH BACON, TOASTED PECANS, AND FRISÉE AND ENDIVE SALAD

Like people, landscapes, and music, food caries a lot of potential for romance. But we seem to outsource much of the romance of food in our culture. We romanticize the foods of other cultures, other kitchens, other cooks. We lust after magazine photos of food on rustic countertops and meals on fine china, forgetting that the food in our own home puts the authenticity back into the romance. We romanticize something when we want it or wished we had it, but we experience romance in the moment. When I made this dish for the first time, I put it all on one plate. Two hungry mouths and a plate of food — it was simply and completely romantic.

This duck goes excellently with a salad of frisée and endive, but really any fresh greens will do. I prefer to use fresh tarragon, but dried is also good.

❖ YIELD: 4 SERVINGS ❖

FOR THE DUCK

- 1½ cups pecans
- 2 pounds duck breasts, with skin
  Salt and coarsely ground black pepper
- 4 tablespoons fresh tarragon or
  4 teaspoons dried
- 6 slices nitrate-free bacon

FOR THE FRISÉE AND ENDIVE SALAD

- 1 head frisée
- 1 small head endive

FOR THE DRESSING

- ½ cup olive oil
- 3 tablespoons red wine vinegar
- 2–3 scallions, chopped
- ⅛ teaspoon salt

I. Preheat the oven to 325°F (170°C).

2. Toast the pecans in a skillet on the stovetop, stirring often, until they start to smell aromatic and begin to darken in color, 3 to 5 minutes. Remove from the heat, let cool, and coarsely chop.

3. Rub both sides of the duck breasts with salt, pepper, and 3 tablespoons of the fresh tarragon (or 3 teaspoons dried). Set aside.

4. Cut the bacon strips into 1-inch pieces. Sauté in an ovenproof skillet over medium heat until crispy. Remove the bacon from the skillet with a slotted spoon and set aside on paper towels to absorb any excess grease.

5. Pour off half of the bacon grease from the skillet and then return the skillet to medium heat. When it's hot, place the duck breasts, fat side down, in the pan. Place them gently where you want them and leave them there; the trick to a good sear is to let the meat be and not move it around a lot. Reduce the heat slightly and cook the duck for 3 minutes on each side.

6. Transfer the skillet to the oven and cook the duck for 5 to 10 minutes (5 minutes will be closer to rare, 10 minutes closer to well done). To assess the doneness of the meat, cut into the thickest part of the breast. Rare will be red in the middle, not fully cooked through, and juicy. Medium will be cooked through, but still pink in the center and juicy. When it's done to your liking, remove the skillet from the oven and let the duck rest for 3 to 5 minutes before serving.

7. While the duck is cooking and resting, prepare the salad: Cut the frisée into 1-inch pieces. Remove the outer leaves of the endive and cut the whole head into ¼-inch strips, then cut the rounds in half. Toss the frisée and endive together.

8. Prepare the dressing: Combine the oil, vinegar, scallions, and salt in a jar and shake well.

9. When you're ready to serve, dress the greens and arrange them on a plate. Set the duck alongside, garnished with the pecans, bacon, and the remaining 1 tablespoon fresh tarragon or (1 teaspoon dried). Any leftover dressing can be stored at room temperature for about a week.

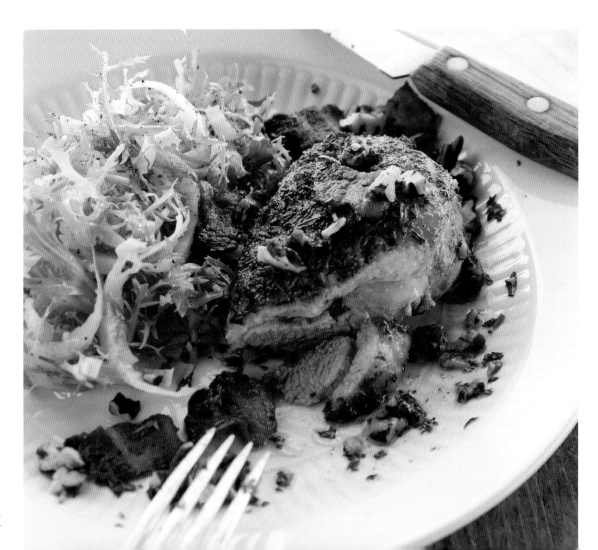

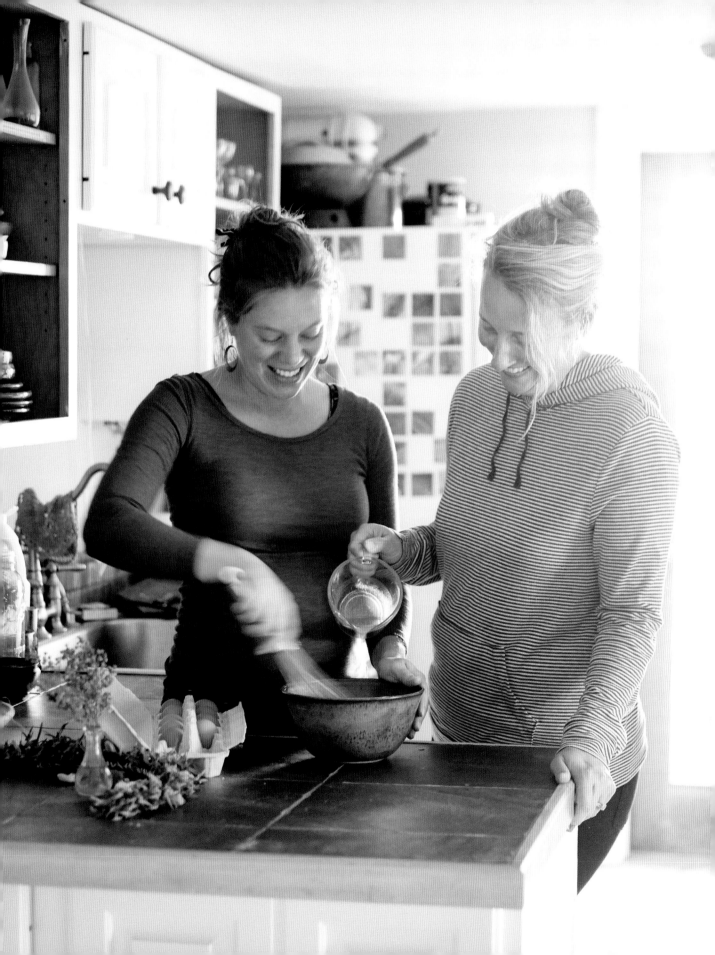

GARLICKY BRAISED LAMB

Braising uses a low temperature and long cooking time to break down cartilage and connective tissues, rendering tough pieces of meat more tender. This process of transformation is one of the gifts of cooking; it makes the food both more digestible and more enjoyable. Braising is traditionally used with larger cuts of meat, like this leg of lamb, which lends itself well to feeding groups. Eating from the same pot can be a powerful ritual, gathering people together to be nourished by the food and by one another. It becomes a way to share in celebration and connect with others, even if it is just to celebrate togetherness and the presence of food.

Serve the lamb with rice or couscous, or in a bowl au jus.

◆ YIELD: 6 SERVINGS ◆

1   (3-pound) bone-in leg of lamb or half leg of lamb

Salt and freshly ground black pepper

1   teaspoon ground coriander

8–10   ounces garlic scapes, 6–8 heads green garlic (bulbs and green tops), or 2 heads cured garlic

2   cups white wine

1½   pounds root vegetable, cut into 2-inch chunks

I. Preheat the broiler.

2. Generously coat all sides of the lamb with salt and pepper, then dust evenly with the coriander. Place the lamb in a roasting pan. Position the oven rack so the meat will be about 4 inches from the broiler. Broil the lamb for 6 to 10 minutes on each side, until it is golden brown and sizzling.

3. While the lamb is searing, prep the garlic: If you're using scapes, cut the tip from the flower; if you're using green garlic, trim off the ends; if you're using regular garlic, separate and peel the cloves. Put the garlic in a food processor and blend until finely chopped.

4. Remove the lamb from the oven and set the oven heat to 350°F (180°C).

5. Transfer the lamb to a plate. Pour the wine into the hot roasting pan. It will sizzle and steam. Scrape up and mix in any bits stuck to the bottom of the pan. Return the meat to the pan, add the garlic and root vegetables around the edges, and sprinkle these additions with salt.

6. Cover the pan and roast for 2 hours. Then flip the meat and cook another 1 to 2 hours, until the meat is tender and falling off the bone. Serve the lamb warm, alongside the roasted garlic and root vegetables, with plenty of tasty drippings from the pan.

VARIATIONS

In early spring, I usually make this dish with green garlic and carrots or overwintered parsnips. In summer, I use garlic scapes and tender new potatoes, carrots, or beets. And in winter, I use cured garlic and sweet potatoes, potatoes, turnips . . . you get the idea. Use whatever roots you have available and that sound good to you! The lamb, the pungency of the garlic (which mellows as it cooks), and the sweetness of the roots complement each other wonderfully.

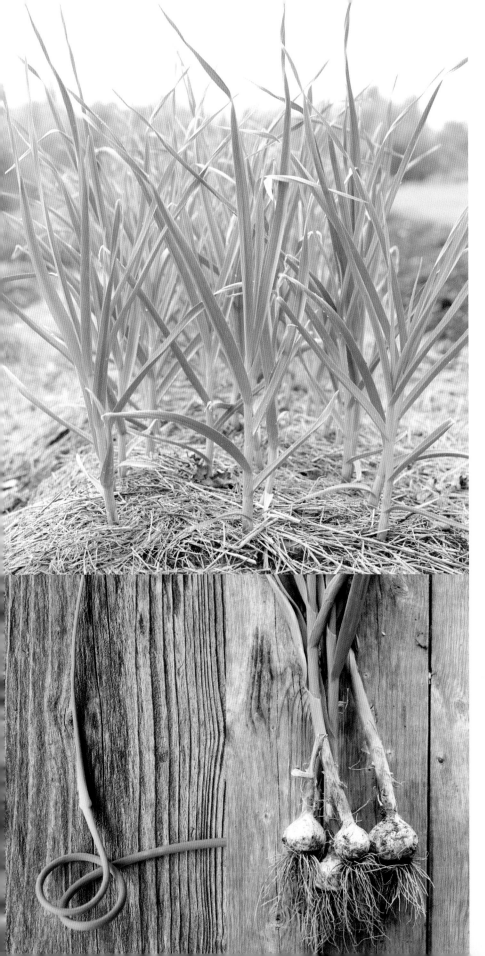

STAGES OF GARLIC

Garlic is one of the oldest cultivated plants in the world. And it is not hard to see why, as it makes a superb food and medicine during all stages of growth.

Garlic is a bulb. Individual cloves are planted in the fall and allowed to overwinter. In spring it sends up a bladelike shoot looking something like a scallion, and at this stage the entire plant — "green garlic" — can be used, including the leaves. In late spring and early summer the scape forms; this is the flower bud on a curly stem determined to spiral as many times as possible before blooming. The scape is usually removed (and can be eaten!) to encourage the plant to put its energy into the bulb. The bulb is ready to harvest when the lower leaves begin to brown and die back, in mid to late summer. After being pulled from the ground, the bulb is generally cured (dried) and stored.

HERBED PIZZA DOUGH

Simply put, pizza is a piece of dough with stuff on it. But homemade pizza is a process: you have to make the dough and let it rise, then decorate your pizza with a variety of toppings. It is a fun project to do with kids or friends at a pizza party, where you prep a lot of toppings and then have a free-for-all and see what kinds of creative results emerge. Turning the pizza pie into a communal activity where we can share in making *and* eating is in stark contrast to the grab-and-go mentality of the modern relationship with pizza. It reunites us with the work and processes of the kitchen and helps us develop a deeper appreciation for our food.

Start the dough 2 to 3 hours before baking the pizza, or even the day before.

◆ YIELD: 6-8 SERVINGS ◆

2	teaspoons active dry yeast
½	cup lukewarm water
2½	cups white wheat or spelt flour
1	cup whole wheat or spelt flour or rye flour
1	teaspoon salt
¾	cup cold water
½	cup packed fresh herbs
4–6	garlic cloves
¼	cup olive oil
	Pinch of cornmeal
	Pizza toppings of your choice

1. Combine the yeast with the lukewarm water in a large bowl. Then mix in ½ cup of the white flour and let sit until bubbly, 20 to 30 minutes.

2. While the yeast mixture is proofing, combine the remaining 2 cups white flour and the whole wheat flour with the salt in separate bowl, mix well, and set aside. Combine the cold water in a food processor with the fresh herbs and garlic and blend until smooth.

3. Once the yeast mixture is bubbly, add the flour mixture, the herb slurry, and the oil, and stir until the mixture forms a dough. Turn the dough out onto a floured surface and knead for 3 to 5 minutes. Place the dough in an lightly oiled bowl, cover with a moist towel, and set aside to rise in a warm place until it has doubled in volume, 1½ to 2 hours.

4. Once the dough has risen, if you're making it well ahead of time, punch the dough down and form it into a ball. Put the dough ball in a plastic bag, squeeze out all the air you can, and put it in the refrigerator. The cold temperature will slow the yeast. Take the dough out and let it warm to room temperature for 1 to 2 hours before baking.

5. When you are ready to make the pizza, preheat the oven to 500°F (260°C). You can bake the pizza on a pizza stone or a baking sheet; if you're planning to use a stone, put it in the oven while it preheats so the stone can slowly come up to temperature.

6. Roll the dough out on a floured surface to fit the shape of whatever stone or baking sheet you are using. Sprinkle cornmeal over the stone or baking sheet before putting down the dough. Decorate the dough with the toppings of your choice.

7. Bake for 10 to 12 minutes if you use a pizza stone, often longer if you use a baking sheet, until the crust is golden brown and cooked through. Keep an eye on the bottom of the crust to make sure it doesn't burn.

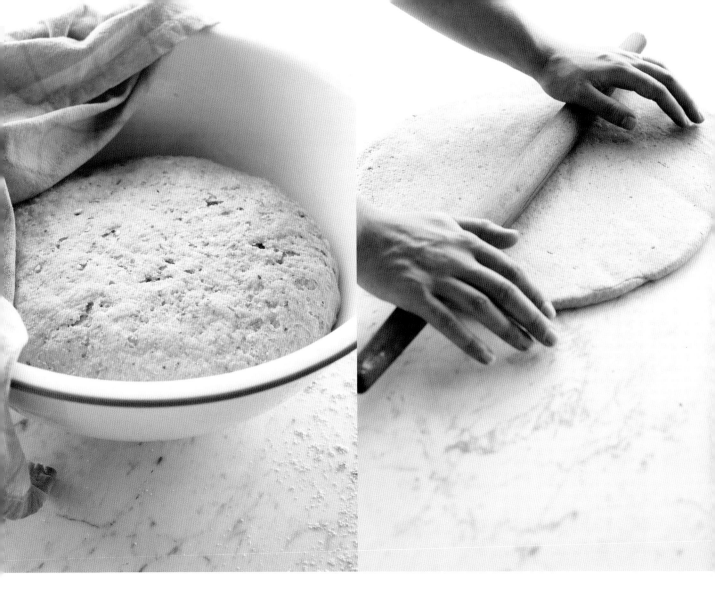

HERBS AND TOPPINGS

For the herbs in this crust, I like to use some combination of parsley, rosemary, thyme, sage, and oregano, but you can use any herbs and spices you like. Keep the quantities roughly the same to maintain good flavor and texture. Fresh herbs are better, but you can use dried herbs if that is all you have.

For the toppings, I like to use more fresh herbs and garlic, plus pesto and/or tomatoes or tomato sauce. I love mushrooms, olives, bell peppers, chiles, chicken, and sausage. In summer, I often fall for the simplicity of fresh tomato and mozzarella. In winter, I enjoy sautéed greens on my pizza with bits of meat, nuts, dried fruit, or hard cheese. Sometimes pizza can even be a good place to use leftovers! There are no limits or right answers; just have fun.

ROSEMARY-OLIVE OIL TEA CAKE

Someone once told me that if you want to sell a house, you should bake a loaf of bread. When you walk into a home where something is baking, feelings of comfort and warmth immediately surface. Home cooking is a sign of sharing, of giving, of nurturing one's self and others. These qualities are the grounding point of the home and the emotions of the heart. As the expression goes, "Home is where the heart is." It is important to our physiology too. It has been proven that up to 20 percent of digestive secretions associated with digesting a meal are released before food even hits the stomach. This is called the cephalic phase, and it is stimulated by thoughts, tastes, and smells of food. Cooking does far more than create delicious food. It connects us to the processes of our body and helps create a feeling of home for ourselves and our loved ones.

◆ YIELD: 1 LOAF ◆

1½ cups unbleached white wheat or spelt flour

¾ cup whole wheat or whole spelt flour

¾ cup raw cane sugar

1½ teaspoons baking powder

1 teaspoon salt

3 eggs

1 cup olive oil

¾ cup whole milk

¼ cup finely chopped fresh rosemary

I. Preheat the oven to 350°F (180°C). Grease a 4½- by 13-inch loaf pan with olive oil.

2. Combine the flours, sugar, baking powder, and salt in a large bowl and stir well, pressing out any lumps.

3. Whisk the eggs together in a separate bowl, then add the oil, milk, and rosemary. Add the egg mixture to the flour mixture, gently folding until combined.

4. Pour the batter into the prepared pan, smoothing the top so it is relatively even. Bake for 70 to 80 minutes, or until the top is golden and a toothpick inserted into the center comes out clean.

5. Remove the bread from the oven. You can eat it hot from the pan, or you can let it cool in the pan, then remove it, wrap it in plastic, and store it in the refrigerator, where it will keep for 3 to 4 days.

OLIVE OIL

The type of olive oil you use will influence the flavor; any olive oil that has a flavor you like will be excellent. However, don't use refined or "light" olive oil, as it lacks flavor and depth.

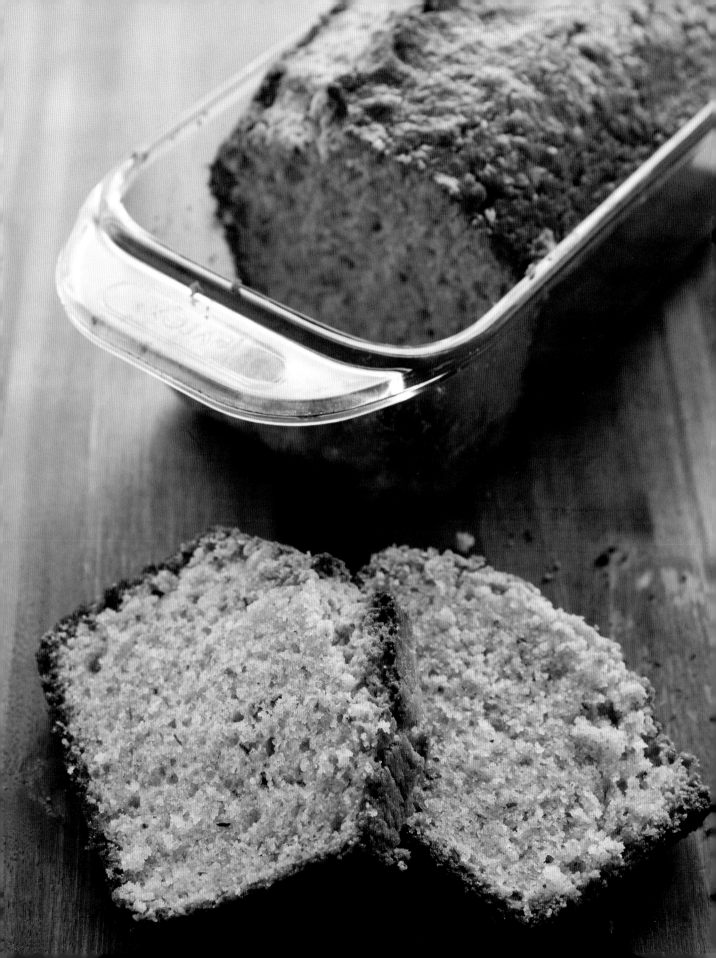

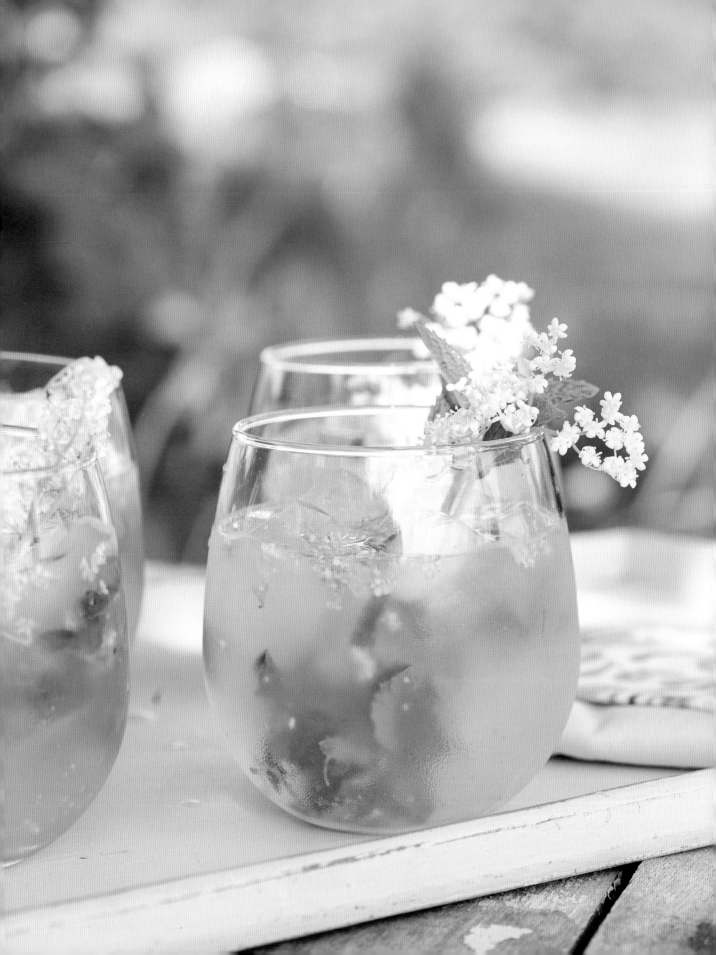

ELDERFLOWER
AND MINT MOJITO

Elderflowers have the most subtle yet magical scent, like pure pollen: flowery, sweet, dusty, and serene. The pollen itself is copious and gets everywhere. Make sure to bury your face deep enough in the flowers that you let some of it settle on your nose! Magical lore about the elder tree goes back hundreds of years, and it's no wonder, with such a sensuous smell and generous healing properties. Among its many gifts, the elder tree is said to bestow blessings — gently yet assertively, like a wise elder.

✦ YIELD: 4 SERVINGS ✦

1 handful fresh mint (try a mild mint, like spearmint or mountain mint, rather than peppermint)

1 large handful fresh elderflowers, large stems removed

2 tablespoons honey

Juice of 1 lime

4 ounces white rum (optional)

1 tray ice cubes

24 ounces sparkling water

I. Set aside four mint leaves and four elderflowers for garnish.

2. Combine the rest of the mint and elderflowers in a quart-size pitcher or clean widemouthed 1-quart mason jar. Add the honey, lime juice, and rum, if using, and muddle with a wooden spoon, bruising the herbs to release their juices and aromas and dissolving the honey. Empty half a tray of ice cubes over this mixture. Pour the sparkling water over it all and stir gently to mix.

3. Divide the remaining ice cubes among four glasses, pour the drink into each glass, and garnish each glass with the reserved mint and elderflower.

ELDERFLOWER ICE CUBES

If you don't have fresh elderflowers, you can still enjoy the fragrance and flavor of the plant; just use ice cubes made from dried elderflower tea. Pour 2 cups hot water over ½ cup dried elderflowers, cover, and let steep for 10 minutes. Strain, cool, and then freeze in an ice cube tray.

BASIL-LAVENDER TEA

I love serving tea at parties. Having hot tea to offer people as they arrive, particularly if the weather is cold, wet, or gray, generates an immediate feeling of warmth. On warmer days, serve tea at room temperature, or iced. This tea creates a lovely atmosphere to start a social occasion, reducing any stress, anxiety, tension, or preoccupations that may be lingering from the day and helping everyone settle into the moment.

◆ YIELD: ABOUT 3 CUPS ◆

½ cup packed fresh basil leaves and stems

2 teaspoons fresh lavender leaves or flowers or 1 teaspoon dried

3–4 cups boiling water

Combine the basil and lavender in a teapot or glass jar and pour the boiling water over them. Cover and let steep for 10 to 15 minutes. Pour and enjoy.

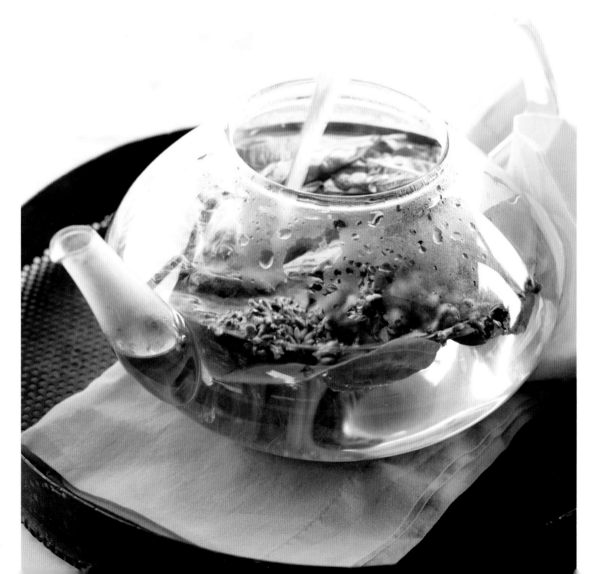

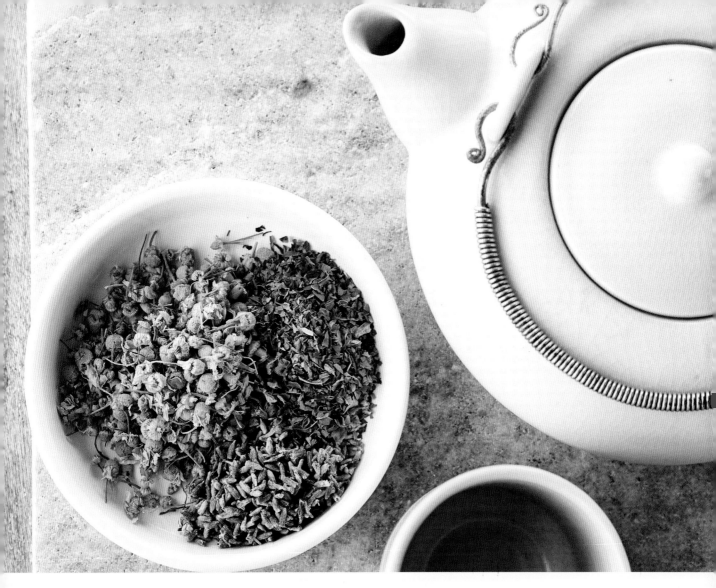

THE TEAPOT

The teapot is a perfect vessel for tea to steep in. It holds in heat and steam, which makes the tea stronger and more medicinal, and it makes handling and pouring hot liquids easy. Teapots are also beautiful in their shape and their function. Picture a teapot being poured, with a hand placed gently on the lid as the pot is tipped and a steaming stream of healing, aromatic, colorful liquid gracefully arcs its way into the cup. The whole process is one of elegance and ritual — it makes you want whatever is inside.

The teapot provides a way for people to gather around an activity that unites without preoccupying. The teapot symbolizes a desire to gather, collect, commune, and be together. Importantly, it also teaches us to share. It teaches us that to drink from the same pot is to experience love, connection, and community alongside cooperation, communication, and compromise: we each may have our own mug, but our tea all comes from the same pot. The teapot exudes the healing magic inherent in sharing before you even fill the kettle.

METRIC CONVERSION CHARTS

Unless you have finely calibrated measuring equipment, conversions between US and metric measurements will be somewhat inexact. It's important to convert the measurements for all of the ingredients in a recipe to maintain the same proportions as the original.

GENERAL FORMULA FOR METRIC CONVERSION

Ounces to grams	multiply ounces by 28.35
Grams to ounces	multiply grams by 0.035
Pounds to grams	multiply pounds by 453.5
Pounds to kilograms	multiply pounds by 0.45
Cups to liters	multiply cups by 0.24
Pints to liters	multiply pints by 0.473
Quarts to liters	multiply quarts by 0.946
Fahrenheit to Celsius	subtract 32 from Fahrenheit temperature, multiply by 5, then divide by 9
Celsius to Fahrenheit	multiply Celsius temperature by 9, divide by 5, then add 32

APPROXIMATE METRIC EQUIVALENTS BY WEIGHT

US	Metric
¼ ounce	7 grams
½ ounce	14 grams
1 ounce	28 grams
1¼ ounces	35 grams
1½ ounces	40 grams
2½ ounces	70 grams
3½ ounces	100 grams
4 ounces	112 grams
5 ounces	140 grams
8 ounces	228 grams
10 ounces	280 grams
15 ounces	425 grams
16 ounces (1 pound)	454 grams

APPROXIMATE METRIC EQUIVALENTS BY VOLUME

US	Metric
1 teaspoon	5 milliliters
1 tablespoon	15 milliliters
¼ cup	60 milliliters
½ cup	120 milliliters
1 cup	230 milliliters
1¼ cups	300 milliliters
1½ cups	360 milliliters
2 cups	460 milliliters
2½ cups	600 milliliters
3 cups	700 milliliters
4 cups (1 quart)	0.95 liter
4 quarts (1 gallon)	3.8 liters

Acknowledgments

The words "thank you" don't even begin to reflect the gratitude that I feel at the dusk of completing this book and the dawn of sharing it with the world. An endeavor such as this requires the support, commitment, and skills of many people and many resources. I feel enormously blessed and humbly grateful for the support I have been shown throughout this process.

Thank you to my agent, Sally Ekus, for your interest, care, and encouragement from that first day we met at my kitchen table. Thanks also to the rest of the team at the Lisa Ekus Group, and to Samantha, for your support, guidance, and genuine interest.

Thank you to the truly amazing staff at Storey Publishing for all the support, love, and care you put into the book and for your commitment to making it such a true expression of my work, inside and out. Thank you specifically to Deborah Balmuth and Dan Reynolds for recruiting me so thoughtfully and gracefully; Carolyn Eckert for bringing so much talent and intuition to the design process; Margaret Sutherland for asking more of me and making the book an even richer expression of my passions; and Nancy Ringer for being such a supportive, open-minded wordsmith. Great thanks to the photo team who helped craft these gorgeous photographs — Joe, Alexandra, Sally, and Ginger.

My thanks to the incredibly rich community food system I am surrounded by for keeping me so well fed and inspiring me to cook and cook some more. Particular thanks to the bright-spirited crew at Old Friends Farm.

Of the many influences that have inspired my work over the years, I am grateful for *The Sun* magazine interviews; the writings and teachings of Lewis Mehl-Madrona and John O'Donoghue; my

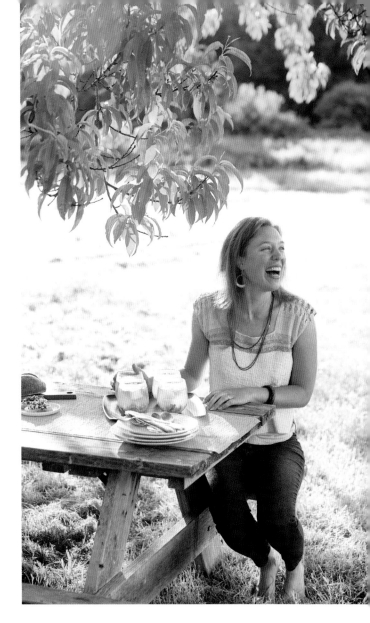

continued study of Ayurveda, Chinese medicine, and Western herbalism; and my mentors, colleagues, students, and clients.

For all my friends and family who have continually expressed excitement and anticipation throughout this process — your momentum has fed my own. I thank my family for being so fantastic, fun, and supportive and for loving me unconditionally. With deepest gratitude, I thank my husband, Casey, who lovingly and faithfully staffs his post as QB Lead Support Coordinator (Extraordinaire!).

INDEX

Page numbers in *italic* indicate photos.

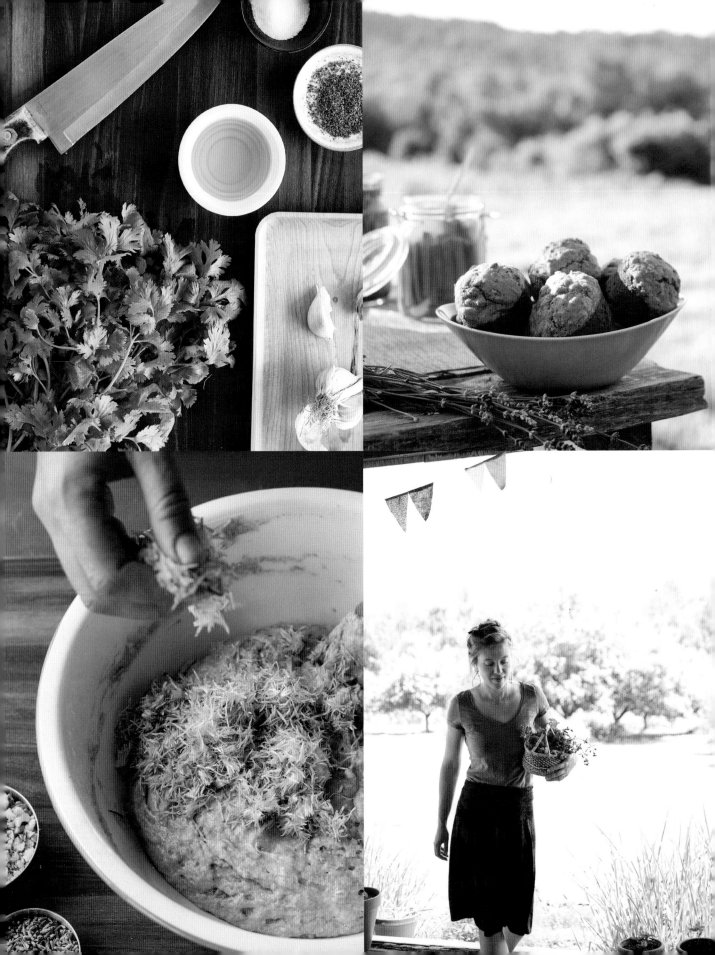

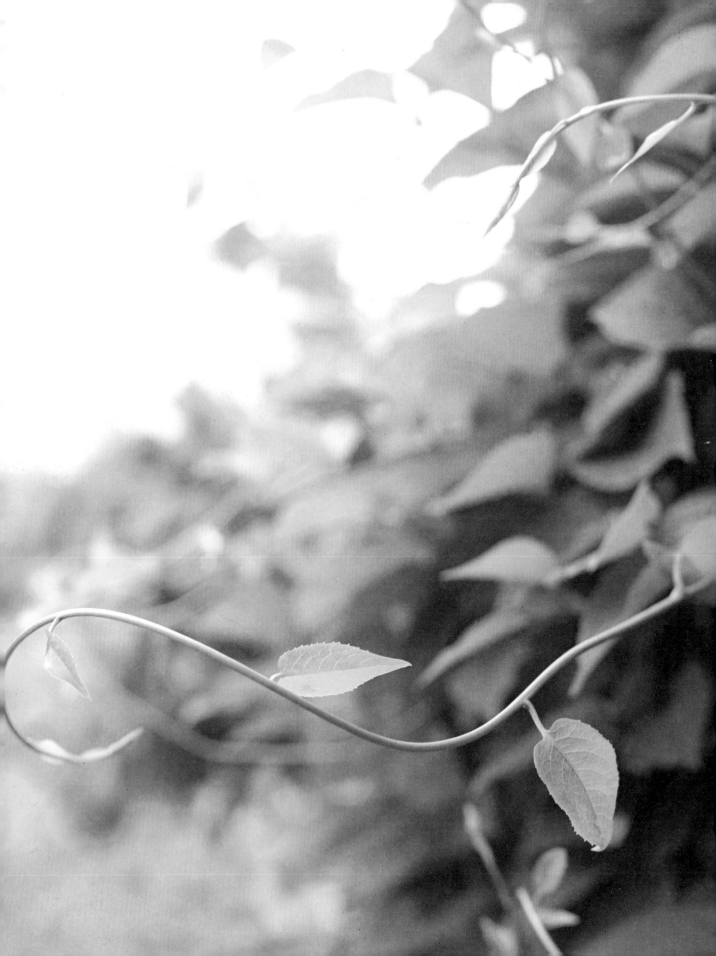

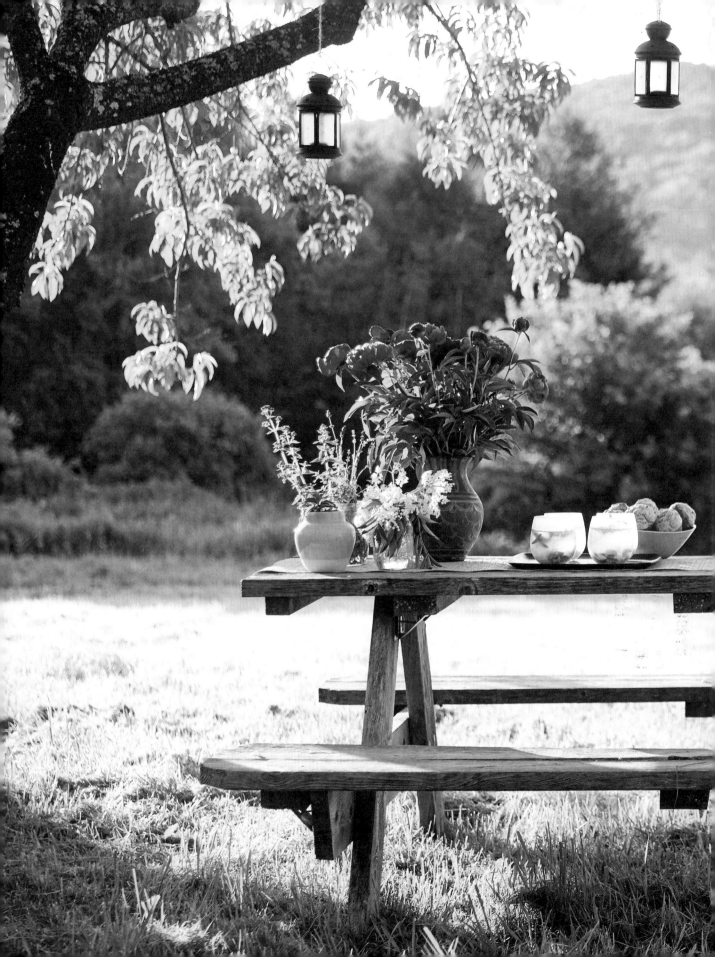